Pediatric Neurology

Editors

GARY D. CLARK
JAMES J. RIVIELLO Jr

NEUROLOGIC CLINICS

www.neurologic.theclinics.com

Consulting Editor
RANDOLPH W. EVANS

August 2021 • Volume 39 • Number 3

ELSEVIER

1600 John F. Kennedy Boulevard • Suite 1800 • Philadelphia, Pennsylvania, 19103-2899

http://www.theclinics.com

NEUROLOGIC CLINICS Volume 39, Number 3
August 2021 ISSN 0733-8619, ISBN-13: 978-0-323-83570-1

Editor: Stacy Eastman
Developmental Editor: Hannah Almira Lopez

Neurologic Clinics (ISSN 0733-8619) is published quarterly by Elsevier Inc., 360 Park Avenue South, New York, NY 10010–1710. Months of issue are February, May, August, and November. Periodicals postage paid at New York, NY, and additional mailing offices. Subscription prices are $333.00 per year for US individuals, $881.00 per year for US institutions, $100.00 per year for US students, $408.00 per year for Canadian individuals, $938.00 per year for Canadian institutions, $461.00 per year for international individuals, $938.00 per year for international institutions, $210.00 for foreign students/residents, and $100.00 for Canadian students/residents. To receive student/resident rate, orders must be accompanied by name of affiliated institution, date of term, and the *signature* of program/residency coordinator on institution letterhead. Orders will be billed at individual rate until proof of status is received. Foreign air speed delivery is included in all *Clinics* subscription prices. All prices are subject to change without notice. **POSTMASTER:** Send address changes to *Neurologic Clinics*, Elsevier Health Sciences Division, Subscription Customer Service, 3251 Riverport Lane, Maryland Heights, MO 63043. **Customer Service: Telephone: 1-800-654-2452 (U.S. and Canada); 314-447-8871 (outside U.S. and Canada). Fax: 314-447-8029. E-mail: journalscustomerservice-usa@elsevier.com (for print support); journalsonlinesupport-usa@elsevier.com (for online support).**

Reprints. For copies of 100 or more of articles in this publication, please contact the Commercial Reprints Department, Elsevier Inc., 360 Park Avenue South, New York, New York, 10010-1710; Tel.: +1-212-633-3874; Fax: +1-212-633-3820, and E-mail: reprints@elsevier.com.

Neurologic Clinics is also published in Spanish by Nueva Editorial Interamericana S.A., Mexico City, Mexico.

Neurologic Clinics is covered in *Current Contents/Clinical Medicine, MEDLINE/PubMed (Index Medicus), EMBASE/Excerpta Medica, and PsycINFO, and ISI/BIOMED.*

Contributors

CONSULTING EDITOR

RANDOLPH W. EVANS, MD
Clinical Professor, Department of Neurology, Baylor College of Medicine, Houston, Texas, USA

EDITORS

GARY D. CLARK, MD
Professor of Pediatrics and Neurology, Department of Pediatrics, Division of Neurology and Developmental Neuroscience, Blue Bird Endowed Chair for the Chief of Neurology and Developmental Neuroscience, Baylor College of Medicine, Chief of the Neurology Service, Texas Children's Hospital, President of the Texas Neurological Society, Houston, Texas

JAMES J. RIVIELLO Jr, MD
Associate Section Head for Epilepsy, Neurophysiology, and Neurocritical Care, Section of Pediatric Neurology and Developmental Neuroscience, Department of Pediatrics, Professor of Pediatrics and Neurology, Baylor College of Medicine, Texas Children's Hospital, Houston, Texas

AUTHORS

SAMIYA F. AHMAD, MD
Assistant Professor, Department of Pediatrics, Baylor College of Medicine, San Antonio, Texas

IRFAN ALI, MD
Texas Children's Hospital, Houston, Texas

ANNE E. ANDERSON, MD
Department of Pediatrics, Section of Pediatric Neurology and Developmental Neuroscience, Baylor College of Medicine, Jan and Dan Duncan Neurologic Research Institute, Texas Children's Hospital, Houston, Texas

ASHURA W. BUCKLEY, MD
Director, Sleep and Neurodevelopmental Service, Pediatrics and Developmental Neuroscience Branch, National Institute of Mental Health, National Institutes of Health, Magnuson Clinical Center, Bethesda, Maryland

GARY D. CLARK, MD
Professor of Pediatrics and Neurology, Department of Pediatrics, Division of Neurology and Developmental Neuroscience, Blue Bird Endowed Chair for the Chief of Neurology and Developmental Neuroscience, Baylor College of Medicine, Chief of the Neurology Service, Texas Children's Hospital, President of the Texas Neurological Society, Houston, Texas

ROHINI COORG, MD
Section of Pediatric Neurology and Developmental Neuroscience, Department of Pediatrics, Baylor College of Medicine, Department of Neurology and Developmental Neuroscience, Texas Children's Hospital, Houston, Texas

BRIAN D. CORDASCO, MHSA, FACHE
Director of Neurology and Genetics, Houston, Texas

GLORIA DIAZ-MEDINA, MD
Assistant Professor, Departments of Pediatrics and Neurology, Baylor College of Medicine, Texas Children's Hospital, Houston, Texas

DAN DIPRISCO, MHA
Executive Vice President, Texas Children's Hospital, Houston, Texas

LISA EMRICK, MD
Pediatric Neurogenetics Clinic, Blue Bird Circle Clinic for Pediatric Neurology, Section of Pediatric Neurology and Developmental Neuroscience, Texas Children's Hospital, Baylor College of Medicine, Houston, Texas

JENNIFER ERKLAUER, MD
Medical Director of Neurocritical Care, Section of Pediatric Neurology and Developmental Neuroscience, Medical Director of the Neurointensive Care Unit, Section of Pediatric Critical Care Medicine, Department of Pediatrics, Assistant Professor of Pediatrics, Baylor College of Medicine, Department of Pediatrics, Texas Children's Hospital, Houston, Texas

DANIEL G. GLAZE, MD
Professor, Departments of Pediatrics and Neurology, Baylor College of Medicine, Houston, Texas

J. LLOYD HOLDER Jr. MD, PhD
Department of Pediatrics, Section of Pediatric Neurology and Developmental Neuroscience, Baylor College of Medicine, Jan and Dan Duncan Neurologic Research Institute, Texas Children's Hospital, Houston, Texas

KIM HOUCK, MD
Texas Children's Hospital, Houston, Texas

AKSHAT KATYAYAN, MD
Assistant Professor, Departments of Pediatrics and Neurology, Baylor College of Medicine, Texas Children's Hospital, Houston, Texas

YI-CHEN LAI, MD
Department of Pediatrics, Section of Pediatric Critical Care Medicine, Baylor College of Medicine, Jan and Dan Duncan Neurologic Research Institute, Texas Children's Hospital, Houston, Texas

MICHAEL LAROSE, MHA, MBA
Practice Administrator, Texas Children's Hospital, Houston, Texas

TIMOTHY E. LOTZE, MD
Professor of Pediatrics and Neurology, Department of Pediatrics, Division of Neurology and Developmental Neuroscience, Baylor College of Medicine, Program Director of Child Neurology, Division of Neurology and Developmental Neuroscience, Texas Children's Hospital, President of the Professors of Child Neurology, Houston, Texas

NIKITA MALANI SHUKLA, MD
Assistant Professor, Department of Neurology and Developmental Neuroscience, Texas Children's Hospital, Baylor College of Medicine, Houston, Texas

FATEMA MALBARI, MD
Assistant Professor, Department of Pediatrics, Division of Pediatric Neurology and Developmental Neurosciences, Texas Children's Hospital, Baylor College of Medicine, Houston, Texas

LUIS A. MARTINEZ, PhD
Department of Pediatrics, Section of Pediatric Neurology and Developmental Neuroscience, Baylor College of Medicine, Jan and Dan Duncan Neurologic Research Institute, Texas Children's Hospital, Houston, Texas

EYAL MUSCAL, MD
Assistant Professor, Department of Pediatrics, Texas Children's Hospital, Baylor College of Medicine, Co-appointment in Department of Neurology and Developmental Neuroscience, Houston, Texas

JAMES J. RIVIELLO Jr, MD
Associate Section Head for Epilepsy, Neurophysiology, and Neurocritical Care, Section of Pediatric Neurology and Developmental Neuroscience, Department of Pediatrics, Professor of Pediatrics and Neurology, Baylor College of Medicine, Texas Children's Hospital, Houston, Texas

ROA SADAT, MMSc, CGC
Pediatric Neurogenetics Clinic, Blue Bird Circle Clinic for Pediatric Neurology, Section of Pediatric Neurology and Developmental Neuroscience, Texas Children's Hospital, Baylor College of Medicine, Houston, Texas

ELAINE S. SETO, MD, PhD
Section of Pediatric Neurology and Developmental Neuroscience, Department of Pediatrics, Baylor College of Medicine, Department of Neurology and Developmental Neuroscience, Texas Children's Hospital, Houston, Texas

Contents

a diagnostic and supportive field into an interventional one. Training child neurology residents in clinical research and therapeutic intervention is increasingly important to assure the ongoing ability to support research discoveries and treatment.

Drug-resistant epilepsy warrants referral to an epilepsy surgery center for consideration of alternative treatments including epilepsy surgery. Advances in technology now allow for minimally invasive neurophysiologic monitoring and surgical interventions, approaches that are attractive to families because large craniotomies and associated morbidity are avoided. This work reviews the presurgical evaluation process and discusses the use of invasive stereo-electroencephalography monitoring to localize seizure onset zones. Minimally invasive surgical techniques are described for the treatment of focal and generalized epilepsies. These approaches have expanded our capacity to palliate and cure epilepsy in the pediatric population.

The presence of unprovoked, recurrent seizures, particularly when drug resistant and associated with cognitive and behavioral deficits, warrants investigation for an underlying genetic cause. This article provides an overview of the major classes of genes associated with epilepsy phenotypes divided into functional categories along with the recommended work-up and therapeutic considerations. Gene discovery in epilepsy supports counseling and anticipatory guidance but also opens the door for precision medicine guiding therapy with a focus on those with disease-modifying effects.

Epilepsy can now be diagnosed even in the presence of one unprovoked seizure or if the diagnosis of an epilepsy syndrome can be made. Epilepsy syndromes represent a specific set of seizure types and electroencephalographic and imaging features that tend to have age-dependent features, triggers, and prognosis. Epilepsy syndromes are the third and final level of epilepsy diagnosis, after classification of seizure and epilepsy types. Some epilepsy syndromes are self-limiting and pharmacoresponsive and others are pharmacoresistant and associated with poor developmental outcomes (epileptic and developmental encephalopathy). Features and management of 7 common age-dependent pediatric epilepsy syndromes are described.

Neuromodulation alters neuronal activity with electrical impulses delivered to the targeted neurologic sites. The various neuromodulation options available today for epilepsy management have proven efficacy primarily in adult trials. These include open-loop stimulation with invasive vagus nerve stimulation and deep brain stimulation, as well as closed-loop responsive neurostimulation. The use of neurostimulation therapy to treat intractable epilepsy in children is growing. This article reviews the literature, historical background, and current principles in pediatric patients.

Pediatric neuroinflammatory conditions are a complex group of disorders with a wide range of clinical presentations. Patients can present with a combination of focal neurologic deficits, encephalopathy, seizures, movement disorders, or psychiatric manifestations. There are several ways that pediatric neuroinflammatory conditions can be classified, including clinical presentation, pathophysiologic mechanism, and imaging and laboratory findings. In this article, we group these conditions into acquired demyelinating diseases, immune-mediated epilepsies/encephalopathies, primary rheumatologic conditions with central nervous system (CNS) manifestations, CNS vasculitis, and neurodegenerative/genetic conditions with immune-mediated pathophysiology and discuss epidemiology, pathophysiology, clinical presentation, treatment, and prognosis of each disorder.

Central nervous system (CNS) tumors are the most common solid tumor in pediatrics and represent the largest cause of childhood cancer–related mortality. With advances in molecular characterization of tumors, considerable developments have occurred impacting diagnosis and management, and refined prognostication. Advances in management have led to better survival, but mortality remains high and significant morbidity persists. Novel therapeutic approaches targeting the biology of these tumors are being investigated to improve overall survival and decrease treatment-related morbidity. Further molecular understanding of pediatric CNS tumors will lead to continued refinement of tumor classification, management, and prognostication.

The goal of neurocritical care (NCC) is to improve the outcome of patients with neurologic insults. NCC includes the management of the primary brain injury and prevention of secondary brain injury; this is achieved with standardized clinical care for specific disorders along with neuromonitoring. Neuromonitoring uses multiple modalities, with certain modalities better suited to certain disorders. The term "multimodality monitoring" refers to using multiple modalities at the same time. This article reviews pediatric NCC, the various physiologic parameters used, especially continuous electroencephalographic monitoring.

> Healthy sleep, including proper amounts in the 24-hour day/night period, is crucial for developing children. Sleep development in infants and children is characterized by increased amounts of sleep, including rapid eye movement and non–rapid eye movement (NREM) slow-wave sleep. Expected changes as well as deviations may contribute to sleep problems, which are common in typically developing children and very common in those with neurodevelopmental disorders and often are chronic. Periodic screening of children for sleep problems is important for timely and effective management of these.

> Medical care has become more complex as the scientific method has expanded medical knowledge. Medicine is also now practiced across different medical systems of varying complexity, and creating standard treatment guidelines is one way of establishing uniform treatment across these systems. The creation of guidelines ensures the delivery of quality medical care and improved patient outcomes. Evidence-based medicine is the application of scientific research to produce these treatment guidelines. This article shall focus on the current treatment guidelines used for inpatient pediatric neurology.

NEUROLOGIC CLINICS

ISSUES OF RELATED INTEREST

Neurosurgery Clinics
https://www.neurosurgery.theclinics.com/
Neuroimaging Clinics
https://www.neuroimaging.theclinics.com/
Psychiatric Clinics
https://www.psych.theclinics.com/
Child and Adolescent Psychiatric Clinics
https://www.childpsych.theclinics.com/

THE CLINICS ARE AVAILABLE ONLINE!
Access your subscription at:
www.theclinics.com

Preface

Memento Akademia: Introduction and Editorial Regarding the State of Child Neurology

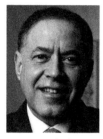 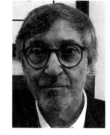

Gary D. Clark, MD   James J. Riviello Jr, MD
Editors

Memento Mori, "remember death," was whispered into the ears of victorious generals in ancient Rome as a reminder of their mortality and fallibility. The title of this article is meant to summon similar reminders, but of an academic mission. This mission is difficult to sustain in current health care systems, thus making this call timely and important.

Akademia (named after Akedemos, the owner of the property near Athens) was the location of many of Plato's lectures and where he developed much of what became the foundation for modern western education, religion, and political thought. He did most of his writing and teaching here, and thus, this is the Greek root of academics. Importantly, his student, Aristotle, developed what would become the scientific method of posing hypotheses and testing these through impartial observations and experiments. Remarkably, the Greeks knew that the earth was not flat, but spherical, because their measurements of distances and angles of cast shadows could only fit that hypothesis. Their contemporary, Hippocrates, incorporated some of this academic thought, moved medicine into its own distinct field with a body of knowledge, and promoted disease causation as an explainable phenomenon, not a curse by the gods. It would take a millennium for the traditions of medicine and of academics and of science to reach a confluence. That juxtaposition of science, scientific method, and medicine resulted in the advent of academic medical centers and academic medicine. Academics and academic medicine herein refer to current studies of disease, educating students and residents, cutting-edge clinical care, basic and clinical research, and publishing of new knowledge.

Doctor derives from Latin for teacher. As doctors, we teach our patients and their families about disease, and we are called upon to teach our profession to learners.

Neurol Clin 39 (2021) xiii–xv
https://doi.org/10.1016/j.ncl.2021.05.006
0733-8619/21/© 2021 Published by Elsevier Inc.

neurologic.theclinics.com

To remain current, we read, attend meetings, practice evidence-based medicine, and seek maintenance of certifications; as such, all of us are academic to some degree. An increasing majority of child neurologists work in academic medical centers or in some way are sponsored by affiliate hospitals.

Academic medical centers are the life blood of medicine in this country. These centers serve as the educators of our students, residents, and fellows; these are the innovation engines of medicine, changing our professions profoundly through research, new technologies, expertise, and skills. Yet, these institutions are under considerable stress owing to financial pressures that few of us understand. Hospital systems control revenue streams that could be and have been brought to bear to assist medical schools, residencies, and research programs. Yet, it seems that the money in health care, at least for now, is completely under control of the hospitals and not with the doctors who generate the margins and make the systems famous. No margin, no mission as is commonly said, and let there be no doubt, physicians and academic medical centers have little say in how margin is spent. And there is a healthy friction that arises from this separation. But as Dr Lilly Marks[1] so brilliantly stated in a recent editorial in *The Pharos*, the journal of the Alpha Omega Alpha Honor Medical Society: "Can academic medicine survive if margin is sought not as support for missions, but as the mission?" Should we, as margin generators, be able to have a say in how margin is spent, especially in not-for-profit academically affiliated systems?

"Damn it, Jim, I'm a doctor not a..." businessperson, manager, chief executive officer (although some are), or a lawyer as Dr McCoy from *Star Trek* might have said to Captain Kirk. That approach may work in the twenty-fourth century, but it will not suffice for now. If today's academic medicine is to progress, then some of us must be all the things in the first sentence of this paragraph. But we must all understand the finances of today's medicine or we will never be able to advocate for ourselves, our patients, our learners, and the research that makes deadly and disabling disease treatable.

Child Neurology began in the 1950s as a National Institutes of Health–funded spinoff of adult neurology programs. Our first 50 years or so were spent characterizing and naming diseases affecting the nervous system of children. We then moved into the genetic and immunologic characterization of neurologic disease, found the root cause of neurologic disease, modeled these diseases in mice and other animal systems, and learned a great deal in so doing about the nervous system, its development, and the pathogenesis of nervous system disease. These studies have led to treatments aimed at the root causes of neurologic disease in children; diseases heretofore thought to be untreatable and fatal are now commonly treated. We have seen a profound transformation of child neurology from a diagnostic and symptomatic treatment profession to one in which interventions are made to change a disease trajectory. There is much to be done to further this transformation; now is not a time to retreat nor become consumed by relative value units and billing. Nor is it a time to ignore the flat-earth influencers that without scientific rigor promote that immunizations cause autism, hydroxychloroquine can treat COVID-19, and that cannabidiol oil can fix everything.

Yet despite what should be the renaissance period for child neurology, neurologists are facing burnout, are not confident about the future of our field, and are highly dependent upon sponsoring institutions. This *Neurologic Clinics* is meant to change some of that for child neurology. Here, we show the financial power of a fully matured child neurology program for a sponsoring institution. We visit several areas where there are dramatic changes to the field of child neurology. We advocate for a shift in the training of child neurologists, and we publish our evidence-based treatment protocols for complex neurologic conditions.

We hope that this *Neurologic Clinics* can serve as a blueprint for institutions considering robust child neurology programs to develop such programs, and we hope that our evidence-based protocols can assist, in some modest way, the treatment of children with complex conditions. Furthermore, we call for courage in the face of the current forces in health care. Memento Akademia; remember academics (remember you are academic).

Gary D. Clark, MD
Baylor College of Medicine
Texas Children's Hospital
6701 Fannin Street, Suite MWT 1250
Houston, TX 77030, USA

James J. Riviello Jr, MD
Baylor College of Medicine
Texas Children's Hospital
6701 Fannin Street, Suite MWT 1250
Houston, TX 77030, USA

E-mail addresses:
gdclark@texaschildrens.org (G.D. Clark)
jjriviel@texaschildrens.org (J.J. Riviello)

REFERENCE

1. Marks L. The Pharos. Spring 2020;4–8.

The Finances of Neurology in a Major Children's Hospital

Michael LaRose, MHA, MBA[a],*, Brian D. Cordasco, MHSA[b], Dan DiPrisco, MHA[c], Gary D. Clark, MD[d]

KEYWORDS

- Net revenue/expense ratio • Relative value units • RVU • Downstream revenue

KEY POINTS

- Relative value units (RVUs) are heavily skewed for child neurology and are influenced by proceduralists (EEG readers, prolonged EEG readers, intraoperative monitoring readers, and so forth).
- Most outpatient neurologists cannot achieve the mean RVU expectation and are usually around the median.
- Yet the finances for individual neurologists in a major children's hospital are very positive, with a net revenue/expense ratio of 1.97.
- Downstream revenue from the practice of a single neurologist is about $2,000,000.00 per year.

Child neurology programs in large, academic settings can be characterized by demanding services with significant admissions, consultations, procedures, imaging, diagnostic testing, therapies, and surgical interventions necessary to provide care to a complex patient population. The accompanying outpatient physician practice enterprises, while busy with significant work relative value unit (wRVU) production, are devoid of ancillary revenue streams. Outpatient practices are reliant on volume in physician professional charges and bear significant salary and benefit expense. However, when viewed in aggregate and considering the related downstream revenues in departments such as radiology, surgery, oncology, and pharmacy, neurology programs are a significant contributor to a hospital's margin, allowing institutions to reinvest those margins toward supporting less margin generating, but equally critical service lines. These interdependencies are what makes a child neurology program an integral service in the pediatric outpatient, acute care, critical care, and surgical setting in a large children's hospital.

---

[a] Texas Children's Hospital, 6701 Fannin Street, Suite MWT 1250, Houston, TX 77030, USA; [b] 6701 Fannin Street, Suite MWT 1250, Houston, TX 77030, USA; [c] Texas Children's Hospital, 6701 Fannin Street, Houston, TX 77030, USA; [d] Baylor College of Medicine, Texas Children's Hospital, 6701 Fannin Street, Suite MWT 1250, Houston, TX 77030, USA
* Corresponding author.
E-mail address: mllarose@texaschildrens.org

Neurol Clin 39 (2021) 689–697
https://doi.org/10.1016/j.ncl.2021.05.001
0733-8619/21/© 2021 Elsevier Inc. All rights reserved.

The child neurology program at Texas Children's Hospital (TCH) in Houston, Texas, consists of 75 Baylor College of Medicine faculty members; 49 are child neurologists. There are 20 epilepsy specialists, 16 subspecialists (neurocritical care [NCC], movement disorders, sleep, neuro-oncology, neuromuscular, neuro-inflammatory [immunology], headache, neurogenetics, and so forth), and 20 advance practitioners, and there are 19 generalists in the community. In 2020, there were 45,000 outpatient neurology encounters, and 13,500 new patients entered the Texas Children's Hospital clinical enterprise through child neurology.

There are 16 inpatient neurology services: three consult services (West Campus, the Woodland Campus, and Main Campus), NCC (now two services), inpatient neurology (primary), neuro-oncology, neonatal neurology consult services, epilepsy monitoring units (3 services, including a dedicated invasive service), epilepsy consult services, Electroencephalogram (EEG), intraoperative monitoring, magnetoencephalography, and neuro-ICU monitoring services. Inpatient encounters in 2020 were down by 12%, but NCC volumes were up by 8% over 2019 volumes and up by more than 50% since 2018. This makes sense in the context of coronavirus disease 2019; early in the pandemic, many elective admissions were deferred. Long-term EEGs were up by 13% from 2019. There is a large clinical research enterprise, and there is a large basic science enterprise in child neurology at our institution that pays for themselves and brings in considerable indirect costs to pay for their infrastructure costs. These are revenue neutral for this analysis.

In this system, a general child neurologist, subspecialist, or epileptologist collectively bill for 1.6 times their salaries, but collection is approximately 70% to 85% of their salaries. This is due to payor mix, government-based reimbursement rates, and bad debt accounts. The remainder of the salary comes from hospital revenue by cost sharing via a physician service organization. The true financial picture for child neurology can best be understood when one considers the whole clinical enterprise.

RELATIVE VALUE UNITS

The wRVU productivity and distribution in our system are similar to those reported in national surveys (**Figs. 1–3**). A general child neurologist and a subspecialist can be expected to generate about 3700 RVUs per full-time equivalent (FTE). An epileptologist can be expected to generate about 4000 RVUs per FTE (prior to the recent decreased RVUs for long-term EEG). This results in skewing of aggregate data of all child neurologists such that means are 3850, yet medians are 3700. The means are not mathematically achievable for general child neurologists with a typical outpatient template (**Table 1**).

An analysis of RVU data from Medical Group Management Association (MGMA) (2014, see **Fig. 1**) showed a heavily skewed data set with a minority of high-productivity providers that are presumably proceduralists—EEG, long-term EEG, sleep, intraoperative monitoring, and magnetoencephalography. For the MGMA data set, the mean wRVU per clinical FTE was 4040; presumptively, the mean was influenced by the skewing from proceduralists (skewness .5). The median was 3666; most providers were in the range of the median (see **Fig. 1**).

Our wRVU data from the year 2018 are similar in skewing and in distribution. Our mean was 4103, which puts the section of neurology at the 50th percentile. Our distribution is slightly more skewed with a skewness of 1.5, but amazingly like other child neurology data, and in our case, it was definitely influenced by high-productivity proceduralists (EEG, sleep). Yet most provider productivity is aggregated around the median of 3538, with those higher than the median at the main campus generally. Those

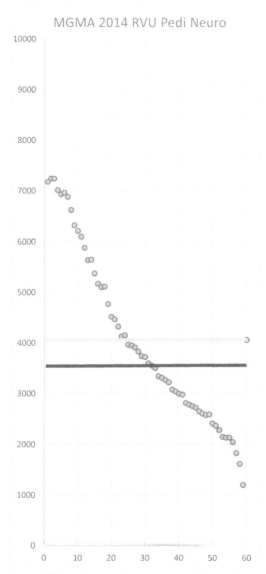

Fig. 1. MGMA data from 2014 analysis derived from available individual productivity measures for an FTE. The y-axis is RVU data, and the x-axis is rank order from highest to lowest RVUs. The yellow bar is the mean, and the blue bar is the median. Note the majority of neurologists are at or below the mean.

main campus general neurology providers are on heavy RVU-generating services (NCC, consult service, and inpatient services). Those in the community have no opportunity to generate RVUs on busy services, have no opportunity to be proceduralists (general child neurology providers), and, when on services to our community hospitals, must be available to the hospital and, therefore, cannot generate high volumes of RVUs. Thus, general child neurologists must solely generate RVUs from seeing patients in outpatient settings.

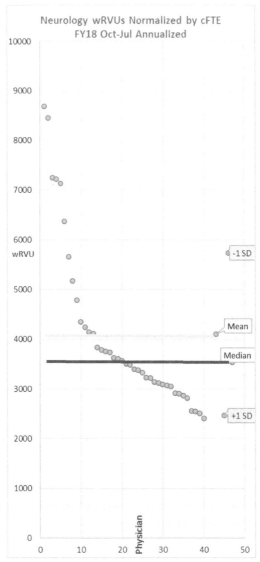

Fig. 2. Child neurologist RVU productivity for Texas Children's Hospital in 2018. Note similarities to MGMA data from 2014. Most providers are at or below the median. There appears to be few high-productivity providers that skew the data even more than the MGMA data set.

The demand for child neurology far exceeds capacity. Our program is one of the largest ones in the United States, and we have the capacity to see 13,500 new patients per year. There are about 2,000,000 children in Houston, and estimates are that 14% of those children will need to see a neurologist. If those 280,000 children only needed to see a neurologist once in their 18 years of life, that would be 15,500 patients per year, still exceeding our capacity to see new patients. We have evidence that the demand is greater than this, and given the financial impact of neurology, perhaps, programs need to be larger than the present size, or systems such as ours will have to

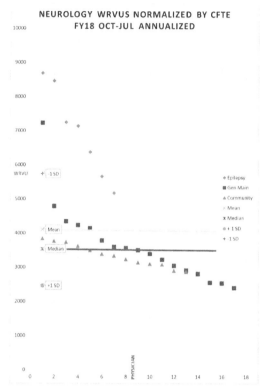

Fig. 3. RVU productivity of Texas Children's Hospital child neurologists by location and by epilepsy specialty. Note that epileptologists generate more RVUs because of highly rewarded EEG, long-term EEG, and epilepsy monitoring reads. Community-based neurologists have little opportunity to participate in high-RVU-generating services and procedures.

treat our population to be served with a population health strategy, so as not to miss important, treatable conditions in child neurology.

The general child neurologist is the entry point to our system, and the last year brought ∼13,500 unique patients into the TCH system. Some of these patients had MRI scans (80% of MRI scans at TCH are ordered by neurologists), hospitalizations, EEGs, sleep studies, intraoperative monitoring, and other highly reimbursed and highly RVU-rewarded activities for other providers.

COMMUNITY NEUROLOGY

Child neurology cannot be practiced with 10-min visits, and the standard visits are 30 minutes for a return visit and 1 hour for a new patient visit. For our practice, 8 clinic sessions per week are expected from a full-time child neurologist.

The current mathematically achievable RVU productivity for our community providers (general neurologist) is 3025 RVUs at the 23rd percentile. The analysis in **Table 1** incorporates our 10% same-day cancellations and 18% no-shows. The analysis also incorporates call availability to the hospital in the community. We have an expectation that our providers are available for hospital consults within an hour. Availability and productivity are inversely related, so with an average of 2 consults per day,

Table 1		
Excel spreadsheet calculation of predicted RVUs for a general child neurologist in an outpatient-only environment		
Practice Management Variables		
cFTE		1.00
Current Slot (New)		16
Current Slot (Return)		32
Total Slots		48
%, New		33%
%, Return		67%
Duration (Min)—New		60
Duration (Min)—Return		30
wRVU/Visit (New)		3.17
wRVU/Visit (Return)		1.77
Number of Weeks		34
No-Show Rate		18.0%
Average NPR (New)	$	218.16
Average NPR (Return)	$	110.34
Template Util, %		90%
Predictive Performance (FY18 Bench)		**Optimized (Added)**
Weekly wRVUs (New)—Templated		51
Weekly wRVUs (Return)—Templated		57
Total Weekly wRVUs—Templated		107
Clinic wRVUs Annualized—Templated		2694
% Inpatient wRVUs		10.00%
% Other Outpatient/Surgical wRVUs		0.00%
Total Annualized wRVUs		**3025**
Percentile Ranking		**22.5%**

Abbreviations: util, utilization; NPR, net patient revenue.
This model assumes an average of 3.17 RVUs for a new patient and 1.77 RVUs for a return patient. Ten weeks of inpatient activity is assumed, with vacation and meeting time incorporated.

productivity is low while being available to the hospital for consults in the community. If we allow community providers to see a few patients while on the consult call, productivity rises to an achievable 3421 wRVUs at the 27th percentile, but availability declines (**Table 2**).

Finally, if a system begins to address no-shows and same-day cancellations and cut these rates in half, we can conservatively estimate that productivity will rise to 3911 wRVUs at the 42nd percentile (**Table 3**). We feel that there needs to be a recognition of the value of the input into the system that general child neurologists bring and of a reason why providers who serve to bring patients into the system cannot meet productivity expectations with current deficiencies in scheduling, call responsibilities, no-show rates, and same-day cancellations. All of these factors are not under the control of general child neurologists in the community.

When considering community neurology, the benefit to the neurology enterprise derives from new patients entering the system. If one considers child neurology as a

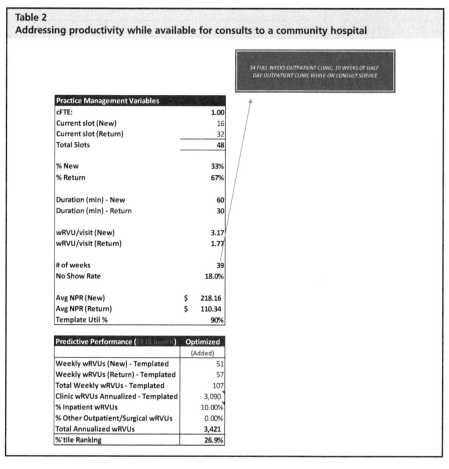

Table 2
Addressing productivity while available for consults to a community hospital

34 FULL WEEKS OUTPATIENT CLINIC, 10 WEEKS OF HALF-DAY OUTPATIENT CLINIC WHILE ON CONSULT SERVICE

Practice Management Variables	
cFTE:	1.00
Current slot (New)	16
Current slot (Return)	32
Total Slots	48
% New	33%
% Return	67%
Duration (min) - New	60
Duration (min) - Return	30
wRVU/visit (New)	3.17
wRVU/visit (Return)	1.77
# of weeks	39
No Show Rate	18.0%
Avg NPR (New)	$ 218.16
Avg NPR (Return)	$ 110.34
Template Util %	90%

Predictive Performance (FY18 Bench)	Optimized
	(Added)
Weekly wRVUs (New) - Templated	51
Weekly wRVUs (Return) - Templated	57
Total Weekly wRVUs - Templated	107
Clinic wRVUs Annualized - Templated	3,090
% Inpatient wRVUs	10.00%
% Other Outpatient/Surgical wRVUs	0.00%
Total Annualized wRVUs	3,421
%'tile Ranking	26.9%

practice, patients tend to remain with the child neurologist well into their early adult years and sometimes longer if afflicted by complex and rare congenital disease. The true metrics that general and community neurology should be gauged are how many new patients are entering the system and the downstream care that they receive. This is a much more fiscally responsible way to look at the benefit that community neurologists bring to the clinical enterprise rather than RVUs.

The RVU expectations for child neurologists are flawed, and given the financial impact discussed in the following paragraphs, need reforms. Child neurologists have some of the highest wRVU expectations of pediatric subspecialists, although all bill the same codes for outpatient visits. An important consideration should be the financial impact that a neurologist brings to a clinical enterprise. Neurology could not exist with only high-RVU-generating proceduralists; general child neurologists feed the whole neuroscience enterprise. This is not a lost-leader scenario, rather generalists are an essential part of the corpus of neurology.

COMPLETE FINANCIAL ANALYSIS OF THE CHILD NEUROLOGY ENTERPRISE AT TEXAS CHILDREN'S HOSPITAL

Importantly, the downstream revenue for a general neurologist is estimated nationally at about $2,000,000 per year (Merritt Hawkins—2019 Physician Inpatient/Outpatient

Table 3 Addressing no-show and scheduling issues can dramatically improve productivity of child neurologists		
Practice Management Variables		
cFTE		1.00
Current slot (New)		16
Current slot (Return)		32
Total Slots		48
% New		33%
% Return		67%
Duration (Min)—New		60
Duration (Min)—Return		30
wRVU/Visit (New)		3.17
wRVU/Visit (Return)		1.77
Number of Weeks		39
No-Show Rate		10.0%
Avg NPR (New)	$	218.16
Avg NPR (Return)	$	110.34
Template Util %		95%
Predictive Performance (FY18 Bench)		**Optimized (Added)**
Weekly wRVUs (New)—Templated		51
Weekly wRVUs (Return)—Templated		57
Total Weekly wRVUs—Templated		107
Clinic wRVUs Annualized—Templated		3580
% Inpatient wRVUs		10.00%
% Other Outpatient/Surgical wRVUs		0.00%
Total Annualized wRVUs		3911
Percentile Ranking		41.9%

Abbreviations: util, utilization; NPR, net patient revenue.

Revenue Survey). Neurologists order the majority of all MRI scans (80%) and genetic testing, participate in the care of 25% of all children's hospital admissions, and are responsible for not only ordering but also the interpretation of almost all neurophysiology studies. When looking at these components, it is evident that investment in a child neurology practice impacts critically important facets of care in the hospital.

Direct revenue (excluding downstream revenue) for neurology can be accounted for by considering that part of the hospital operation in which neurology is solely responsible: outpatient clinics, outpatient diagnostic procedures (EEG and sleep laboratory), functional diagnostics (Magnetoencephalography [MEG] and Transcranial Magnetic Stimulation [TMS]), outpatient treatments (Botox, nerve blocks, and so forth), epilepsy monitoring units, inpatient physician services, and neuro-ICU monitoring units. Although areas such as outpatient clinics have traditionally had minor losses for operations, these losses are more than compensated for by the direct revenue that the enterprise receives in all these areas. This results in a net revenue/expense ratio of approximately 1.97 averaged over 3 years. This means every dollar invested in a child neurology program yields nearly two dollars in net revenue after collections. This is very dependent on the child neurology program's payor mix, contracted private insurance rates, and government-based reimbursements. Unfortunately, Texas has one of the lower Medicaid reimbursement rates, with a Medicaid/Medicare ratio of 0.64, or is the 37th in the country and below the national average of 0.72.[1] This means that the net revenue/expense ratio of 1.97 ratio would likely increase in states with more favorable reimbursement ratios. If one were to include downstream revenue, this financial impact is even more impressive for neurology.

The breakdown of our child neurology revenue is 36% in outpatient services, 31% in neurophysiology (90% of neurophysiology's revenues are recognized in the inpatient setting), 30% in inpatient services, and approximately 3% in treatment procedures. More than 60% of the child neurology program's effort in total clinical time is in the outpatient setting, whereas the other 40% is equally divided between diagnostics and inpatient services. Thus, 40% of the clinical effort generates 60% of the revenue in our operation. This means that investing in inpatient and neurophysiology clinical services yields a greater margin per unit of time for a child neurology program.

Thus, it is really the complex, inpatient care that generates the majority of the revenue in child neurology. Yet, for us, the inpatient activities have closely followed the volumes in the outpatient clinics, which is an interesting and potentially important correlation. It does make sense that the more the patients in a clinical enterprise, the larger the need for inpatient activities.

Large, mature child neurology programs can greatly enhance the financial picture of children's hospitals. These programs generate a margin that appears to be scalable. But it is important to consider the aggregate picture of neurology as a clinical enterprise. In other words, billing on the professional side is not where the financial margins are generated. The inpatient activities, directly attributable to the neurologist, are where the positive margins are generated; the downstream revenue is another positive aspect (but is not essential in considering the financial power of neurology). Interestingly, it is the more academic activities that generate the highest margins, those touched by learners and involving the most complex and cutting-edge care. Yet, without outpatient activities, there may not be patients to be hospitalized and generate the larger margins. Therefore, all are important—outpatient, inpatient, teaching services, complex care, epilepsy, NCC, research, and so forth.

Here, we demonstrate the positive margin that a large, complex, academic child neurology program can generate. It is hoped that this can be duplicated in other systems, not only to improve hospital margins but also to support child neurology program growth because this support can result in a mutually beneficial relationship.

DISCLOSURE

The authors have nothing to disclose.

REFERENCE

1. Kaiser Family Foundation. Medicaid-to-Medicare Fee Index. 2016. Available at: https://www.kff.org/medicaid/state-indicator/medicaid-to-medicare-fee-index/?currentTimeframe=0&sortModel=%7B%22colId%22:%22All%20Services%22,%22sort%22:%22desc%22%7D. Accessed February 22, 2021.

Neurology in a Pandemic

Gary D. Clark, MD[a],*, Timothy E. Lotze, MD[b]

KEYWORDS

• Telemedicine • Teleneurology • Virtual meetings • Online • COVID-19

KEY POINTS

- COVID-19 pandemic: there has been rapid adaption of online technologies to serve child neurology.
- Virtual meetings: professional meetings have moved from in person to online (virtual).
- Online interviews: because of restrictions on travel, interviews for residency and for faculty positions have become virtual only.
- Telemedicine or teleneurology: the rapid adaption of teleneurology has transformed care in child neurology.

We are an adaptable species, and child neurologists have proved to be some of the most adaptable of physicians. Time in the field of child neurology can be considered as prepandemic, currently pandemic, and hopefully, postpandemic soon. Our adaptions are virtual professional meetings, virtual interviews, audio and visual telemedicine, and virtual multidisciplinary clinics (**Fig. 1**). And while we have served our patients, met educational needs, and kept operations functioning, how much of this virtual world will persist postpandemic?

VIRTUAL PROFESSIONAL MEETINGS

The coronavirus disease 2019 (COVID-19) pandemic, the need to socially isolate, and the asymptomatic spread of severe acute respiratory syndrome coronavirus 2 (SARS-CoV-2) has necessarily limited in-person meetings and travel. This limitation has led to adaptions of multiple different meeting types, all of which happen to be computer based. Content in such meetings can be quite robust and may even exceed prepandemic meeting content. However, speakers complain that there is no audience feedback and that it is difficult to maintain a speaking style while looking at one's laptop computer. Knowing that there is quite an extensive audience connected to that laptop is a peculiar feeling, and those of us that try to use a little humor in our educational

[a] Neurology and Developmental Neuroscience, Baylor College of Medicine, Neurology Service, Texas Children's Hospital, Texas Neurological Society, 6701 Fannin St., Suite MWT 1250, Houston, TX 77030, USA; [b] Baylor College of Medicine, Child Neurology, Division of Neurology and Developmental Neuroscience, Texas Children's Hospital, Child Neurology, 6701 Fannin St., Suite MWT 1250, Houston, TX 77030, USA
* Corresponding author.
E-mail address: gclark@bcm.edu

Neurol Clin 39 (2021) 699–704
https://doi.org/10.1016/j.ncl.2021.05.002
0733-8619/21/© 2021 Elsevier Inc. All rights reserved.

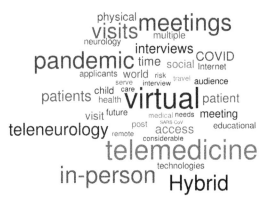

Fig. 1. Word representation in this article by size of the word. Prepandemic, many of these terms were not in common use in neurology publications.

content find these virtual formats to be quite challenging. At present, in most professional meetings the content is recorded before the meeting date. Content is then delivered, and the speaker is available for a question-and-answer session. Often a synopsis of the speech or talk is given before the question-and-answer session. Eligibility for continuing medical education is often determined by an honor system in which the audience member seeking continuing medical education reviews the content and criticizes the speaker.

These virtual meeting formats, while offering considerable advantages in terms of content and time away from offices, often suffer from lack of social contact and collegiality. The so-called virtual social hours and other mechanisms used to try to make up for some of this lack of collegiality and social interaction often feel too artificial, perhaps for now in a pandemic world. However, one can imagine that busy practitioners unable to leave their practice and perhaps bearing the considerable cost of travel from remote locations would really prefer this sort of content delivery even in a postpandemic world. As of the time of this content development, meetings are all virtual. However, multiple societies are considering in-person meeting formats in the near future, and at the time of publication of this article in-person meetings will probably again be the norm.

Hybrid meetings are being considered by multiple societies. Hybrid meetings would have in-person content, availability of social interactions, live audience interaction with speakers, and live question-and-answer periods. The meeting would also have the option for remote viewing of content and remote availability of question-and-answer interaction with a live speaker. In addition, content could be recorded for asynchronous or at a time of convenience of the remote audience to review content and to benefit from the educational activities. Such meetings are a considerable expense for sponsoring societies and may not be able to be maintained. Alternatively, hybrid meetings may be the meetings of the future. When one considers the number of attendees that may be available for a hybrid meeting, the attendance may exceed prepandemic in-person meetings; the impact on travel, hotel, and sponsorship of such meetings has yet to be determined. The only limitations seem to be our own imagination and the work that will be necessary to put forth both an in-person and a virtual format in the future.

Virtual Interviews

Virtual interviews during the pandemic have taken the place of in-person interviews for both the educational (residency and fellowship) programs and the faculty recruitments. The limitations of a virtual interview have significant disadvantages, yet the expense of a virtual interview is essentially nothing. In the setting of a virtual interview, the advantage seems to go to the sponsoring institution because the applicant neither gets to see the physical plant nor must endure long days of movement from one location to another. Certainly, during the pandemic all of us have made recruitment decisions based on virtual interviews. We have piloted tours of the physical plant during interviews, and this has been well received by applicants to training programs. Yet it is our impression that applicants are resistant to choose to train in distant locations without setting foot in the city in which the programs are located.

In some ways, the virtual interview is an extension of a social media presentation. Aside from the somewhat typical interviews between recruitment committee members and the applicant, programs are challenged to capture the applicants' interests with videos displaying their city, recorded testimonials from current residents, and social events using platforms that better appeal to younger generations. It is unclear as to how the technological savvy of an individual program influences the individual applicant, but applicants are certainly closely looking at the ease in navigation of program web sites, Twitter posts, and online reviews of experiences with programs by fellow applicants.

The travel expense savings during the pandemic have been considerable. One begins to wonder if a virtual interview in the future may be sufficient for a first round, and then an invitation for an in-person visit could be offered to a limited pool of applicants. This option would be problematic for training program applicants, but efficient for faculty applicants.

Audio and Visual Telemedicine

There is no doubt that the COVID-19 pandemic has jump started efforts to apply telemedicine to child neurology. By now all of us have participated in telemedicine (teleneurology). Federal and state regulations have eased this remarkably fast transition to online visits; one hopes that regulations will allow these visits to continue. Yet, as we consider the place of telemedicine or teleneurology[1,3,7,9,10] in a postpandemic world, when and who should be offered these visits?

In the postpandemic world, it is our intent to offer teleneurology visits to new patients at some distance from our outpatient facilities for certain low-risk conditions. The limitation of the physical and neurologic examinations via telemedicine gives one pause when considering higher-risk conditions. Likely this sort of risk assessment will be made on an individual basis and will likely differ between institutions. There are publications regarding telemedicine assistive technologies such as retinal scans, stethoscopes, and other screens without a physical examination via telemedicine.[4,0,0] In addition, enlisting the family's assistance in doing parts of the neurologic examination, such as briskly tapping the patellar tendon, not only can provide useful information but also can be a useful way for the patient and parents to better understand how the nervous system works. Yet, there will always be conditions in which a physical and neurologic examination in person will be essential. For those patients with a nonprogressive, low-risk condition, return visits could be considered by teleneurology. For instance, a patient with well-controlled epilepsy who has had a normal magnetic resonance imaging (MRI) may have some visits by telemedicine, whereas the patient with tuberous sclerosis and a giant cell astrocytoma, even with excellent seizure control, will need a physical examination and therefore an in-person visit.

Telemedicine is the new physician house call allowing us to better understand how neurologic conditions affect the patient in their home environment. In addition, the ability of most online telemedicine platforms to allow the neurologist to share their screen allows for display and discussion of an MRI or other laboratory result as well as guiding parents to online resources. Follow-up visits for patients doing well are shorter, allowing clinicians to have more clinic visits or spend time on other academic pursuits.

When considering a mix of teleneurology and in-person visits, there are considerations regarding the length of time it takes to room a patient, especially for children. In our experience, telemedicine visits almost always occur at the scheduled time. The latency between arrival at a front desk in a clinic and rooming of a patient can be up to 20 minutes, and therefore patients in person almost never are in a room at the time of their scheduled visit. So, one may follow a group of teleneurology visits with in-person visits, but not vice versa.

Other considerations, which were not anticipated at the beginning of the pandemic, have been the new social determinants of health, such as Internet access and technology access.[2] Before the pandemic there were few discussions regarding Internet access as a social determinant of health, but now Internet access is considered a social determinant of health. During the pandemic, patients without Internet access and without technologies to access health care through telemedicine were faced with only in-person visits. Although in-person visits were likely safe with proper precautions, the perception of the public was that health care institutions harbored SARS-CoV-2 and therefore should be avoided. Many of our less fortunate citizens chose not to access the health care system because of the risks perceived. Lack of Internet access and technology also impacted the education of our less fortunate citizens and probably still leads to some vaccine hesitancy among them.

Other surprising considerations have been the setting in which telemedicine visits could occur. In general, early morning visits are difficult for most families, and with school conflicts, most families would prefer their children to be in school instead of visiting with the doctor via telemedicine. We have had to modify our initial script discussing the mechanism of a telemedicine visit to quite simply say that the patient needs to be present, the parent cannot be driving during the telemedicine visit, and if a patient family is in a car during the visit, they cannot be in line at the drive through ordering at a fast-food restaurant. Current camera systems used by parents and caregivers for telemedicine appointments have limitations in their ability to allow the clinician to really "see" the patient. In addition, the correct camera angles to watch gait, eye movements, and other parts of the examination are not intuitive for many caregivers and often result in the need for redirection by the clinician. This speaks to the potential benefit of scripted and detailed examination instructions that might be provided to the patient and caregiver before the appointment, customized to specific complaints and conditions.

Multidisciplinary Clinics

There is little doubt that multidisciplinary clinics offer great value to patients and families; the ability to make one visit to a medical center and see multiple specialists needed to care for the complex child is of great value. The movement of such children often takes ambulances, special vans, beds or electric wheelchairs, oxygen tanks, pumps for G-button feeds, oxygen saturation monitors, and ventilators. To care for our most complex patients it was necessary to replicate this in a telemedicine world. Although multiple technologies can be used to accomplish this, we chose to use Microsoft Teams where multiple disciplines could discuss a patient in a secure, HIPPA-compliant manner and then leave the common "room" and accomplish individual visits via telemedicine. When considering a postpandemic world, some complex patients may be best served by continuing an online format such as described earlier.

Telemedicine might even eventually allow for a child neurologist to be "in the office" with the pediatrician and patient having urgent neurologic issues for real-time consultation.

SUMMARY

The novel coronavirus pandemic of 2019, 2020, and 2021, has forced the medical profession to very quickly adapt and change dramatically to serve our patients, our educational needs, and our recruitment needs. Although necessary steps were taken to develop virtual meetings, virtual interviews, telemedicine, and other technologies to serve child neurology, postpandemic we should not allow the progress that has been made to be squandered. Intelligent adaptions of the aforementioned technologies will best serve our patients, our learners, and our profession as we move forward. Some forms of virtual meetings are likely here to stay, and some form of virtual interviews should be smartly applied. Telemedicine can serve large portions of our patient population and can be intelligently applied for screening situations and other not fully realized purposes. Although we believe that in-person meetings, traditional physical and neurologic examinations, and in-person interviews are all especially important, the technology that we all have very quickly adapted in this pandemic can be used for a better future for child neurology.

CLINICS CARE POINTS

- Although online technologies have been applied to meetings, to interviews, and to clinical care during the COVID-19 pandemic, the use of these technologies in a postpandemic world will have advantages and disadvantages.

- In some situations, virtual technologies will not substitute for in-person meetings and clinical assessments.

- Child neurologists have been adaptable during the pandemic and may soon face decisions regarding the application of online technologies in a postpandemic world.

DISCLOSURE STATEMENT

The authors have nothing to disclose.

REFERENCES

1. Al Kasab S, Almallouhi E, Holmotodt CA. Optimizing the Use Of Teleneurology During the COVID-19 Pandemic. Telemed J E Health 2020;26(10):1197–8.
2. Benda NC, Veinot TC, Sieck CJ, et al. Broadband Internet Access Is a Social Determinant of Health! Am J Public Health 2020;110(8):1123–5.
3. Klein BC, Busis NA. COVID-19 is catalyzing the adoption of teleneurology. Neurology 2020;94(21):903–4.
4. Lakhe A, Sodhi I, Warrier J, et al. Development of digital stethoscope for telemedicine. J Med Eng Technol 2016;40(1):20–4.
5. Li Z, Wu C, Olayiwola JN, et al. Telemedicine-based digital retinal imaging vs standard ophthalmologic evaluation for the assessment of diabetic retinopathy. Conn Med 2012;76(2):85–90.
6. Maa AY, Wojciechowski B, Hunt KJ, et al. Early Experience with Technology-Based Eye Care Services (TECS): A Novel Ophthalmologic Telemedicine Initiative. Ophthalmology 2017;124(4):539–46.

7. McGinley MP, Ontaneda D, Wang Z, et al. Teleneurology as a Solution for Outpatient Care During the COVID-19 Pandemic. Telemed J E Health 2020;26(12): 1537–9.
8. Noda A, Saraya T, Morita K, et al. Evidence of the Sequential Changes of Lung Sounds in COVID-19 Pneumonia Using a Novel Wireless Stethoscope with the Telemedicine System. Intern Med 2020;59(24):3213–6.
9. Roy B, Nowak RJ, Roda R, et al. Teleneurology during the COVID-19 pandemic: A step forward in modernizing medical care. J Neurol Sci 2020;414:116930.
10. Zha AM, Chung LS, Song SS, et al. Training in Neurology: Adoption of resident teleneurology training in the wake of COVID-19: Telemedicine crash course. Neurology 2020;95(9):404–7.

Genetic Testing and Counseling and Child Neurology

Roa Sadat, MMSc, CGC[a],*, Lisa Emrick, MD[b]

KEYWORDS

- Channelopathies - epilepsy, movement disorders, neuromuscular
- Structural proteins - muscle, synapses, neurodevelopment
- Enzymes - metabolic disorders, cell function
- Epigenetic modifiers - downstream effect on genes and proteins
- Genetic counseling

KEY POINTS

- Gene discovery and a better understanding of the pathophysiology for neurological disorders.
- There has been an increase in targeted therapeutic options based on a better understanding of genetic mechanisms of disease.
- Genetic counseling with pretest and post-test counseling is important to understand diagnosis and recurrence risks.
- Genetic disorders remain undiagnosed secondary to unknown genes and mechanisms for disorders.

INTRODUCTION

The knowledge of neurology in the 21st century was based on understanding of anatomy, physiology, and biochemistry. Localization of neurologic disorders to the brain, cord, nerve, or muscle was based on history taking and physical examination,

[a] Pediatric Neurogenetics Clinic, Blue Bird Circle Clinic for Pediatric Neurology, Section of Pediatric Neurology and Developmental Neuroscience, Texas Children's Hospital | Baylor College of Medicine, 6701 Fannin St., Suite 1250.07, Houston, TX 77030, USA; [b] Pediatric Neurogenetics Clinic, Blue Bird Circle Clinic for Pediatric Neurology, Section of Pediatric Neurology and Developmental Neuroscience, Texas Children's Hospital | Baylor College of Medicine, Houston, TX, USA
* Corresponding author.
E-mail address: Roa.Sadat@bcm.edu

Neurol Clin 39 (2021) 705–717
https://doi.org/10.1016/j.ncl.2021.05.003
0733-8619/21/© 2021 Elsevier Inc. All rights reserved.

including a thorough neurologic examination. Advancements in ancillary tests such as neuroimaging with magnetic resonance imaging (MRI) have led to a better understanding of structural lesions and biochemical function/dysfunction of the brain with newer imaging techniques. Electrophysiology studies aid the provider with understanding function of the cortex, peripheral nerves, and muscles. The publication of the human genome draft in 2000 and advances in genetic technologies have led to better characterization of genomic mechanisms for neurologic disorders and the field of neurogenetics.

Neurogenetics is the study of genetics involving the development and formation of the central nervous system (brain and spine), peripheral nerves, and muscle. Disorders include structural brain malformations, disorders of brain connectivity involved in epilepsy, movement disorders, and neurodevelopmental disorders. Brain disorders can also be caused by disruptions of genes involved in other systems. This can be seen with *COL4A* vasculopathies causing brain malformations and microgliopathies and interferonopathies causing leukoencephalopathies.[1] Advancing technology has allowed for more gene discovery and better understanding of the underlying pathophysiology involved in disorders of the nervous and neuromuscular systems. In addition to better understanding of the genes and pathophysiology has also come a shift in management from solely symptomatic care toward new precision-based treatment options. The scope of this article is to review genetic concepts to understand the underlying etiologies and pathophysiology of neurogenetic disorders in addition to the counseling and ethical implications. The topic of neurogenetics is too broad and large to tackle in 1 article; therefore the scope of this article is to provide a framework for neurologists to learn and build on with advances in genetic technology.

What is Medical Genetics?

Medical genetics is the field of medicine working to better understand how genes and their products interact normally and form disorders and diseases when they do not. Genetic medicine encompasses an understanding of how the genome evolves with variation and expression of the genome in response to environmental factors and the impact on cellular function.

To better understand how genes lead to diseases, one must first review the basic concepts related to human genetic makeup, variability, and the impact on cellular function. The human genome is made up of approximately 20,000 coding genes, and the central dogma of biology outlines that deoxyribonucleic acid (DNA) is transcribed into ribonucleic acid (RNA) then finally translated into a protein product. The genome also includes approximately another 20,000 genes that are transcribed into noncoding RNA (ncRNA). These do not form a protein product, but may help with regulatory elements of gene expression. The sections of DNA that make up the coding regions are exons and are only about 1% of the genome; this is the majority of what is covered in exome sequencing.

The exonic portions of DNA are interspersed between intronic DNA throughout the genome. DNA is transcribed into RNA and then a mechanism called splicing works via identification of a specific RNA code to cut out the intronic noncoding RNA sequences and place together the exons to form messenger RNA (mRNA). The mRNA will then be translated into amino acids that will form a protein product.

Most of the DNA in cells is in the nucleus and is called nuclear-encoded DNA. In addition to nuclear-encoded DNA, there is a small amount of DNA located in the mitochondria. Mitochondria (mt) is a unique organelle because it has its own genome and therefore there are also disorders secondary to pathogenic variants in the mtDNA genome. Most primary mitochondrial disorders are caused by pathogenic variants from nuclear encoded DNA.

Nuclear-encoded genes are located on 22 paired autosomal chromosomes and 1 pair of sex chromosomes (XX for females and XY for males). The genes are located at a precise location on the chromosomes. Genes provide the code to make protein products for the cells to function in people. In addition to the nucleus that houses the DNA, the cell has multiple organelles in place to function properly. Cell systems need an infrastructure to help with trafficking molecules through the cell (endoplasmic reticulum, ribosomes, and golgi apparatus). Cells need a place to recycle their by-products (lysosomes and peroxisomes) and energy to support these processes (mitochondria). Protein products can be placed in various categories. These include enzymes that help metabolize a product, infrastructure for cells, and channels that help transport ions and small molecules in and out of a cell system. Disruption of the function of proteins involved in cellular homeostasis leads to metabolic conditions, epilepsy, movement disorders, neurodevelopmental disabilities, and neuromuscular disorders.

The human genome has almost the same number of coding genes as the mouse with about 20,000 genes and a fly with around 15,000 genes. So why are people more complex in their systems and advanced in their development? The human genome has complex mechanisms involving the ncRNA to differentiate genes into more than 1 product and add more variation into gene expression. The 20,000 genes can encode for hundreds of thousands of proteins called the proteome. For example, only certain genes should be turned on in a tissue at a time. The expression of genes both in quantity and location of tissue depends on multiple factors to turn on and off genes. The amount of expression of a gene depends on multiple regulatory factors called promotors, enhancers, insulators, and locus control regions. These are influenced by factors depending on the tissue-specific gene expression and gene-gene interaction.[2]

GENETIC TESTING OVERVIEW
Common Genetic Studies

Table 1 lists various types of genetic tests with the pros, cons, and limitations for detecting these variants.

Microdeletions or microduplications, also known as copy number variants (CNVs) have been reported in patients with diagnoses of neurologic disorders. Previous studies have reported a detection rate of 10 to 12% of likely pathogenic CNVs in patients with developmental delay.[3]

Genetic variations can also occur secondary to single nucleotide variants (SNVs) that can be detected with DNA sequencing methods such as Sanger sequencing or next generation sequencing.[4] Variants are classified as benign, likely benign, pathogenic, likely pathogenic, or of unknown significance. The term variants with the qualifying statements ranging from benign to pathogenic replaced the previous terms such as mutations. Next generation sequencing (NGS) may be used in phenotype-specific panels such as epilepsy, movement disorders, migrational anomalies, or neuropathies. An advantage of sending phenotype-specific panels with only a few known genes is lower cost; most cover both SNVs and CNVs for the genes on the panel, are less likely to have an unexpected incidental finding, and in some cases may have better coverage of the genes than exome sequencing. Gene panels have a disadvantage of lower detection rates in less specific phenotypes such as hypotonia,

Table 1
Genetic testing options

Genetic Test	Indications	Pros	Cons/Limitations
Karyotype	• Specific dysmorphic features • History of multiple miscarriages in mother	• Trisomies • Large chromosomal deletions/duplications • Balanced chromosomal rearrangement • Ring chromosomes	• Does not detect microdeletions or microduplications
Chromosome microarray (CMA)	• Dysmorphic features • Multiple congenital anomalies • Associated developmental delay • Nonspecific phenotype	• Microdeletions/duplications • SNP arrays – detect areas of homozygosity (AOH) and uniparental disomy (UPD)	• Does not detect small deletions or insertions • Does not detect balanced rearrangements or ring chromosomes • Variants of unknown significance
Gene panel/single gene	• Specific phenotypes	• Better coverage than ES • Limited detection of mosaicism	• Limited number of genes
Exome sequencing	• Nonspecific phenotype	• Broad coverage of genes • Medically actionable findings • Gene discovery	• Variants of unknown significance • Incidental findings • Limited CNVs or repeat expansions
Whole Genome Sequencing	• Nonspecific phenotype	• Detect single base variant (SNV) • Microdeletion/duplication • Repeat expansions • Gene discovery	• Insurance coverage • Variants of unknown significance • Incidental findings
mtDNA	• Mitochondrial DNA-specific conditions	• Specific to mtDNA genome	• Heteroplasmic difference in blood and other tissues • Variants of unknown significance
Repeat expansion panels – ataxia panel	• Specific disorder	• No variants of unknown significance	• Limited number of genes if panel or single-gene testing

developmental delay, or in conditions with recent gene discovery such as hereditary spastic paraplegia (HSP). Exome or whole genome sequencing (WGS) may have a higher diagnostic yield for less specific phenotypes, such as hypotonia and HSP compared to panel.[5]

Exome sequencing (ES) is DNA sequencing of the part of the genome that encodes for protein-producing genes, the exons and a small portion of the intronic sequences. As noted previously, the coding region of the genome only covers about 1% of the genome. ES became clinically available in 2011, and since that time, the number of genes associated with a known Mendelian disorder has increased from approximately 2000 to currently over 4000 and is still increasing. In addition to new genes being discovered, researchers also now see about 4% to 5% of patients undergoing ES can have more than 1 diagnosis,[6] and autosomal-recessive conditions may arise from a pathogenic variant in 1 allele and a deletion in the other allele.[7,8] The analysis of ES results also found a higher rate of de novo autosomal-dominant conditions when using a trio based format of sequencing the patient (the proband) and both parents.[8] The detection rate for making a genetic diagnosis is improving with better sequencing methods, more robust genetic bioinformatic programs to analyze the data, and gene discovery. However, as of 2020 the detection rates range from 25% to 40%.[9,10] Genetic testing may show variants of unknown significance (VUS) that can be difficult to prove to be pathogenic secondary to lack of functional testing such as a metabolic marker or in vitro assay. Other reasons for the lower detection rate include pathogenic variants in noncoding regions, repeat expansions, or small deletions or duplications that may be present but were not detected on the previous testing platforms. WGS and RNA sequencing can detect many of those variants that are not detected with exome sequencing.

WGS is DNA-based sequencing of the intronic and exonic sequences of the genome but is not currently at 100% coverage of the genome. WGS can detect SNVs, CNVs, and repeat expansions. It became more clinically available by some commercial labs in 2019 but is still expensive and not covered by most insurances. The costs of testing will decrease over time with the development of newer faster technologies. Bioinformatic tools to analyze the data will most likely develop in the coming years to assist with interpreting and storing the data.[11]

RNA-sequencing (RNA-seq) is a tool to assist with the study of gene expression and alternate splicing effects. As noted earlier in the chapter, levels of gene expression vary based on tissue. RNA-seq performed on skin fibroblasts have proven to be more sensitive than blood for the detection of neurological and neurodevelopmental disorders.[12,13] If the expression level of a gene is significantly less than normal, then it would be worthwhile to look closer at that gene for possible variants that were not previously detected. Variants may be within the promoter or enhancer region, intronic variants, small indels or affect splicing. For example, RNA-seq can assist with analyzing a known gene with autosomal recessive inheritance when only one pathogenic variant was detected. RNA-seq may also show an abnormal pattern of expression of multiple genes if the pathogenic variant is in a gene such as a transcription factor that has the ability to affect expression of multiple genes downstream.

Common Metabolic Studies

Mutations in genes that affect cell metabolism can disrupt normal cellular function and cause metabolic disorders. Inborn errors of metabolism can be the cause of developmental delays, regression, epilepsy, and movement disorders. The list of treatable disorders is increasing with developments of precision-related therapies and improved delivery mechanisms to get the treatments to the central nervous system (CNS). Many of the disorders can be detected with either screening metabolic tests or more specific tests of enzyme function.

Initial metabolic tests that cover many of the more common inborn errors of metabolism include plasma amino acids, acylcarnitine profile, and urine organic acids. Plasma amino acids detect aminoacidurias, urea cycle disorders, and some organic acidurias. Acylcarnitine profile is a blood test for fatty acid oxidation disorders. The acylcarnitine profile can also assist in diagnosing aminoacidurias and organic aciduria disorders with the assistance of urine organic acid tests.

There is a spectrum of clinical indications ranging from acute encephalopathy, seizures, motor regression, and more mild deficits affecting behavior and mental health in adolescents. The severity of the clinical features depends on how much activity the gene product has based on the pathogenic variant. Hypomorphic variants lead to a less severe phenotype and are frequently overlooked because providers are not often testing for metabolic conditions in adolescents or adults. The clinical history may be positive for symptoms that worsen with illness or stress and leads to a catabolic state. In these situations, the patient may be self-restricting certain foods because they feel worse when they eat these foods. An example of this is ornithine transcarbamylase (OTC) deficiency, which is one of the most common urea cycle disorders. OTC deficiency is an X-linked condition but female carriers can also be affected.

Many of the disorders detected with these initial metabolic screening tests are now detected in the United States as a part of state newborn screening tests. However, newborn screening tests vary by state and are updated through the years. Therefore, the metabolic conditions a child has been screened for depends on where and when they were born.

Additional metabolic testing may be indicated depending on the patient's clinical presentation. Cerebrospinal fluid (CSF) studies can be helpful alone or with comparison of blood samples obtained around the same time to compare ratios for relatively low levels in the CSF for transporter defects such as GLUT1 deficiency or compared with plasma amino acids for nonketotic hyperglycinemia. CSF neurotransmitters are classified into 2 main categories: biogenic amines and amino acids. Dopamine, serotonin, epinephrine, and norepinephrine are examples of biogenic amines. Individuals with disorders in these pathways often present with movement disorders classified as either too much or too little movement. These can also affect autonomic function and present with abnormal eye movements, such as oculogyric crisis. In addition to biogenic amines, CSF neurotransmitters are useful in the detection of amino acid neurotransmitters such as gamma aminobutyric acid (GABA).

Historically, metabolic tests for inborn errors of metabolism focused on targeting certain metabolites that may be increased or decreased based on specific metabolic pathways. Plasma amino acids focus on looking for a limited number of amino acids based on the assay used. In 2017, untargeted metabolomic profiling became clinically available and has led to new biomarkers for known conditions, ability to monitor therapy for some conditions, and diagnose metabolic dysfunction in less severe hypomorphic forms of some metabolic disorders.[14]

GENETIC COUNSELING CONSIDERATIONS
Modes of Inheritance

The patterns of inheritance for single-gene disorders, also called Mendelian inheritance, are essential in understanding disease transmission. The basic modes of inheritance are autosomal dominant, autosomal recessive, X-linked (dominant and recessive), and mitochondrial.

There are of course exceptions and other considerations that complicate the basic principles of these inheritance patterns. One example is genetic heterogeneity, which refers to locus heterogeneity, where variants at different loci cause a same or similar phenotype. Locus heterogeneity can be seen in channelopathies such as autosomal-dominant nocturnal frontal lobe epilepsy (ADNFLE), which is caused by variants in *CHRNA4* (OMIM 600513), *CHRNB2* (OMIM 605375), *CHRNA2* (OMIM 610353), *KCNT1* (OMIM 615005), or *DEPDC5* (OMIM 604364). ADNFLE is characterized as a cluster of motor seizures during drowsiness or sleep originating from the frontal lobes, but it can also present with but reduced intellect and psychiatric comorbidity. Most individuals with ADNFLE inherit a genetic variant from a parent who may not have any symptoms, as penetrance is estimated to be between 60% to 80%.[15] Penetrance refers to the proportion of individuals in a population who have a pathogenic variant and express the phenotype. A thorough family history is needed to detect the inheritance pattern with ADNFLE, because the nocturnal seizures are often mistaken for nightmares. This can be compared with allelic heterogeneity, where the same or similar phenotype is caused by different variants at a single gene locus. This can be seen in ciliopathies such as Meckel-Gruber syndrome (MKS) (OMIM 607361) and Joubert syndrome (JBTS) (OMIM 610688), which are both autosomal-recessive conditions caused by pathogenic variants in *TMEM67* (also known as *MKS3*). MKS is a lethal and rare condition characterized by a triad of symptoms: occipital encephalocele, large polycystic kidneys, and postaxial poly-dactyly.[16] Classical JBTS is characterized by a distinctive cerebellar vermis hypoplasia and brainstem anomalies known as the molar tooth sign, hypotonia, and developmental delays. Individuals with JBTS can have additional features that may not be seen in all patients, such as retinal dystrophy, renal disease, ocular colobomas, occipital encephalocele, hepatic fibrosis, polydactyly, and other abnormalities.[16] This is known as variable expressivity, where individuals with the same condition may express different symptoms. The variability seen in these conditions between individuals may be a result of gene-gene and gene-environment interactions.

Some families may have more than 1 affected offspring even in the absence of family history and negative parental testing. This type of inheritance may be explained by gonadal or somatic mosaicism, where the parent has a de novo variant that occurs in a prezygotic mutational event during his or her early embryonic development. Because of parental mosaicism, the recurrence risk for apparently de novo variants is never 0%; instead 1% to 3% is often quoted as the recurrence risk, but it is being learned that this may actually be much higher as seen in with *SCN1A*-related epilepsy, Dravet syndrome,[17] and Duchenne muscular dystrophy.[18]

Family History

Medical genetics focuses not only on the patient but also the entire family. Family history is an important piece in the analysis of any condition and differential diagnosis. A detailed pedigree can help elicit inheritance, natural history, reduced penetrance, and variable expressivity. A pedigree can also provide a visual of a family's social structure. When obtaining a pedigree, it is important to use the standard symbols and configuration[19] so that others may accurately read the pedigree. Obtaining a detailed pedigree can also help identify patients and family members who may be at risk for certain genetic conditions so that proper management, prevention, and counseling can be offered to the patient and the family. When collecting a pedigree, relevant and specific questions such as those in **Table 2** can help identify potential modes of inheritance and direct best genetic testing strategies.

Table 2
Relevant questions in obtaining a family history

Question	Genetic Testing Implications	Genetic Test
Is there a family history of similar motor delay?	Autosomal-dominant conditions	Focused testing based on family history
Is there a family history of other neurodevelopmental disorders?	Neurodevelopmental condition with phenotypic heterogeneity	Focused testing based on family history
Is there a possibility of shared ancestry between parents?	Consanguinity increases risk for at least 1 if not more than 1 autosomal-recessive condition	SNP-based chromosomal microarrays can detect chromosomal regions of loss of homozygosity Prefer broad sequencing testing such as exome or whole-genome sequencing based on risk for multiple recessive disorders
If there is a family history of multiple miscarriages?	Increased risk for chromosomal anomaly (ie, unbalanced translocation in patient)	Chromosomal testing – chromosomal microarray to detect microdeletions or duplications + karyotype to see if there is a translocation. Karyotype in parents to detect balanced translocations
Is there a family history of other possible conditions such as early cancer, stroke, or cardiac conditions?	Possibility of detecting other genetic conditions that may be treatable or medically actionable for the patient Decrease the chance of unsuspected incidental findings if sending exome or genome sequencing	Recommend sending exome or genome sequencing for the most complete genetic testing for the patient based on phenotype and family history of other possible dominantly inherited condition

Pre- and Post-test Counseling

Pretest counseling

With the increasing accessibility and complexity of genetic testing, it is important that health care providers know the benefits, limitations, and risks of the various genetic tests offered. Obtaining an informed consent or assent for children who are old enough is essential for the patient and parents to fully understand the benefits, risks, and limitations, and make an informed decision. Pre- and post-test counseling should be done in a nondirective, clear, and objective manner. The patient should be given the option to decline any or all genetic tests offered. Pretest consent and counseling for genetic testing should include

- A description of the test and its purpose (what genetic test is being done and what is being detected)
- What type of sample is needed for the test (blood, buccal, saliva)
- Possible test results
  - o Positive
  - o Negative
  - o Variant of uncertain significance
  - o Incidental findings, which may include medically actionable conditions related to heart disease and cancer, and variants related to pharmacogenetics
- Potential psychosocial, insurance, and employment risks
  - o The Genetic Information Nondiscrimination Act of 2008 (GINA) protects individuals from health insurance and employment discrimination and harassment; GINA does not apply to life, disability, and long-term care
  - o Some genetic tests, like exome sequencing may detect nonpaternity
  - o Risks to other family members or future offspring
  - o Feelings of guilt and shame
  - o Anxiety and uncertainty of the outcomes
  - o Detection of consanguinity (with tests such as chromosome microarray) and nonpaternity
- When and to whom results will be reported
- If a health care provider does not have knowledge or expertise to counsel a patient appropriately, a referral to a genetic counselor of geneticist should be considered

Post-test counseling

Genetic testing results for patients in a pediatric neurology setting can have devasting effects on families, alter a patient's medication management, allow the option of gene therapy or lifesaving therapeutics, and determine heritability and risks to other family members. Genetic counselors can assist in interpreting results and providing appropriate follow-up. Without proper genetic counseling, results misinterpretation, inappropriate medical management, and adverse psychosocial outcome have been reported.[20] In a pre-COVID-19 (coronavirus 2019) world, telegenetics was underutilized;[21] however, telemedicine is now commonly utilized to return sensitive genetic results. A systematic review by Kubendran and colleagues reported high patient satisfaction with telegenetics that was comparable to in-person counseling. Results disclosure should be done sensitively and allow time to evaluate psychological response, answer questions, and provide support resources. Post-test counseling should include

- Management options (clinical trials, research options)
- Implications for relatives and reproductive risks
- Emotional impact of results and additional counseling referrals if warranted
- Discussion of additional testing or screenings if applicable

Ethical and Policy Issues

Many neurogenetic conditions are inherited, and positive test results may have significant implications for family members. This can often raise difficult ethical issues and be complicated by a family's social structure. A positive test result may provide an answer for the child's main clinical symptoms but can also provide information that the child or parent may be at risk for later adult-onset symptoms.

This can be seen with X-linked adrenoleukodystrophy (X-ALD). X-ALD presents with variable expressivity and reduced penetrance and can be difficult to track in a family history. It is estimated that over 95% of cases are inherited[22] and can present in 3 different forms: childhood cerebral onset with leukodystrophy and death in early childhood, Addison disease with adrenal insufficiency, and the adult-onset form known as adrenomyeloneuropathy (AMN),.[22] With effective bone-marrow transplant treatment for the early childhood form and potentially gene therapy, X-ALD has recently been added to the newborn screening (NBS) recommended uniform screening panel (RUSP). The NBS identifies carrier females and affected males. There is great inter- and intrafamilial variability with X-ALD and no clear genotype-phenotype correlation.[22] Infant boys who have a positive NBS and are confirmed to be positive may develop any of the 3 forms or remain asymptomatic. Additionally, carrier infant girls and mothers may be at risk for the adult-onset AMN. This results in unintentional predictive testing. Cases such as these present with difficulty in counseling and require sensitivity and consideration of the psychosocial and clinical effects of testing. It is recognized that with the increasing treatments available for pediatric neurogenetic conditions, more conditions may be added to the RUSP in the near future, which may raise concerns of autonomy.

Genetic testing in children is widely accepted for diagnostic purposes; however, many parents of affected children may want other asymptomatic children tested for risk estimate and carrier status. Many parents are seeking relief from anxiety that their children or future grandchildren are not at risk. The National Society of Genetic Counselors, The American College of Medical Genetics and Genomicsand the American Academy of Pediatrics do not support testing asymptomatic minors. The recommendation is to defer testing until adulthood.[23]

Because of the heritability of genetic conditions, especially autosomal-recessive and X-linked conditions, other relatives may have an increased risk of having affected offspring, and there is a duty to warn them. Parents are encouraged to share their carrier status with at-risk relatives. The failure to do this can prevent the at-risk relatives of making informed decisions for their own health and reproductive management. The 4 principles of medical ethics consist of beneficence, nonmaleficence, autonomy, and justice.[24] These principles may be viewed differently according to the stakeholder (ie, patient, family member, medical provider, or society). With the increasing accessibility of genetic testing, it is important to be mindful of the ethical issues that arise to reduce the potential for patient harm.

Management Strategies

Discussion/application: how to approach a neurogenetic workup

Every neurologist should be able to describe the clinical phenotype. The phenotype should include the neurologic features, extraneurological features if present, and family history. Neurologic features include the presence of seizures, movement disorders, muscle tone, weakness, and examination findings and neuroimaging findings. Extraneurological features are the presence of other system-related issues that may assist with a diagnosis and treatment plans/referrals for symptomatic management. Examples of extraneurological features include adrenal insufficiency for X-ALD or cardiac rhabdomyomas for patients with tuberous sclerosis complex (TSC) that if present may assist with making a clinical diagnosis.

There are different approaches for sending genetic testing in patients with a diagnosis of a neurologic disorder. If the patient's clinical history including family history and neuroimaging has a specific phenotype, then start with targeted testing based on that phenotype. If the features are nonspecific but there are dysmorphic features or other congenital anomalies or multiple miscarriages in the mother, then a CMA would be a good test to send. If there is a history of developmental regression, then metabolic testing and an urgent referral to a specialist is recommended. Metabolic testing can also assist in characterizing a patient's phenotype and assist with more specific testing when indicated.

If the patient's phenotype is nonspecific such as hypotonia, then one should consider sending a broad test based such as exome sequencing if SMA, myotonic dystrophy, and chromosomal abnormalities have been ruled out based on clinical history or negative testing. There are gene panels for many specific phenotypes such as ataxia, CNS migrational disorders, neuromuscular disorders, and treatable disorders. There is a Web site called the Genetic Testing Registry, www.ncbi.nlm.nih.gov/gtr, that may be helpful in choosing a panel or a laboratory to select for genetic testing. The yield of genetic testing will likely continue to improve with advances in technology such as genomic sequencing and most likely other mechanisms such as mosaic, epigenetic mechanisms like imprinting or other multifactorial disorders that have yet to be discovered. Functional assays to assist in determining if a variant is benign or pathogenic, however, continue to lag behind the sequencing technology and will hopefully also improve in the future to assist with variants of unknown significance.

What if testing is nondiagnostic? Providers can request a reanalysis of a patient's previous ES at least 1 year after the report date or an updated exome or panel if a significant number of years has passed. Updated genetic testing can also be considered if the patient's symptoms or family history has changed. A reanalysis may lead to a diagnosis if a new gene was discovered after the initial or previous testing or if a variant of unknown significance was reclassified as pathogenic. Reanalysis, research tools, functional analysis, RNA-sequencing, and other emerging tools can also help provide a diagnosis, as genetics is a dynamic specialty with updates occurring on a regular basis.

SUMMARY

As understanding of genetics increases, so does the availability of therapeutic interventions for neurogenetic conditions. It is becoming increasingly important to identify a patient's genotype to tailor treatment or management to his or her condition, avoid contraindicated medications, or confirm eligibility for clinical trials. These molecular therapies represent 1 facet of the important paradigm embraced by the concept of precision medicine.

It is also understood that the concept of genetics applies to more than just the symptomatic patient, but instead the entire family unit. Genetic testing and diagnoses come with great ethical considerations and implications. Neurologists can work together with genetics professionals to ensure proper genetic testing and counseling for patients and families.

As the field of genetics continues to advance, new genes and mechanisms for genetic disorders will be discovered.

DISCLOSURE STATEMENT

The authors have nothing to disclose.

REFERENCES

1. Cavallin M, Mine M, Philbert M, et al. Further refinement of COL4A1 and COL4A2 related cortical malformations. Eur J Med Genet 2018;61(12):765–72.
2. Nussbaum RL, McInnes RR, Willard HF. Thompson & Thompson genetics in medicine. 8th editionxi. Elsevier; 2016. p. 546.

3. Borlot F, Regan BM, Bassett AS, et al. Prevalence of pathogenic copy number variation in adults with pediatric-onset epilepsy and intellectual disability. JAMA Neurol 2017;74(11):1301–11.

4. Richards S, Aziz N, Bale S, et al. Standards and guidelines for the interpretation of sequence variants: a joint consensus recommendation of the American College of Medical Genetics and Genomics and the Association for Molecular Pathology. Genet Med 2015;17(5):405–24.

5. Kim A, Kumar KR, Davis RL, et al. Increased diagnostic yield of spastic paraplegia with or without cerebellar ataxia through whole-genome sequencing. Cerebellum 2019;18(4):781–90.

6. Posey JE, Harel T, Liu P, et al. Resolution of disease phenotypes resulting from multilocus genomic variation. N Engl J Med 2017;376(1):21–31.

7. Yang Y, Muzny DM, Reid JG, et al. Clinical whole-exome sequencing for the diagnosis of mendelian disorders. N Engl J Med 2013;369(16):1502–11.

8. Yang Y, Muzny DM, Xia F, et al. Molecular findings among patients referred for clinical whole-exome sequencing. JAMA 2014;312(18):1870–9.

9. Stranneheim H, Lagerstedt-Robinson K, Magnusson M, et al. Integration of whole genome sequencing into a healthcare setting: high diagnostic rates across multiple clinical entities in 3219 rare disease patients. Genome Med 2021;13(1):40.

10. Vissers L, van Nimwegen KJM, Schieving JH, et al. A clinical utility study of exome sequencing versus conventional genetic testing in pediatric neurology. Genet Med 2017;19(9):1055–63.

11. Biesecker LG, Green RC. Diagnostic clinical genome and exome sequencing. N Engl J Med 2014;371(12):1170.

12. Cummings BB, Marshall JL, Tukiainen T, et al. Improving genetic diagnosis in Mendelian disease with transcriptome sequencing. Sci Transl Med 2017; 9(386). https://doi.org/10.1126/scitranslmed.aal5209.

13. Murdock DR, Dai H, Burrage LC, et al. Transcriptome-directed analysis for Mendelian disease diagnosis overcomes limitations of conventional genomic testing. J Clin Invest 2021;131(1). https://doi.org/10.1172/JCI141500.

14. Alaimo JT, Glinton KE, Liu N, et al. Integrated analysis of metabolomic profiling and exome data supplements sequence variant interpretation, classification, and diagnosis. Genet Med 2020;22(9):1560–6.

15. Steinlein OK, Hoda JC, Bertrand S, et al. Mutations in familial nocturnal frontal lobe epilepsy might be associated with distinct neurological phenotypes. Seizure 2012;21(2):118–23.

16. Hartill V, Szymanska K, Sharif SM, et al. Meckel-Gruber syndrome: an update on diagnosis, clinical management, and research advances. Front Pediatr 2017; 5:244.

17. de Lange IM, Koudijs MJ, van 't Slot R, et al. Assessment of parental mosaicism in SCN1A-related epilepsy by single-molecule molecular inversion probes and next-generation sequencing. J Med Genet 2019;56(2):75–80.

18. Helderman-van den Enden AT, de Jong R, den Dunnen JT, et al. Recurrence risk due to germ line mosaicism: Duchenne and Becker muscular dystrophy. Clin Genet 2009;75(5):465–72.

19. Bennett RL, French KS, Resta RG, et al. Standardized human pedigree nomenclature: update and assessment of the recommendations of the National Society of Genetic Counselors. J Genet Couns 2008;17(5):424–33.

20. Buchanan AH, Rahm AK, Williams JL. Alternate service delivery models in cancer genetic counseling: a mini-review. Front Oncol 2016;6:120.

21. Kubendran S, Sivamurthy S, Schaefer GB. A novel approach in pediatric telegenetic services: geneticist, pediatrician and genetic counselor team. Genet Med 2017;19(11):1260-7.
22. Wiesinger C, Eichler FS, Berger J. The genetic landscape of X-linked adrenoleukodystrophy: inheritance, mutations, modifier genes, and diagnosis. Appl Clin Genet 2015;8:109-21.
23. Ross LF. Ethical and policy issues in newborn screening of children for neurologic and developmental disorders. Pediatr Clin North Am 2015;62(3):787-98.
24. Beauchamp TL. The 'Four Principles' Approach to Health Care Ethics. In: Richard E,, Ashcroft AD, Draper H, et al, editors. Principles of health care ethics. 2nd Edition. John Wiley & Sons, Ltd; 2006.

Novel Treatments and Clinical Research in Child Neurology

Gary D. Clark, MD, Timothy E. Lotze, MD*

KEYWORDS

- Child neurology clinical research • Child neurology residency training
- Antisense oligonucleotide • Enzyme replacement • Gene therapy

KEY POINTS

- Research into therapeutics for neurologic disorders in children has markedly increased due to greater molecular understanding of the pathogenic mechanisms of disease.
- Child neurology residency programs should provide trainees with experiences that build interest and skill in clinical research.
- Novel treatments for heretofore untreatable and fatal disorders promise to change the field of Child Neurology.

INTRODUCTION

Child neurology has transformed into a field of novel therapies aimed at the root cause of disease. In this article, the authors cover some of the recent treatments that turned degenerative and fatal disorders into chronic conditions. The future for therapy in child neurology is very bright, and the practicing child neurologist will have to understand the principles of these novel therapies.

The molecular understanding of the pathogenic mechanisms responsible for neurologic diseases of children has led to a remarkable period of research that addresses the root causes of diseases. The promise of this research has been realized with cures and treatments that correct underlying deficiencies. The breakneck rate at which new research is being proposed promises to usher in a transformation of child neurology from a diagnostic and supportive field into an interventional one.

ENZYME REPLACEMENT

Somatic diseases resulting from enzyme deficiencies can be treated with intravenous infusions of enzyme, such that enzyme replacement is relatively common for somatic

Department of Pediatrics, Division of Neurology and Developmental Neuroscience, Baylor College of Medicine, 6701 Fannin Street Suite 1250, Houston, TX 77030, USA
* Corresponding author.
E-mail address: tlotze@bcm.edu

Neurol Clin 39 (2021) 719–722
https://doi.org/10.1016/j.ncl.2021.05.004
neurologic.theclinics.com

disorders. The brain remains a challenging organ for enzyme replacement because most proteins do not cross the blood-brain barrier.

Therefore, enzyme replacement for brain disease is and will be challenging. Cerliponase alfa, a recombinant tripeptidyl peptidase (actually manufactured as a proenzyme), is the first of the enzyme replacement strategies to have received full approval for a human neurologic disorder, late infantile neuronal ceroid lipofuscinosis (*CLN2*-related Batten disease).[1] In a remarkable achievement, this treatment, inspired by a treatment of a spontaneously occurring Beagle model[2] of late infantile neuronal ceroid lipofuscinosis, is an enzyme replacement given every 2 weeks via a ventricular port in humans. It leads to an arrest of the disorder that is a rapidly progressive neurodegenerative disorder. Because the treatment has only been in existence for about 5 years, it is not known if this will prevent only brain disease and allow disease to progress in the eyes or even other tissues. Because this is an enzyme replacement, reactions are common, as seen in other enzyme replacements. Premedication with diphenhydramine and methylprednisolone is often used. Because enzyme deficiency is often a cause for neurologic disease, this strategy may be used in other disorders.

ANTISENSE OLIGONUCLEOTIDES

Antisense oligonucleotides (ASOs) are small DNA molecules that can modify RNA and protein expression, target mutant allele expression, prevent DNA silencing, and produce dosage effects.[3] The targeting and design of these ASOs is beyond the scope of this chapter and have been the subject of much study. However, the human benefits of these small molecules have been demonstrated in spinal muscular atrophy, muscular dystrophy, and in an N-of-1 study, *CLN7*-related Batten disease.

In spinal muscular atrophy, children lack the ability to make enough survival motor neuron (SMN) protein for their anterior horn cells to survive. This protein can be produced via transcription from *SMN1* and less efficiently from *SMN2*. Nusinersen modifies the transcripts (modifies splicing) from *SMN2* to make the SMN protein more efficiently, thereby preventing disease progression and in some cases improving neurologic function.[4,5]

Duchenne muscular dystrophy results from loss-of-function variants in *Dystrophin*. This gene is long (79 exons), and disease results often from premature stops owing to various mutations. ASOs designed to treat Duchenne have had success by skipping exons in a personal mutation-specific manner, thereby leading to the production of some protein.

Pointing to a possible future for ASOs, a child affected by *CLN7*-related neuronal ceroid lipofuscinosis (*CLN7*-related Batten disease) was found to have a splice-altering intron insertion in one allele of *CLN7* and a pathogenic variant in the other allele. A personalized ASO was designed to alter the transcripts from the intron-inserted variant, thereby enhancing production of an intact *CLN7* transcript.[6] This treatment has been rendered intrathecally via a lumbar puncture every 3 months, similar to that of nusinersen.

Clinical trials for other ASOs to unmask imprinted (silenced) genes in Angelman syndrome, dosage effects from duplication syndromes, and other personalized ASO strategies are underway.

VIRAL VECTORS TO INTRODUCE GENES

Adeno-associated viruses (AAV) to introduce genes into the central nervous system (CNS) has been a strategy for several recent clinical trials, including a transformational one to treat spinal muscular atrophy. The efficiency of these vectors to introduce genes into neurons has been the subject of much of the criticism of this approach. Although this remains debated, the efficacy of an AAV-9 introduction of *SMN* into the CNS of patients with spinal muscular atrophy has been dramatically established.[7]

Pharmacologic Agents to Modify Signaling Pathways in Disease

At this point, nearly every signaling pathway in humans has been targeted by pharmaceutical companies, and new agents have been brought to treat neurologic disorders based on the disturbed signaling pathways.

For example, the mammalian target of rapamycin (mTOR) has been inhibited in conditions in which it is upregulated. Tuberous sclerosis is one such disorder that results from hemizygous loss of either *TSC1* or *TSC2*, resulting in upregulation of mTOR. In patients with tuberous sclerosis, the treatment with everolimus has been shown to shrink giant cell astrocytomas and angiomyolipomas and to lessen seizure burden.[8–11]

Neurofibromatosis 1 results from loss-of-function mutations in *NF1* that results in upregulation of the Ras–mitogen-activated protein kinase (MAPK) pathway. Selumetinib, a selective MAPK 1 and 2 inhibitor, shrinks inoperable plexiform neuromas in patients with neurofibromatosis type 1.[12]

CLINICAL RESEARCH IN CHILD NEUROLOGY

The few examples of dramatic, innovative treatments for child neurologic disorders point to the possibilities that transformational clinical research in our field will lead to a bright future for our patients. However, who will do this research? Are there enough child neurologists trained for clinical research to provide the throughput necessary to realize this future?

The regulatory components, the care of the vulnerable child in an experimental trial, the time constraints on the practicing child neurologist, and money, all conspire to make the charge of accomplishing the necessary research to transform our field challenging. Yet, we must train the next generation of child neurologists to do clinical research, to understand the basis of new and transformational clinical trials, and we must become an interventional field for our patients.

DISCLOSURE

The authors have nothing to disclose.

REFERENCES

1. Schulz A, Ajayi T, Spo008io N, et al. Study of Intraventricular Cerliponase Alfa for CLN2 Disease. New Engl J Med 2018;378(20):1898–907.
2. Vuillemenot BR, Katz ML, Coates JR, et al. Intrathecal tripeptidyl-peptidase 1 reduces lysosomal storage in a canine model of late infantile neuronal ceroid lipofuscinosis. Mol Genet Metab 2011;104(3):325–37.
3. Rinaldi C, Wood MJA. Antisense oligonucleotides: the next frontier for treatment of neurological disorders. Nat Rev Neurol 2018;14(1):9–21.
4. Finkel RS, Chiriboga CA, Vajsar J, et al. Treatment of infantile-onset spinal muscular atrophy with nusinersen: a phase 2, open-label, dose-escalation study. Lancet 2016;388(10063):3017–26.
5. Chiriboga CA, Swoboda KJ, Darras BT, et al. Results from a phase 1 study of nusinersen (ISIS-SMN(Rx)) in children with spinal muscular atrophy. Neurology 2016;86(10):890–7.

6. Kim J, Hu C, Moufawad El Achkar C, et al. Patient-Customized Oligonucleotide Therapy for a Rare Genetic Disease. New Engl J Med 2019;381(17):1644–52.

7. Mendell JR, Al-Zaidy S, Shell R, et al. Single-Dose Gene-Replacement Therapy for Spinal Muscular Atrophy. New Engl J Med 2017;377(18):1713–22.

8. Bissler JJ, Kingswood JC, Radzikowska E, et al. Everolimus for angiomyolipoma associated with tuberous sclerosis complex or sporadic lymphangioleiomyomatosis (EXIST-2): a multicentre, randomised, double-blind, placebo-controlled trial. Lancet 2013;381(9869):817–24.

9. Curatolo P, Franz DN, Lawson JA, et al. Adjunctive everolimus for children and adolescents with treatment-refractory seizures associated with tuberous sclerosis complex: post-hoc analysis of the phase 3 EXIST-3 trial. Lancet Child Adolescent Health 2018;2(7):495–504.

10. Franz DN, Belousova E, Sparagana S, et al. Everolimus for subependymal giant cell astrocytoma in patients with tuberous sclerosis complex: 2-year open-label extension of the randomised EXIST-1 study. Lancet Oncol 2014;15(13):1513–20.

11. Franz DN, Belousova E, Sparagana S, et al. Efficacy and safety of everolimus for subependymal giant cell astrocytomas associated with tuberous sclerosis complex (EXIST-1): a multicentre, randomised, placebo-controlled phase 3 trial. Lancet 2013;381(9861):125–32.

12. Dombi E, Baldwin A, Marcus LJ, et al. Activity of Selumetinib in Neurofibromatosis Type 1-Related Plexiform Neurofibromas. New Engl J Med 2016;375(26):2550–60.

Epilepsy Surgery
Monitoring and Novel Surgical Techniques

Elaine S. Seto, MD, PhD[a,b,*], Rohini Coorg, MD[a,b]

KEYWORDS

- Drug-resistant epilepsy • Stereo-electroencephalography
- Minimally invasive surgery • Laser interstitial thermal therapy

KEY POINTS

- Patients with drug-resistant epilepsy should be referred to epilepsy surgery centers as soon as possible.
- The epilepsy presurgical evaluation may include multiple testing modalities, including neurophysiology, imaging, and functional studies.
- Stereo-electroencephalography (SEEG) is often preferred over subdural electrodes due to decreased morbidity and the ability to sample multiple anatomic regions including depth of sulci and deep brain structures.
- There is increasing evidence for the efficacy and safety of minimally invasive surgical treatments for epilepsy, including laser ablation, thermo-SEEG, gamma knife, and endoscopic surgery.

INTRODUCTION

Drug-resistant epilepsy, defined as the persistence of seizures despite 2 appropriately trialed medications, occurs in approximately one-third of epilepsy cases.[1] Given the potential for morbidity and mortality over a lifetime, it is important to consider additional therapeutic options. It is recommended that patients with drug-resistant epilepsy be evaluated at an epilepsy surgery center, particularly patients with surgically amenable brain lesions.[2,3] Despite this, epilepsy surgery represents an underutilized treatment, often with significant delays between seizure onset and surgical intervention.[4] Traditional surgical techniques include potentially curative approaches such as craniotomy with lobectomy, lesionectomy, anatomic or functional hemispherectomies, and resections further tailored with invasive monitoring techniques. Traditional

[a] Section of Pediatric Neurology and Developmental Neuroscience, Department of Pediatrics, Baylor College of Medicine, Houston, TX, USA; [b] Department of Neurology and Developmental Neuroscience, Texas Children's Hospital, 6701 Fannin Street, Suite 1250, Houston, TX 77030, USA
* Corresponding author. Texas Children's Hospital, 6701 Fannin Street, Suite 1250, Houston, TX 77030.
E-mail address: esseto@bcm.edu

Neurol Clin 39 (2021) 723–742
https://doi.org/10.1016/j.ncl.2021.04.001
0733-8619/21/© 2021 Elsevier Inc. All rights reserved.

palliative surgical approaches include craniotomy with corpus callosotomy and vagus nerve stimulator implantation. These traditional approaches, although efficacious, are subject to significant corridor-related morbidity, namely the morbidity associated with craniotomy, opening of the dura, and accessing the intended tissue.

Advances in technology use a minimally invasive approach both in defining the epileptogenic zone and proceeding with surgical treatment. These techniques reduce corridor-related morbidity and are often more attractive to potential surgical candidates who otherwise decline to proceed with surgical evaluation due to the perceived risks of a large operation. The approaches described in this article in conjunction with a thorough epilepsy center evaluation may help to reduce this treatment gap.[5,6]

PRESURGICAL EVALUATION

The presurgical evaluation, often referred to as "Phase I," is central to determining the underlying etiology of the patient's epilepsy, localization of seizure-onset zones, and most appropriate surgical approach. Features of the history, including handedness, risk factors for epilepsy, age of seizure onset, presence or absence of infantile spasms, and clinical semiology, provide important details about whether the patient's epilepsy represents a focal, multifocal, or generalized process. Curative or palliative goals (such as reducing total seizure burden or targeting a specific debilitating seizure type) should be discussed with the patient or relevant caregivers to establish realistic expectations before embarking on a thorough and potentially expensive evaluation. Neuroimaging and electroencephalogram (EEG) monitoring are considered mandatory in the presurgical evaluation but additional ancillary testing may be necessary on an individualized basis.[7]

MRI of the brain is critical for identification of structural etiologies and may provide prognostic information. Epilepsy with mesial temporal sclerosis, for example, is associated with increased high risk of drug resistance but higher chances of surgical success.[8,9] In the absence of abnormalities on initial imaging, high-resolution MRI with thin slices is recommended, as well as 3T imaging if available, to increase the likelihood of detecting subtle focal cortical dysplasias (FCDs).[9] Infants, who are in the process of myelination, may require serial MRI to identify FCDs.

The neurophysiology portion of the evaluation is paramount to localizing seizure onset. Interictal and ictal abnormalities on continuous EEG-video may identify regions of cortical irritability and probable seizure onset while precisely documenting semiologic features that may not have previously been observed or reported by the patient or family. Notably, however, when arising from deep structures within the frontal lobes, parietal lobes, or near locations involved in prior brain surgery, the ictal onset may be nonexistent, diffuse/bilateral, or merely lateralized to a hemisphere on scalp EEG.

In the absence of concordant clinical, imaging, and neurophysiologic data, additional diagnostic testing may provide additional insight into the seizure-onset zone. Subtraction interictal-ictal single-photon emission computed tomography (SISCOM or Ictal-SPECT) may be performed during continuous EEG-video. Focal seizures are associated with increased blood flow at the site of seizure onset such that a radiotracer injected at seizure onset will accumulate in the region of cerebral hyperperfusion, thereby visualizing the seizure onset.[10] Subtle differences in radiotracer uptake can be enhanced by subtraction of a scan taken in the interictal state. Brain electrical source analysis can be used to analyze EEG interictal and ictal waveforms and model their 3-dimensional localization. Magnetoencephalography (MEG) can be performed to visualize tangentially oriented sources in the interhemispheric region or along sulci, which are typically poorly visualized on surface EEG.

Functional studies are used in conjunction with neurophysiologic studies to clarify eloquent regions and clarify risks of functional deficits with surgery. Fluorodeoxyglucose-positron emission tomography (FDG-PET) identifies areas of hypometabolism that regionalize brain dysfunction, although often greater in volume than the actual epileptogenic zone.[11] Task-based and resting state functional MRI are used to localize language and motor regions. MEG also can be used to map sensory and motor areas in pediatric patients and language areas in adults.[12,13] Transcranial magnetic stimulation is useful to identify eloquent motor regions.[14] In selected cases in which language or memory is unable to be noninvasively identified, a Wada test may assist with hemispheric localization of language and memory functions. Last, but arguably most important, a comprehensive neuropsychology evaluation provides insight into current focal cognitive deficits, the risk for further deficits with surgery, and comorbidities, such as autism, attention-deficit/hyperactivity disorder, and mood disorders, which may impact surgical decision making for the patient and family.[15]

Following completion of these studies, results are discussed in a multidisciplinary epilepsy surgery conference to develop an individualized treatment plan. Some surgical options may be recommended based on the noninvasive data alone. If the data implicate several regions potentially amenable to surgery or if the surgical solution is unclear, invasive monitoring is often recommended to further localize seizure onset and guide a surgical plan.

INVASIVE MONITORING BY STEREO-ELECTROENCEPHALOGRAPHY

Bancaud and Talarach used subdural and depth electrodes as early as 1959 to study the onset and early propagation of seizures. Stereo-EEG (SEEG) as a localizing tool in the setting of inconclusive noninvasive data became established in the Montreal Neurologic Institution in 1972. The minimally invasive nature of this monitoring method is attractive to families and has the benefit of decreased tissue distortion and the ability to localize deeper seizure onsets. SEEG electrodes can be placed through small twist drill holes using a conventional stereotactic frame, frameless stereotactic apparatus, or more recently, robotic assistance (**Fig. 1**). In our experience at Texas Children's Hospital, SEEG electrodes may be successfully placed in children as young as 12 months, although limited skull thickness challenges the security of bolts and SEEG electrodes. Precise electrode placement is crucial for neurophysiologic sampling, as well as to avoid injury to vascular structures. The most common complication associated with SEEG is intracranial hemorrhage, with a reported risk of 0.075% to 0.15% per electrode.[16] Depending on the number of SEEG electrodes placed, the risk of hemorrhage may be comparable to the 4% risk reported for monitoring with subdural grids.[17] The risk of infection, however, is only 1% for SEEG compared with 3% for grids.[16,17]

Having well-defined hypotheses to guide placement of SEEG electrodes is important. Strategies for electrode placement are dependent on the presence or absence of lesions and the proposed epileptic network based on clinical seizure semiology and electrographic evolution on surface EEG.[18] SEEG monitoring is helpful in cases of bitemporal epilepsy or distinguishing between frontal or temporal epilepsy, especially in nonlesional cases.[19] A common case may include confirming mesial temporal sclerosis as the source of seizure onset in the presence of discordant history of diagnostic features (often referred to as "temporal-plus" scenarios).[18,20] To explore this, mesial temporal structures in addition to lateral temporal and extratemporal (anterior cingulate, orbitofrontal, and insular) regions may be sampled. More recently, SEEG

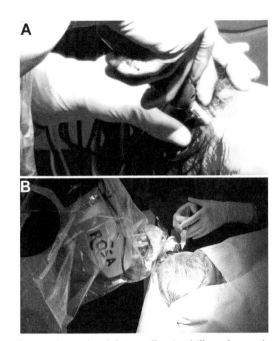

Fig. 1. Placement of SEEG electrodes. (*A*) A small twist drill can be used to generate craniostomies of ~3-mm diameter lining up with the planned electrode trajectory. (*B*) Frameless stereotaxy in combination with robotic assistance (eg, ROSA system shown) allows for more rapid in placement of depth electrodes.

has been used to identify the most epileptogenic region in cases of multifocal, disparate lesions.[21] At our institution, we aim to target the entire network of the seizure in our coverage to include anatomic regions implicated in both the onset and propagation of the seizure. Wide coverage is favored and possible through the minimally invasive nature of the recording electrodes.

SEEG implantation can also be used as part of a staged surgical process to narrow down to a more focused hypothesis that may require further invasive exploration or mapping before surgical treatment.[18] In our center, for complex cases, SEEG is sometimes seen as an "extension" of the noninvasive presurgical workup to regionalize the seizure-onset zone. If extensive coverage is needed due to complex epileptic networks or multiple targeted seizure types, limitations in amplifier size may occur. In these cases, recording from every other contact of the SEEG electrode in areas deemed less likely to be implicated in the ictal onset may be a useful strategy. As coverage is limited with SEEG, recording scalp EEG simultaneously may be beneficial to help distinguish nonepileptic events that may be similar to their ictal semiology (eg, behavioral inattentiveness or nocturnal arousals).

Case Example

A 3-year-old boy with refractory epilepsy due to tuberous sclerosis complex (TSC) had daily seizures of 2 semiologies: focal hypermotor and gelastic seizures. This genetic condition caused the development of cortical tubers in multiple brain regions (**Fig. 2**A, B). Discordant results during the Phase I presurgical evaluation guided placement of 14 SEEG electrodes in regions of both the right and left hemispheres (**Fig. 2**C).

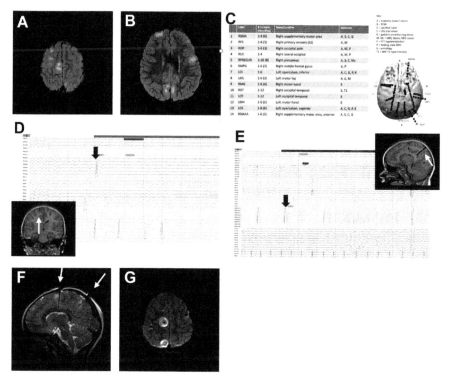

Fig. 2. Case example of SEEG characterization of seizures in TSC. (*A, B*) MRI brain, axial T2 fluid-attenuated inversion recovery images show multifocal tubers, including a prominent tuber in the right central midline region (*A*) and multiple tubers in the bilateral mesial occipital, right frontal, and left frontal regions (*B*). (*C*) SEEG electrode list and 3-dimensional brain reconstruction. (*D*) SEEG onset (*black arrow*) in RSMA2-4 with focal hypermotor seizures, corresponding to a cortical tuber in the right midline region, near the supplementary motor region (indicated in red on MRI brain coronal T1 image). (*E*) SEEG onset (*black arrow*) in RPRECUN2-6 with gelastic seizures. This corresponded to a cortical tuber in the right precuneus region (indicated in red on MRI Brain sagittal T1 image). (*F*) Intraoperative MRI brain sagittal T2 image shows trajectories through 2 implicated tubers. (*G*) MRI brain axial diffusion weighted image following laser ablation of 2 tubers.

Electrocorticography (ECoG) revealed that the habitual seizure types arose from distinct tubers (**Figs. 2**D, E) and the patient underwent MRI-guided stereotactic laser ablation of both seizure foci using 2 trajectories (**Fig 2**F, G). The patient remained seizure-free at 2-year follow-up (Engel 1A outcome).

Role of high-frequency oscillations in stereo-electroencephalography

There is emerging evidence that high-frequency oscillations (HFOs) may be useful as markers of the epileptogenic zone. HFOs can be subdivided into ripples and fast ripples. Definitions vary between studies, generally 80 to 200 or 80 to 250 Hz activity for ripples and 200 to 500 or 250 to 500 Hz activity for fast ripples. HFO identification requires a high sampling rate (≥2000 Hz) and good signal-to-noise ratio. Visual analysis is time-consuming, so automated detection is commonly used, frequently focusing on non–rapid eye movement sleep when HFOs are more abundant.[22]

HFOs detected by macroelectrodes have been described independent and coincident of interictal epileptiform discharges, occurring more frequently in seizure-onset zones in adults (**Fig. 3**).[23] Ictally, studies of small patient cohorts have shown localized brief or prolonged runs of HFOs near the time of seizure onset in regions that correspond to the ECoG seizure-onset zone in both adults and children.[24,25] Some studies suggest that removal of HFO-generating regions is associated with better surgical outcomes.[25,26] Although these data are intriguing, HFOs also can be seen physiologically, for example, over the motor cortex during finger movements,[27] and physiologic HFOs are morphologically similar to HFOs occurring in seizure-onset regions. Given this, a 2014 Cochrane review found that there is insufficient evidence for the use of HFOs to guide epilepsy surgery decision making at this time, and larger, randomized studies are needed.[28]

Functional mapping with stereo-electroencephalography

The goal of epilepsy surgery is to remove the epileptogenic zone with minimal induced deficits. Although brain regions can be presumed functional based on our understanding of normal brain anatomy, patients can exhibit significant variability, especially in the context of insults at a young age. Electrical stimulation mapping using implanted electrodes can be performed at the bedside or intraoperatively to determine if the epileptogenic region overlaps with eloquent cortex involved in movement, sensation, language, vision, or higher-order brain functions. This mapping technique can induce positive signs (eg, arm movement) or negative signs (eg, interruption of speech) and is dependent on rapid assessment of functional changes while stimulation is applied. For most functions, patient cooperation is also required. Importantly, the absence of clinical signs does not exclude all functions in the stimulated tissue but may reflect functions not acutely tested, functions with broad or bilateral representation, or inadequate stimulation. ECoG is simultaneously monitored for stimulus-induced afterdischarges or seizures.

Technically, using SEEG electrodes for mapping has significant differences from subdural electrodes.[29] SEEG contacts within an electrode are spaced 5 mm apart so bipolar stimulation affects only a focal region in direct proximity to the contacts. Stimulation is, however, efficient, as there is greater surface area in contact with the brain and less dissipation from cerebrospinal fluid. Because of these differences, the maximum stimulation parameters that can be safely used for SEEG electrode mapping are reduced compared with subdural electrodes.

A novel technique for functional mapping involves quantification of high gamma frequency (70–150 Hz) activity evoked during functional tasks such as limb movement, auditory perception, picture naming, and question-answer trials.[30,31] Case studies have shown evoked gamma activity localized to functional regions predicted anatomically or proven by electrical stimulation mapping with good specificity. The region of gamma activity may, however, be broader than indicated by stimulation mapping. This technique has several potential benefits over stimulation mapping in that multiple brain regions can be assessed simultaneously without risk for induced seizures and it may allow for language mapping in patients of a younger age or with delayed processing speed. Further development of paradigms are, however, necessary to validate this approach and increase its sensitivity.

Stimulation-induced seizures

Although spontaneously recorded seizures are ideal for the localization of the ictal onset zone, some centers perform cortical stimulation to activate epileptic networks and elicit seizures. Electrically induced seizures that recapitulate the electrographic

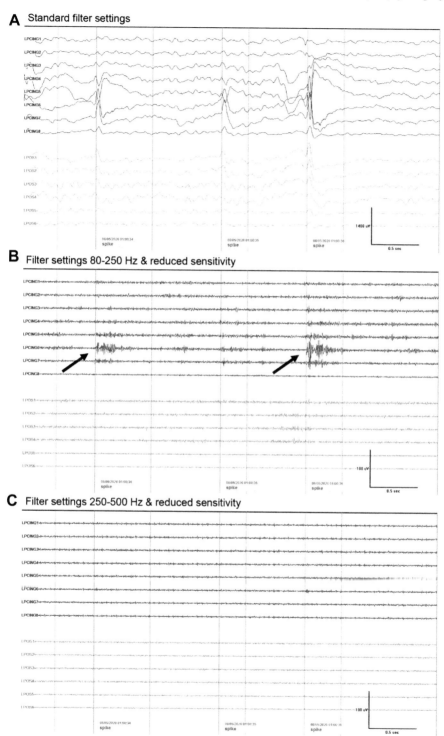

Fig. 3. HFOs. (*A*) Four-second ECoG sample showing 3 spikes maximal at LPCING6-LPCING7 (*pink*) with a field that extends to LPOS1-LPOS2 (*green*). (*B*) Filter settings of 80 to 250 Hz reveals ripples maximal at LPCING6 (*arrow*) coincident with spikes. No ripples are seen at LPOS1-LPOS2. (*C*) Filter settings of 250 to 500 Hz reveals no fast ripples.

spread and semiology of the patient's habitual spontaneous seizures can support a hypothesized ictal onset zone (**Fig. 4**).[32] Induction of nonhabitual seizure semiologies is not beneficial, as stimulation can induce seizures in the absence of underlying irritability. Limited studies from Europe report a 75% to 100% concordance between spontaneous and analogous stimulation-induced seizures with greater concordance seen in mesial temporal lobe epilepsy than lateral temporal or frontal lobe epilepsy.

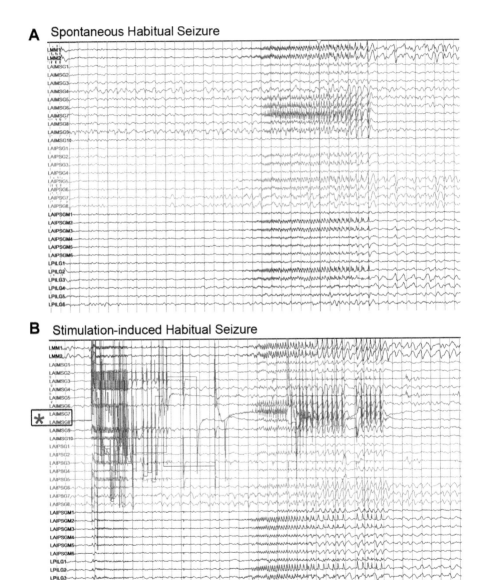

Fig. 4. Stimulation-induced seizures. (*A*) ECoG pattern of patient's habitual seizure; (*B*) 2 mA bipolar stimulation at contacts LAIMSG7-LAIMSG8 (indicated by *box*) induces the patient's habitual seizure semiology and a similar ECoG pattern.

NOVEL SURGICAL INTERVENTIONS
MRI-Guided Laser Interstitial Thermal Therapy

Since Food and Drug Administration (FDA) approval of 2 MRI-guided laser interstitial thermotherapy (LITT) systems, Medtronic Visualase in 2007 and Monteris NeuroBlate in 2009, this minimally invasive technique has been used to treat solid tumors and focal epilepsies.[33,34] These systems involve drilling a small hole, placing a stereotactic bolt, and inserting a saline or CO_2-cooled catheter into the tissue of interest. Because stability of the catheter is dependent on cranial fixation, individuals with thin bone or open cranial vaults, like infants, may require a surgical frame with multiple fixation points. Electrode trajectories used for SEEG monitoring can be used for laser ablation following electrode removal. A fiberoptic with laser tip is inserted to introduce infrared laser energy resulting in increased tissue temperature over time. Using real-time MRI thermographic monitoring, very localized coagulative necrosis can be induced with a small area of surrounding edema (**Fig. 5**). The laser fiber can be moved along the trajectory to produce linear ablation tracts up to 3 cm in diameter. Multiple tracts can be ablated in 1 session and LITT can be performed repetitively if needed. In the Visualase system, protective safety limits to be programmed by the user, shutting off the laser automatically when nearby critical structures show temperature elevation of 50°C (default temperature). One major limitation of LITT is that flowing cerebral spinal fluid or blood, ventricles, and prior resection cavities can lead to heat dissipation, making regions in direct proximity more difficult to ablate. Pathologic tissue samples can be obtained at the time of catheter implantation but may be of insufficient size if a pathologic diagnosis is needed. Postoperative recovery from LITT is generally rapid, usually with discharge the following day.

Use of MRI-guided LITT for the treatment of epilepsy was first described in 5 pediatric patients with lesional epilepsies with all patient becoming seizure-free at last follow-up (2–13 months).[35] Since then, many small case series reporting the use of LITT for pediatric epilepsy have been published. LITT may be preferred to open resection for tissues that are difficult to access surgically (eg, deep brain sites), individuals with multiple anatomically separate seizure-onset zones, and individuals likely to have recurrent epilepsy surgery. LITT also induces less anatomic distortion than open resection. Larger studies are, however, needed to compare the effectiveness and safety of LITT relative to open resection.

Temporal lobe epilepsy

Temporal lobe epilepsy (TLE) is the most common focal epilepsy and is commonly drug resistant. Anterior temporal lobectomies and selective amygdalohippocampectomies have a high rate of seizure freedom (55%–70%) but are often associated with neurocognitive impairments. Several case series have been published using LITT for mesial and neocortical TLE in pediatric and adult patients. In a meta-analysis, only 5 cases of LITT for neocortical TLE with MRI abnormalities were described.[34] All were seizure-free but follow-up was limited (9.0–12.7 months). For mesial TLE, a multicenter trial of 234 patients reported 58% seizure freedom at 1 to 2 years following LITT.[36] The presence of radiographic hippocampal sclerosis did not affect outcomes, but patients with focal to bilateral tonic-clonic seizures were less likely to become seizure-free. A 15% complication rate was reported, which is comparable to resective approaches. The overall seizure freedom rates reported for LITT in TLE are slightly lower than the gold-standard open anterior temporal lobectomy. LITT can, however, be repeated if there are residual mesial structures or followed by an open resection if needed.

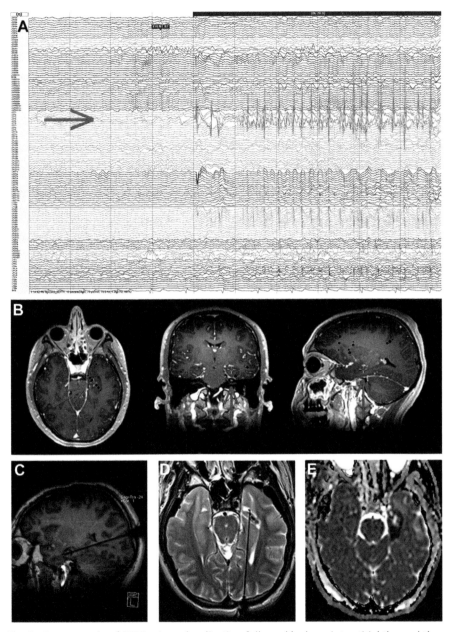

Fig. 5. Case example of SEEG seizure localization followed by laser interstitial thermal therapy. (*A*) SEEG in a patient with multiple FCDs showing habitual seizure onset arising from LOT3-5 (*arrow*). (*B*) Overlay of implanted electrodes on MRI brain T1 images shows localization of electrographic onset in left mesial temporal lobe focal cortical dysplasia (*arrow*). (*C, D*) MRI brain sagittal (*C*) and axial (*D*) images show positioning of laser applicator with tip in probable seizure-onset zone. (*E*) MRI brain axial apparent diffusion coefficient image obtained during the ablation shows region of thermal damage.

Dominant and nondominant temporal lobe resections are associated with neurocognitive impairments. Better naming, verbal fluency, and object recognition following LITT amygdalohippocampotomy has been reported compared with anterior temporal lobectomy.[37] Studies have shown variable impairments in memory function,[33,38] and further studies investigating memory function are needed.

Focal cortical dysplasias

FCDs are malformations of brain developmental frequently with epileptogenic potential. FCDs can be overt or indistinguishable from normal tissue on MRI. Several case reports documenting the use of LITT for the treatment of FCDs have been published, the largest by Lewis and colleagues.[39] In their case series,[39] 12 patients had drug-resistant epilepsy and presumed FCDs treated with LITT following video-EEG seizure characterization; 3 of the 12 were later determined to have biopsy-proven tumors. Of the remaining 9, 6 patients had a reduction in seizures with 2 seizure-free at 11 to 35-month follow-up. There was a complication in 1 patient with catheter misplacement resulting in hemorrhage and hydrocephalus. The seizure outcome for LITT treatment of FCDs performed by Lewis and colleagues[39] is inferior to the 60% seizure freedom after open resection,[40] likely due to incomplete ablation of the seizure-onset zone. More complete resection may be achieved by either repeat SEEG monitoring or intraoperative ECoG of the surgical boundaries, followed by further LITT or open resection.[41]

Tuberous sclerosis complex

TSC is a genetic disease that causes tumors in the brain and other organs. Cortical tubers often lead to seizures, developmental delay, and intellectual disability. Use of LITT for treatment of epilepsy in patients with TSC was first described in 2012 and has since been reported in several small series with nearly all patients experiencing a meaningful reduction in seizures.[35,39,42–45] A few patients were also reported to have developmental and neuropsychological improvements.[44,45] No complications occurred. Although results are encouraging, these studies are limited by small patient numbers, differences in seizure-onset zone identification (surface EEG or SEEG), and overall short duration of follow-up. Use of LITT in TSC warrants further investigation, as these individuals are likely to develop new seizure networks over time and may require recurrent epilepsy surgery.

Hypothalamic hamartoma

Hypothalamic hamartomas (HHs) are congenital malformations associated with gelastic seizures that occur in isolation or syndromically. Due to their location in the center of the brain, resection by traditional surgical approaches can be associated with corridor-related morbidity.[46,47] A case series of 14 patients treated with LITT reported 86% seizure freedom at a mean of 9 months' follow-up and a good safety profile with only 1 patient experiencing an asymptomatic subdural hemorrhage.[48] Our program at Texas Children's Hospital has performed surgery on 125 patients. Subsequent studies have similarly reported good efficacy and rare complications, such as memory deficit and worsening diabetes insipidus.[49,50]

Corpus callosotomy

Traditionally, corpus callosotomies for palliation of drug-resistant epilepsy have been performed by open craniotomies. In 2016, LITT of the splenium was used to complete an anterior callosotomy in an adult patient with persistent generalized seizures, resulting in a >50% reduction in seizures at 4-month follow-up.[51] Since then, LITT has been reported in pediatric and adult patients for anterior two-thirds callosotomies and completions with seizure outcomes similar to open craniotomies.[52–55] Rare complications were reported, including hemorrhage, asymptomatic thalamic ablation, and disconnection syndrome.[52,54]

Stereo-Electroencephalogram–Guided Radiofrequency Thermocoagulation

SEEG-guided radiofrequency thermocoagulation (also known as thermo-SEEG) uses the SEEG electrodes initially used for seizure characterization to lesion the seizure-onset zones.[56] The French Clinical Neurophysiology Society and French chapter of the International League Against Epilepsy have established guidelines for thermo-SEEG, recommending its consideration when conventional surgery is not feasible and for deep heterotopias or HHs.[57] Thermo-SEEG is performed intraoperatively during wakefulness without anesthesia to allow for clinical monitoring. A radiofrequency (RF) generator is connected to an SEEG electrode and RF current is delivered between 2 contacts in the seizure-onset zone. This creates an electric field and an oscillatory ionic current density field that causes frictional heating. Initially, a short direct stimulation is applied before to test for eloquent cortex. If nonfunctional, a more prolonged ablative stimulation of ∼50 V is applied to heat the tissue to 78 to 82°C. Higher voltage is associated with larger lesions up to 5 to 7 mm in diameter. Unlike LITT, temperature is not monitored, but coagulation of tissue proteins is associated with a sudden change in resistance such that further current does not produce a larger lesion. Multiple lesions can be induced in a single session. Recovery is rapid, typically with discharge the next day. Patients may experience transient improvement or worsening of seizures before stabilizing. Thermo-SEEG can be performed repetitively in the same patient or followed by other surgical approaches if needed.

A meta-analysis of 296 patients showed significant variability in seizure outcomes, possibly due to technical differences across centers. Overall, 23% were seizure-free and 58% with ≥50% reduction in seizures at 1 year.[56] Notably, patients with periventricular nodular heterotopias had a favorable responder rate, while TLE had inferior outcomes compared with open resection. Thermo-SEEG had a very low unanticipated complication rate due to the functional mapping before thermocoagulation. Only 1 patient in the series had an unanticipated deficit (thumb hypoesthesia).

Gamma Knife Radiosurgery

Gamma knife (GK) is a noninvasive technique that targets convergent small gamma rays on the epileptogenic zone with each beam inducing minimal radiation to surrounding tissues along each track. Although the procedure itself can be completed within a day, the radiation-induced neuromodulation and necrosis can take months to years. In adults, GK for mesial TLE has resulted in significant reduction in seizures after 2 years that is comparable to traditional surgical approaches.[58] There are also limited data for GK treatment of cavernous malformations as well as palliative corpus callosotomies. GK targeted to the anterior or posterior corpus callosum in children and adults leads to significant improvement in drop attacks and/or generalized tonic-clonic seizures in a median of 3 months.

In a prospective trial of GK for the treatment of HH, 69% of 57 patients had significant improvement in seizures with 40% being completely seizure-free after more than 3 years of follow-up[59]; 58% of patients did require a second treatment to achieve these outcomes. Outcome is dependent on lesion size and anatomic localization, with best outcomes seen with small hamartomas within the hypothalamus and third ventricle.[60] Reduction in aggressive behavior was also reported. Giant HHs and those above the floor of the third ventricle may require staged intervention with disconnection of the lower portion followed by GK of the upper part. No permanent neurologic complications were reported. A major disadvantage to this approach, however, is that lasting clinical improvement can take up to 2 to 3 years and is often preceded by periods of fluctuating seizure improvement and exacerbation.

One concern for radiosurgery, especially in the pediatric population, is radiation-induced damage that contributes to tumorigenesis. There is no definite causal relationship seen between radiosurgery and new tumors, and the risk of tumor development following radiosurgery is reportedly far lower than the risk of dying from brain surgery.[60]

Magnetic Resonance–Guided Focused Ultrasound

Originally FDA approved for the treatment of uterine fibroids and pain secondary to bone metastases, MR-guided focused ultrasonography (MRgFUS) is being investigated for the treatment of focal epilepsies.[61,62] This technique uses high-frequency waves to induce a focal increase in tissue temperature. Mild increases in temperature can modulate neuronal activity, whereas high temperatures of ~55°C lead to irreversible cell death. Real-time MRI is used for beam guidance and thermometry for monitoring of the ablation as treatment occurs, thereby minimizing off-target damage.

Although MRgFUS does not require surgical implantation of a laser catheter as in LITT, there are potential complications to this noninvasive technique. Hair underlying the ultrasound transducer must be shaved, as energy absorption by the skin can result in pain and burns. Absorption by the skull can lead to heat damage to the dura and nearby brain parenchyma if cooling is insufficient. In addition, the skull can cause wave distortion and attenuation that impairs targeting and achievement of ablative temperatures. This can be somewhat mitigated by use of specialized ultrasound transducers. High-intensity ultrasound also can affect blood vessels, resulting in bleeding.[63] Additional studies are needed to investigate the feasibility and safety of this technique for the treatment of epilepsy.

Endoscopic Surgery

Another alternative to traditional open resective surgeries makes use of endoscopes. Endoscopes can be introduced through significantly smaller craniotomies and may thereby be associated with reduced intraoperative blood loss and more rapid recovery. Endoscopic approaches are, however, challenging in that tissue visualization and the ability to control bleeding are limited relative to open surgery.

Corpus callosotomy

Endoscopic corpus callosotomies can be performed through a 2 to 3 cm diameter frontal or parietooccipital craniotomy, significantly smaller than the 8 cm × 4 cm incision for the open approach.[64,65] The placement of the craniotomy and length of the endoscopic tools allows the corpus callosum to be reached without brain retraction, one cause of potential complications. Although reported series have limited patient numbers, no complications were reported and the investigators elude to similar seizure outcomes as open procedures. Endoscopic callosotomies can be combined with disconnection of the anterior, posterior, and habenular commissures with improved seizure outcomes, 71.4% with a ≥50% reduction in seizures compared with 53% with callosotomy alone in 1 series of 57 patients.[66] Inclusion of the commissures was not associated with an increase in complications with both treatment groups including infrequent cases of hematoma, hygroma, and hydrocephalus.

Functional hemispherotomy

Expanding on corpus callosotomy disconnections, endoscopic functional hemispherotomies can be performed though craniotomies as small as 4 cm × 2 to 3 cm.[67–69]

Disconnection can be confirmed by intraoperative MRI or postoperative tractography. A case series of 59 patients compared open hemispherotomy with robotic-assisted endoscopic hemispherotomy.[70] Both techniques resulted in similar reductions in seizures at 1 year, but the endoscopic approach was associated with significantly less intraoperative blood loss and modestly shorter hospital stays. Some complications were seen in both treatment groups, the most common being postoperative fever without evidence of infection.

Hypothalamic hamartoma

Trans-ventricular endoscopic disconnection of HHs was first described in 2003.[71] Using a stereotactic robot or neuronavigation system to guide placement, 2 burr-hole incisions are made, one for the endoscope entry to the lateral ventricle and one with a trajectory targeted to the interface between the hamartoma and third ventricle wall.[72] Disconnection is then performed under direct visualization using either a laser probe or ultrasonic aspirator. In a cohort of 112 pediatric patients treated endoscopically, 57% of patients were seizure-free at more than 2-year follow-up with best outcomes seen for small hamartomas located intraventricularly.[73] Notably, 51% of patients required 2 to 4 surgical procedures to achieve these outcomes, with 15 patients having open surgeries to either disconnect or resect residual tissue. An endoscopic complication rate of 7.9% was reported, including cases of memory deficit, motor deficit, meningitis, and transient diabetes insipidus. This rate is acknowledged by the study investigators to be slightly higher than other minimally invasive or noninvasive approaches to address HHs.

Neurostimulation

Neurostimulation for the treatment of epilepsy involves implantation of a battery-operated device that provides nerve or brain stimulation in a programmed or triggered manner. A discussion of these devices can be found in Ali and colleagues' article, "Neuromodulation in Pediatric Epilepsy," in this issue.

DISCUSSION

Epilepsy is the most common chronic neurologic condition in childhood[74] and is associated with increased risk for injury,[75] academic underachievement,[76] social stress,[77] and sudden death. For those with drug-resistant epilepsy, early referral to an epilepsy center is important for consideration of surgical options as well as dietary therapies. This is especially true for patients with lesional epilepsy who are unlikely to undergo spontaneous remission of their seizures over time. In a randomized controlled trial, pediatric patients with drug-resistant epilepsy who underwent epilepsy surgery had a better chance of seizure freedom and better behavior and quality-of-life scores than those who just continued medical therapy.[78] Surgery at a young age also allows for remodeling of functional brain networks, such as relocalization of language following hemispherectomy.[79] Caregivers of pediatric epilepsy surgery patients often wish that epilepsy surgery had happened sooner.[80,81]

Advances in EEG analysis, imaging, and genetic testing allow us to better understand each patient's underlying etiology and seizure types. Working as a multidisciplinary team, neurologists, neurosurgeons, and neuropsychologists can design a treatment plan for each individual. With the development of SEEG monitoring and minimally invasive treatments, patients with multiple seizure types or disparate seizure-onset zones are no longer poor surgical candidates. At our institution, lack of fully concordant presurgical data does not preclude SEEG characterization if reasonable hypotheses can guide the implantation. Early epilepsy surgery and reduction of seizure burden may help maximize developmental potential even in conditions like TSC in which new epileptic networks may develop over time. Reduction of seizure medications following surgery also may have neurocognitive benefits. Given this, successful epilepsy surgery should be measured not only by the percentage of seizure reduction or duration of seizure freedom, but also neuropsychologic and quality-of-life measures. Reduced risk of injury and sudden unexpected death in epilepsy patients are benefits not to be overlooked.

As epilepsy monitoring and surgical intervention become less invasive with lower associated morbidity, our threshold for using these techniques for the treatment of epilepsy will likely decrease. Curing epilepsy remains a goal, but seizure palliation and iterative minimally invasive interventions are becoming increasingly common. In the future, epilepsy surgery indications may expand to include surgical treatment of subtle clinical or subclinical seizures, lesional epilepsies after failure of the first antiepileptic drug, or even well-controlled epilepsy on multiple medications.

CLINICS CARE POINTS

- Consider epilepsy surgery in patients with medically refractory epilepsy
- SEEG serves as a minimally invasive diagnostic tool allowing for the sampling of multiple, bilateral regions to confirm seizure onset
- Epilepsy surgical techniques are increasingly minimally invasive and may increase the number of potential surgical candidates
- Curative and palliative epilepsy surgery goals are equally important in specific clinical scenarios
- Improved developmental outcome measures are needed to guide long-term benefits for palliative epilepsy surgery in children

DISCLOSURE

R. Coorg and E.S. Seto: No commercial or financial conflicts of interest.

REFERENCES

1. Kwan P, Brodie MJ. Early identification of refractory epilepsy. N Engl J Med 2000; 342(5):314–9.
2. Berg AT, Vickrey BG, Testa FM, et al. How long does it take for epilepsy to become intractable? A prospective investigation. Ann Neurol 2006;60(1). https://doi.org/10.1002/ana.20852.
3. Fountain NB, Ness PCV, Swain-Eng R, et al, For the American Academy of Neurology Epilepsy Measure Development Panel and the American Medical Association–Convened Physician Consortium for Performance Improvement Independent Measure Development Process. Quality improvement in neurology: AAN epilepsy quality measures: Report of the Quality Measurement and Reporting Subcommittee of the American Academy of Neurology. Neurology 2011. https://doi.org/10.1212/WNL.0b013e318203e9d1.
4. Blumcke I, Spreafico R, Haaker G, et al. Histopathological findings in brain tissue obtained during epilepsy surgery. N Engl J Med 2017;377(17). https://doi.org/10.1056/NEJMoa1703784.

5. Englot DJ, Ouyang D, Garcia PA, et al. Epilepsy surgery trends in the United States, 1990-2008. Neurology 2012;78(16). https://doi.org/10.1212/WNL. 0b013e318250d7ea.

6. Ravindra VM, Sweney MT, Bollo RJ. Recent developments in the surgical management of paediatric epilepsy. Arch Dis Child 2017;102(8). https://doi.org/10. 1136/archdischild-2016-311183.

7. Jayakar P, Gaillard WD, Tripathi M, et al. Diagnostic test utilization in evaluation for resective epilepsy surgery in children. Epilepsia 2014;55(4). https://doi.org/10. 1111/epi.12544.

8. Obeid M, Wyllie E, Rahi AC, et al. Approach to pediatric epilepsy surgery: state of the art, Part II: approach to specific epilepsy syndromes and etiologies. Eur J Paediatric Neurol 2009;13(2). https://doi.org/10.1016/j.ejpn.2008.05.003.

9. Bernasconi A, Cendes F, Theodore WH, et al. Recommendations for the use of structural magnetic resonance imaging in the care of patients with epilepsy: a consensus report from the International League Against Epilepsy Neuroimaging Task Force. Epilepsia 2019;60(6). https://doi.org/10.1111/epi.15612.

10. Knowlton RC, Lawn ND, Mountz JM, et al. Ictal SPECT analysis in epilepsy: subtraction and statistical parametric mapping techniques. Neurology 2004;63(1). https://doi.org/10.1212/01.wnl.0000132885.83350.45.

11. Obeid M, Wyllie E, Rahi AC, et al. Approach to pediatric epilepsy surgery: state of the art, part I: general principles and presurgical workup. Eur J Paediatric Neurol 2009;13(2). https://doi.org/10.1016/j.ejpn.2008.05.007.

12. Verrotti A, Pizzella V, Trotta D, et al. Magnetoencephalography in pediatric neurology and in epileptic syndromes. Pediatr Neurol 2003;28(4). https://doi. org/10.1016/s0887-8994(03)00017-1.

13. Tierney TM, Holmes N, Meyer SS, et al. Cognitive neuroscience using wearable magnetometer arrays: non-invasive assessment of language function. NeuroImage 2018. https://doi.org/10.1016/j.neuroimage.2018.07.035.

14. Chen R, Classen J, Gerloff C, et al. Depression of motor cortex excitability by lowfrequency transcranial magnetic stimulation. Neurology 1997;48(5). https://doi. org/10.1212/wnl.48.5.1398.

15. Berl MM, Smith ML, Bulteau C. ILAE survey of neuropsychology practice in pediatric epilepsy surgery evaluation. Epileptic Disord 2017;19(2). https://doi.org/10. 1684/epd.2017.0908.

16. Ostergard T, Miller JP. Depth electrodes: approaches and complications. In: Lhatoo SD, Kahane P, Lüders HO, editors. Invasive studies of the human epileptic brain. New York, NY: Oxford University Press; 2019. p. 50–64.

17. Arya R, Mangano FT, Horn PS, et al. Adverse events related to extraoperative invasive EEG monitoring with subdural grid electrodes: a systematic review and meta-analysis. Epilepsia 2013;54(5). https://doi.org/10.1111/epi.12073.

18. Kalamangalam GP, Tandon N. Stereo-EEG implantation strategy. J Clin Neurophysiol 2016;33(6). https://doi.org/10.1097/WNP.0000000000000254.

19. Olivier A, Boling WW, Tanriverdi T. Techniques in epilepsy surgery : the MNI approach. Cambridge medicine. New York, NY: Cambridge University Press; 2012. p. 287, x.

20. Kahane P, Barba C, Rheims S, et al. The concept of temporal 'plus' epilepsy. Revue Neurol 2015;171(3). https://doi.org/10.1016/j.neurol.2015.01.562.

21. Coorg R, Peters J. Tuberous sclerosis complex. In: Schuele S, editor. A practical approach to stereo EEG. New York, NY: Demos Medical; 2020.

22. Staba RJ, Wilson CL, Bragin A, et al. High-frequency oscillations recorded in human medial temporal lobe during sleep. Ann Neurol 2004;56(1). https://doi.org/10.1002/ana.20164.

23. Urrestarazu E, Chander R, Dubeau F, et al. Interictal high-frequency oscillations (100-500 Hz) in the intracerebral EEG of epileptic patients. Brain 2007;130(Pt 9). https://doi.org/10.1093/brain/awm149.

24. Jirsch JD, Urrestarazu E, LeVan P, et al. High-frequency oscillations during human focal seizures. Brain 2006;129(Pt 6). https://doi.org/10.1093/brain/awl085.

25. Ochi A, Otsubo H, Donner EJ, et al. Dynamic changes of ictal high-frequency oscillations in neocortical epilepsy: using multiple band frequency analysis. Epilepsia 2007;48(2). https://doi.org/10.1111/j.1528-1167.2007.00923.x.

26. Jacobs J, Zijlmans M, Zelmann R, et al. High-frequency electroencephalographic oscillations correlate with outcome of epilepsy surgery. Ann Neurol 2010;67(2). https://doi.org/10.1002/ana.21847.

27. Wang W, Degenhart AD, Collinger JL, et al. Human motor cortical activity recorded with Micro-ECoG electrodes, during individual finger movements. Annu Int Conf IEEE Eng Med Biol Soc 2009. https://doi.org/10.1109/IEMBS.2009.5333704.

28. Gloss D, Nolan SJ, Staba R. The role of high-frequency oscillations in epilepsy surgery planning. Cochrane Database Syst Rev 2014;1(1). https://doi.org/10.1002/14651858.CD010235.pub2.

29. Ritaccio AL, Brunner P, Schalk G. Electrical stimulation mapping of the brain: basic principles and emerging alternatives. J Clin Neurophysiol 2018;35(2). https://doi.org/10.1097/WNP.0000000000000440.

30. Sinai A, Bowers CW, Crainiceanu CM, et al. Electrocorticographic high gamma activity versus electrical cortical stimulation mapping of naming. Brain 2005;128(Pt 7). https://doi.org/10.1093/brain/awh491.

31. Brown EC, Rothermel R, Nishida M, et al. In vivo animation of auditory-language-induced gamma-oscillations in children with intractable focal epilepsy. NeuroImage 2008;41(3). https://doi.org/10.1016/j.neuroimage.2008.03.011.

32. Kovac S, Kahane P, Diehl B. Seizures induced by direct electrical cortical stimulation–Mechanisms and clinical considerations. Clin Neurophysiol 2016;127(1). https://doi.org/10.1016/j.clinph.2014.12.009.

33. LaRiviere MJ, Gross RE. Stereotactic laser ablation for medically intractable epilepsy: the next generation of minimally invasive epilepsy surgery. Front Surg 2016. https://doi.org/10.3389/fsurg.2016.00064.

34. North RY, Raskin JS, Curry DJ. MRI-guided laser interstitial thermal therapy for epilepsy. Neurosurg Clin North Am 2017;20(4). https://doi.org/10.1016/j.nec.2017.06.001.

35. Curry DJ, Gowda A, McNichols RJ, et al. MR-guided stereotactic laser ablation of epileptogenic foci in children. Epilepsy Behav 2012;24(4). https://doi.org/10.1016/j.yebeh.2012.04.135.

36. Wu C, Jermakowicz WJ, Chakravorti S, et al. Effects of surgical targeting in laser interstitial thermal therapy for mesial temporal lobe epilepsy: a multicenter study of 234 patients. Epilepsia 2019;60(6). https://doi.org/10.1111/epi.15565.

37. Drane DL. MRI-guided stereotactic laser ablation for epilepsy surgery: promising preliminary results for cognitive outcome. Epilepsy Res 2018;142. https://doi.org/10.1016/j.eplepsyres.2017.09.016.

38. Donos C, Breier J, Friedman E, et al. Laser ablation for mesial temporal lobe epilepsy: surgical and cognitive outcomes with and without mesial temporal sclerosis. Epilepsia 2018;59(7). https://doi.org/10.1111/epi.14443.

39. Lewis EC, Weil AG, Duchowny M, et al. MR-guided laser interstitial thermal therapy for pediatric drug-resistant lesional epilepsy. Epilepsia 2015;56(10). https://doi.org/10.1111/epi.13106.

40. Hauptman JS, Mathern GW. Surgical treatment of epilepsy associated with cortical dysplasia: 2012 update. Epilepsia 2012;53(Suppl 4). https://doi.org/10.1111/j.1528-1167.2012.03619.x.

41. Ellis JA, Mejia Munne JC, Wang SH, et al. Staged laser interstitial thermal therapy and topectomy for complete obliteration of complex focal cortical dysplasias. J Clin Neurosci 2016;31. https://doi.org/10.1016/j.jocn.2016.02.016.

42. Cobourn K, Fayed I, Keating RF, et al. Early outcomes of stereoelectroencephalography followed by MR-guided laser interstitial thermal therapy: a paradigm for minimally invasive epilepsy surgery. Neurosurg Focus 2018;45(3). https://doi.org/10.3171/2018.6.FOCUS18209.

43. Stellon MA, Cobourn K, Whitehead MT, et al. Laser and the tuber": thermal dynamic and volumetric factors influencing seizure outcomes in pediatric subjects with tuberous sclerosis undergoing stereoencephalography-directed laser ablation of tubers. Childs Nerv Syst 2019;35(8). https://doi.org/10.1007/s00381-019-04255-4.

44. Hooten KG, Werner K, Mikati MA, et al. MRI-guided laser interstitial thermal therapy in an infant with tuberous sclerosis: technical case report. J Neurosurg Pediatr 2018;23(1). https://doi.org/10.3171/2018.6.PEDS1828.

45. Tovar-Spinoza Z, Ziechmann R, Zyck S. Single and staged laser interstitial thermal therapy ablation for cortical tubers causing refractory epilepsy in pediatric patients. Neurosurg Focus 2018;45(3). https://doi.org/10.3171/2018.6.FOCUS18228.

46. Abla AA, Rekate HL, Wilson DA, et al. Orbitozygomatic resection for hypothalamic hamartoma and epilepsy: patient selection and outcome. Childs Nerv Syst 2011;27(2). https://doi.org/10.1007/s00381-010-1250-7.

47. Ng YT, Rekate HL, Prenger EC, et al. Transcallosal resection of hypothalamic hamartoma for intractable epilepsy. Epilepsia 2006;47(7). https://doi.org/10.1111/j.1528-1167.2006.00516.x.

48. Wilfong AA, Curry DJ. Hypothalamic hamartomas: optimal approach to clinical evaluation and diagnosis. Epilepsia 2013;54(Suppl). https://doi.org/10.1111/epi.12454.

49. Curry DJ, Raskin J, Ali I, et al. MR-guided laser ablation for the treatment of hypothalamic hamartomas. Epilepsy Res 2018;142. https://doi.org/10.1016/j.eplepsyres.2018.03.013.

50. Zubkov S, Del Bene VA, MacAllister WS, et al. Disabling amnestic syndrome following stereotactic laser ablation of a hypothalamic hamartoma in a patient with a prior temporal lobectomy. Epilepsy Behav Case Rep 2015;4. https://doi.org/10.1016/j.ebcr.2015.07.002.

51. Ho AL, Miller KJ, Cartmell S, et al. Stereotactic laser ablation of the splenium for intractable epilepsy. Epilepsy Behav Case Rep 2016;5. https://doi.org/10.1016/j.ebcr.2015.12.003.

52. Huang Y, Yecies D, Bruckert L, et al. Stereotactic laser ablation for completion corpus callosotomy. J Neurosurg Pediatr 2019. https://doi.org/10.3171/2019.5.PEDS19117.

53. Palma AE, Wicks RT, Popli G, et al. Corpus callosotomy via laser interstitial thermal therapy: a case series. J Neurosurg Pediatr 2018;23(3). https://doi.org/10.3171/2018.10.PEDS18368.

54. Roland JL, Akbari SHA, Salehi A, et al. Corpus callosotomy performed with laser interstitial thermal therapy. J Neurosurg 2019. https://doi.org/10.3171/2019.9. JNS191769.

55. Ball T, Sharma M, White AC, et al. Anterior corpus callosotomy using laser interstitial thermal therapy for refractory epilepsy. Stereotactic Funct Neurosurg 2018; 96(6). https://doi.org/10.1159/000495414.

56. Bourdillon P, Cucherat M, Isnard J, et al. Stereo-electroencephalography-guided radiofrequency thermocoagulation in patients with focal epilepsy: a systematic review and meta-analysis. Epilepsia 2018;59(12). https://doi.org/10.1111/epi. 14584.

57. Isnard J, Taussig D, Bartolomei F, et al. French guidelines on stereoelectroencephalography (SEEG). Neurophysiol Clin 2018;48(1). https://doi.org/10.1016/j. neucli.2017.11.005.

58. McGonigal A, Sahgal A, De Salles A, et al. Radiosurgery for epilepsy: systematic review and International Stereotactic Radiosurgery Society (ISRS) practice guideline. Epilepsy Res 2017;137. https://doi.org/10.1016/j.eplepsyres.2017. 08.016.

59. Régis J, Scavarda D, Tamura M, et al. Gamma knife surgery for epilepsy related to hypothalamic hamartomas. Semin Pediatr Neurol 2007;14(2). https://doi.org/ 10.1016/j.spen.2007.03.005.

60. Régis J, Scavarda D, Tamura M, et al. Epilepsy related to hypothalamic hamartomas: surgical management with special reference to gamma knife surgery. Childs Nerv Syst 2006;22(8). https://doi.org/10.1007/s00381-006-0139-y.

61. Fiani B, Lissak IA, Soula M, et al. The emerging role of magnetic resonance imaging-guided focused ultrasound in functional neurosurgery. Cureus 2020; 12(8). https://doi.org/10.7759/cureus.9820.

62. Abe K, Yamaguchi T, Hori H, et al. Magnetic resonance-guided focused ultrasound for mesial temporal lobe epilepsy: a case report. BMC Neurol 2020; 20(1). https://doi.org/10.1186/s12883-020-01744-x.

63. Hynynen K, Chung AH, Colucci V, et al. Potential adverse effects of high-intensity focused ultrasound exposure on blood vessels in vivo. Ultrasound Med Biol 1996; 22(2). https://doi.org/10.1016/0301-5629(95)02044-6.

64. Smyth MD, Vellimana AK, Asano E, et al. Corpus callosotomy-open and endoscopic surgical techniques. Epilepsia 2017;58(Suppl). https://doi.org/10.1111/ epi.13681.

65. Sood S, Asano E, Altinok D, et al. Endoscopic posterior interhemispheric complete corpus callosotomy. J Neurosurg Pediatr 2016;25(6). https://doi.org/10. 3171/2016.6.PEDS16131.

66. Sufianov AA, Cossu G, Iakimov IA, et al. Endoscopic interhemispheric disconnection for intractable multifocal epilepsy: surgical technique and functional neuroanatomy. Oper Neurosurg (Hagerstown) 2020;18(2). https://doi.org/10. 1093/ons/opz121.

67. Wagner K, Vaz-Guimaraes F, Camstra K, et al. Endoscope-assisted hemispherotomy: translation of technique from cadaveric anatomical feasibility study to clinical implementation. J Neurosurg Pediatr 2018;23(2). https://doi.org/10.3171/ 2018.8.PEDS18349.

68. Sood S, Marupudi NI, Asano E, et al. Endoscopic corpus callosotomy and hemispherotomy. J Neurosurg Pediatr 2015;16(6). https://doi.org/10.3171/2015.5. PEDS1531.

69. Chandra PS, Kurwale N, Garg A, et al. Endoscopy-assisted interhemispheric transcallosal hemispherotomy: preliminary description of a novel technique. Neurosurgery 2015;76(4). https://doi.org/10.1227/NEU.0000000000000675.

70. Chandra PS, Subianto H, Bajaj J, et al. Endoscope-assisted (with robotic guidance and using a hybrid technique) interhemispheric transcallosal hemispherotomy: a comparative study with open hemispherotomy to evaluate efficacy, complications, and outcome. J Neurosurg Pediatr 2018;23(2). https://doi.org/10.3171/2018.8.PEDS18131.

71. Delalande O, Fohlen M. Disconnecting surgical treatment of hypothalamic hamartoma in children and adults with refractory epilepsy and proposal of a new classification. Neurol Med Chir (Tokyo) 2003;43(2). https://doi.org/10.2176/nmc.43.61.

72. Procaccini E, Dorfmüller G, Fohlen M, et al. Surgical management of hypothalamic hamartomas with epilepsy: the stereoendoscopic approach. Neurosurgery 2006;59(4 Suppl 2). https://doi.org/10.1227/01.NEU.0000233900.06146.72.

73. Ferrand-Sorbets S, Fohlen M, Delalande O, et al. Seizure outcome and prognostic factors for surgical management of hypothalamic hamartomas in children. Seizure 2020;75. https://doi.org/10.1016/j.seizure.2019.11.013.

74. Aaberg KM, Gunnes N, Bakken IJ, et al. Incidence and prevalence of childhood epilepsy: a nationwide cohort study. Pediatrics 2017;139(5). https://doi.org/10.1542/peds.2016-3908.

75. Mahler B, Carlsson S, Andersson T, et al. Risk for injuries and accidents in epilepsy. Neurology 2018. https://doi.org/10.1212/WNL.0000000000005035.

76. Mitchell WG, Chavez JM, Lee H, et al. Academic underachievement in children with epilepsy. J Child Neurol 1991;6(1). https://doi.org/10.1177/088307389100600114.

77. WHO | Epilepsy: a public health imperative. WHO. 2019-06-20 15:12:23 2019;Available at: https://nam03.safelinks.protection.outlook.com/?url=https%3A%2F%2Fwww.who.int%2Fmental_health%2Fneurology%2Fepilepsy%2Freport_2019%2Fen%2F&data=04%7C01%7Cm.packiam%40elsevier.com%7Cc9d41e8b774142abf9d508d920bfb88f%7C9274ee3f94254109a27f9fb15c10675d%7C0%7C0%7C637576831178239019%7CUnknown%7CTWFpbGZsb3d8eyJWIjoiMC4wLjAwMDAiLCJQIjoiV2luMzIiLCJBTiI6Ik1haWwiLCJXVCI6Mn0%3D%7C1000&sdata=mPlei562htIL4QT7yMVTC%2B023ZWdKINSkEAevHldIHQ%3D&reserved=0. Accessed October 1, 2020.

78. Dwivedi R, Ramanujam B, Chandra PS, et al. Surgery for drug-resistant epilepsy in children. N Engl J Med 2017;377(17). https://doi.org/10.1056/NEJMoa1615335.

79. Gott PS. Cognitive abilities following right and left hemispherectomy. Cortex 1973;9(3). https://doi.org/10.1016/s0010-9452(73)80004-8.

80. Nguyen T, Porter BE. Caregivers' impression of epilepsy surgery in patients with tuberous sclerosis complex. Epilepsy Behav 2020;111. https://doi.org/10.1016/j.yebeh.2020.107331.

81. Shen A, Quaid KT, Porter BE. Delay in pediatric epilepsy surgery: A caregiver's perspective. Epilepsy Behav 2018;78. https://doi.org/10.1016/j.yebeh.2017.10.014.

Genetics in Epilepsy

Luis A. Martinez, PhD[a,1], Yi-Chen Lai, MD[b,1],
J. Lloyd Holder Jr, MD, PhD[a], Anne E. Anderson, MD[a,*]

KEYWORDS

- Epilepsy syndromes • Epilepsy phenotype • Dravet syndrome
- Early infantile epilepsy • Precision medicine in epilepsy • GLUT-1 deficiency
- Nonketotic hyperglycinemia

KEY POINTS

- Genetic testing should be considered in any child with unexplained epilepsy.
- Repeat analysis or new genetic testing should be considered in children with medically refractory epilepsy where previous genetic testing has not been informative because of continuous discovery of new genetic epilepsies.
- Genetic diagnosis is important to guide prognosis and targeted therapies for specific gene-related epilepsies.

INTRODUCTION

Epilepsy is defined as having 2 or more unprovoked seizures and may arise after acquired brain injury, including traumatic brain injury, or various insults related to inflammation, hemorrhage, and ischemia. In the absence of an acquired cause, the presence of unprovoked, recurrent seizures or idiopathic epilepsy raises a strong suspicion of an underlying genetic abnormality. It has been proposed that genetic causes account for at least 30% of epilepsies.[1] This article focuses on an overview of genetic abnormalities associated with an epilepsy phenotype, the work-up recommended, and therapeutics.

Understanding mechanisms underlying the epilepsy phenotype is critical to guide counseling and therapeutic considerations, including choice of antiepileptic drug (AED) therapy and other personalized therapeutics, such as protein replacement or genetic constructs, as well as consideration for surgical options and devices. With

[a] Department of Pediatrics, Section of Pediatric Neurology and Developmental Neuroscience, Baylor College of Medicine, Jan and Dan Duncan Neurological Research Institute, Texas Children's Hospital, 1250 Moursund Drive, Houston, TX 77030, USA; [b] Department of Pediatrics, Section of Pediatric Critical Care Medicine, Baylor College of Medicine, Jan and Dan Duncan Neurological Research Institute, Texas Children's Hospital, 1250 Moursund Drive, Houston, TX 77030, USA
[1] These authors contributed equally.
* Corresponding author.
E-mail address: annea@bcm.edu

genetic-directed therapeutics on the horizon in pharmaceutical pipelines, identifying specific genetic causes of epilepsy is crucial.

Genetic mutations with a primary phenotype of epilepsy include those involving ion channels, synaptic and signaling proteins, and other molecules. With rapidly evolving sophistication in genetic testing and wider availability, the list of genetic abnormalities with a primary epilepsy phenotype is growing. However, there are additional genetic causes of epilepsy that occur as part of a broad set of phenotypes that may include intellectual disability, dysmorphisms, and malformations of cortical development. This article provides an overview of the major classes of genes associated with epilepsy phenotypes divided into functional categories. Given that this is a rapidly evolving field and gene discovery is ongoing, it is impossible to be fully comprehensive. However, major classes of gene defects associated with epilepsy are described. When available, information related to the function defects associated with the specific gene mutation, phenotype, and specific treatment guidelines are presented.

CLASSES OF DEFINED GENETIC CAUSES

Several genes have been identified as having a clear and causative role in epilepsy. Neuronal excitability may be affected directly by mutations in ion channel genes such as in Dravet syndrome (DS) and KCNQ2 developmental and epileptic encephalopathy or indirectly through gene mutations affecting intracellular signaling pathways, such as in tuberous sclerosis complex (TSC). Other epilepsies may have more complex symptoms without a distinct cause. For example, malignant migrating partial seizures of infancy is characterized by drug-resistant, early-onset polymorphous migrating focal seizures[2] and has a diversity of implicated genes.[3] Next-generation sequencing has hastened the identification of genetic variants associated with epilepsy and widened our appreciation of potential gene modifiers,[4,5] and it is anticipated this information will ultimately lead to earlier diagnosis and improved treatments.[6–9] **Tables 1–5** provide summary lists of the identified genes associated with epilepsy and function.

ION CHANNELS
Sodium Channels

Most genetic epilepsies are associated with mutations in genes encoding subunits of voltage-gated ion channels, particularly in voltage-gated sodium channels (VGSCs). VGSCs are critical to initiation and propagation of action potentials, and their localization and biophysics are crucial to optimal neuronal function. VGSCs are composed of 1 pore-forming, voltage-sensitive α subunit[10] and 2 auxiliary β subunits that modulate channel kinetics and localization.[11,12] Mutations that enhance sodium channel opening in excitatory neurons or that reduce sodium currents in inhibitory interneurons are expected to promote hyperexcitability. VGSC genes implicated in epilepsy include *SCN1A*, *SCN2A*, *SCN3A SCN8A*, *SCN9A*, and *SCN1B* (see **Table 1**). Mutations in the *SCN1A* gene that codes for the α subunit Nav1.1 are associated with the DS phenotype of often severe epilepsy and cognitive disability. The incidence of DS is 1 in 15,000 to 40,000, and it affects boys and girls equally. DS epilepsy is composed of diverse seizure types; however, convulsive seizures are the most common. The first seizure appears at 5 to 8 months of age and can be triggered by a fever or flashes of light. Like many other early-onset epilepsies, seizures are associated with severe neurologic impairment. The cause of DS was identified in 2001 to be mutations in the *SCN1A* gene and 80% to 90% are de novo mutations.

Table 1
Ion channel mutations and associated epilepsy syndromes/seizure types

Ion Channel	Gene	Protein	Function	Epilepsy Syndromes/Seizure Types	Seizure Onset
Sodium					
α Subunit	SCN1A	Nav1.1	Inward Na$^+$ current in interneurons	DS, GEFS+, GTCs	Infancy childhood
	SCN2A	Nav1.2	Inward Na$^+$ current in excitatory neurons	Benign familial neonatal-infantile epilepsy, sporadic infantile spasm, sporadic neonatal epileptic encephalopathy	Neonatal, infancy
	SCN3A	Nav1.3	Inward Na$^+$ current	Cryptogenic focal epilepsy, focal unaware to bilateral GTC, GTC, myoclonic	Neonatal, infancy, childhood
	SCN8A	Nav1.6	Inward Na$^+$ current in axon initial segment & nodes of Ranvier	GTC, tonic, myoclonic	Neonatal, infancy
β Subunit	SCN9A	Nav1.7	Inward Na$^+$ current	Febrile seizures, focal unaware, GTC	Childhood
	SCN1B	β1	Inward Na$^+$ current	GEFS+,	Childhood, adolescence, adulthood

(continued on next page)

Table 1
(continued)

Ion Channel	Gene	Protein	Function	Epilepsy Syndromes/Seizure Types	Seizure Onset
Potassium					
Voltage dependent	KCNA2	Kv1.2	Delayed K$^+$ rectifier current	GTC, focal unaware, alternating hemiclonic seizures, absence, juvenile myoclonic epilepsy	Infancy, Childhood
	KCNB1	Kv2.1	Delayed K$^+$ rectifier current	GTC, focal unaware, infantile spasm, West syndrome, Lennox-Gastaut	Infancy, childhood
	KCND2	Kv4.2	A-type K$^+$ current	GTC, focal unaware	Infancy, adolescence
	KCNQ2	Kv7.2	M-type current	Benign familial neonatal seizures, tonic	Neonatal, infancy
	KCNQ5	Kv7.5	M-type current	Focal unaware, infantile spasm	Infancy, childhood
	KCNH1	Kv10.1	Inward rectifying K$^+$ current	Temple-Baraitser syndrome, GTC, focal unaware, myoclonic, tonic, clonic	Neonatal, infancy
	KCNH5	Kv10.2	Inward rectifying K$^+$ current	GTC, hemiclonic	Infancy
	KCNMA1	K$_{Ca}$1.1	Ca^{2+} and voltage-dependent K$^+$ current	GTC	Childhood
Non–voltage dependent	KCNT1	K$_{Ca}$4.1	Ca^{2+} activated K$^+$ current	MMFSI, ADNFLE	Infancy, childhood
	KCNJ10	Kir4.1	Inward rectifying K$^+$ current in astrocytes	EAST syndrome, idiopathic generalized epilepsies, childhood absence epilepsy	Infancy, childhood
Chloride					
K$^+$/Cl$^-$ cotransporter	CLCN1	CLC-1	Voltage-dependent Cl$^-$ current	Idiopathic generalized epilepsies	Infancy
	CLCN2	CLC-2	Voltage-dependent Cl$^-$ current	Idiopathic generalized epilepsies, childhood absence, juvenile absence, GTC, tonic	Infancy, childhood
	SLC12A5	KCC2	Extrude intracellular Cl$^-$	Epileptic encephalopathy with focal migrating seizures, idiopathic generalized epilepsy, GTC, myoclonic, absence	Infancy

Calcium					
α Subunit	CACNA1H	Cav3.2	T-type Ca^{2+} current	Idiopathic generalized epilepsies,	Infancy, childhood
	CACNA1A	Cav2.1	Presynaptic vesicle release	Epileptic encephalopathy, absence	Infancy
β Subunit	CNCNB4	β4	Modulate Ca^{2+} current, α subunit trafficking	Myoclonic epilepsy, tonic, idiopathic generalized epilepsies	Infancy, childhood

Abbreviations: ADNFLE, autosomal dominant nocturnal frontal lobe epilepsy; EAST, epilepsy, ataxia, sensorineural deafness, and tubulopathy; GEFs+, Genetic epilepsy with febrile seizures plus; GTCs, Generalized tonic-clonic seizures; MMFSI, malignant migrating focal seizures of infancy.

Table 2
Defects in neurotransmitter receptors and associated epilepsy syndromes/seizure types

Receptor	Gene	Protein	Function	Epilepsy Syndromes/Seizure Types	Seizure Onset
GABA	*GABRA1*	GABA$_{A1}$	Postsynaptic ligand-gated Cl$^-$ current	Absence, idiopathic generalized epilepsy, epileptic encephalopathy, juvenile myoclonic epilepsy	Infancy, childhood, adolescence
	GABRB3	GABA$_{\beta3}$	Postsynaptic ligand-gated Cl$^-$ current	Childhood absence, epileptic encephalopathy	Neonatal, infancy, childhood
	GABRG2	GABA$_{\gamma2}$	Postsynaptic ligand-gated Cl$^-$ current	Childhood absence, GEFS$^+$, idiopathic generalized epilepsy, epileptic encephalopathies	Neonatal, infancy
	GABRE	GABA$_{\epsilon3}$	Postsynaptic ligand-gated Cl$^-$ current	Infantile spasm, focal unaware, focal unaware to bilateral GTC, GTC	Infancy
Nicotinic acetylcholine	*CHRNA4*	nACHR$_{\alpha4}$	Acetylcholine-gated nonselective cation currents	ADSHE	Childhood, adolescence
	CHRNB2	nACHR$_{\beta2}$	Acetylcholine-gated nonselective cation currents	ADSHE	Childhood, adolescence
	CHRNA2	nACHR$_{\alpha2}$	Acetylcholine-gated nonselective cation currents	Benign infantile familial seizures	Infancy
Glutamate	*GRIN1*	GluN1	Postsynaptic ligand-gated Ca^{2+} current	Infantile spasm, tonic, atonic, hypermotor, focal dyscognitive, GTC	Neonatal, infancy, childhood
	GRIN2A	GluN2A	Postsynaptic ligand-gated Ca^{2+} current	Childhood focal epilepsy, rolandic epilepsy, epileptic encephalopathy, absence, tonic, myoclonic	Infancy, childhood
	GRIN2B	GluN2B	Postsynaptic ligand-gated Ca^{2+} current	West syndrome, childhood-onset focal epilepsy, epileptic encephalopathy	Infancy, childhood
	GRIN2D	GluN2D	Postsynaptic ligand-gated Ca^{2+} current	Infantile spasm, focal unaware to bilateral GTC, GTC, myoclonic, atypical absence	Neonatal, infancy, childhood

Abbreviation: ADSHE, autosomal dominant sleep-related hypermotor epilepsy.

Table 3
Mutations of synaptic complexes and associated epilepsy syndromes/seizure types

Location	Gene	Protein	Function	Epilepsy Syndromes/Seizure Types	Seizure Onset
Presynaptic	DNM-1	DYN1	Vesicle trafficking	Infantile spasms, absence with eyelid myoclonia, atonic, myoclonic, tonic, focal, GTCs	Neonatal, infancy
	NRXN1	NRXN1	Cell adhesion	Absence, GTCs, myoclonic	Childhood
	SNAP25	SNAP25	Vesicle trafficking	Infantile spasms, GTCs, focal, absence, myoclonic, tonic	Neonatal, infancy, childhood
	STX1B	STX1B	Vesicle trafficking	GTC, partial, absence, tonic, atonic, Ohtahara syndrome, West syndrome	Infancy, childhood, adolescence
	SV2A	SV2a	Vesicle trafficking	Myoclonic, tonic	Infancy
	TBC1D24	TBC1C24	GTP-ase activating, vesicle trafficking	Myoclonic, GTC, partial, absence, infantile spasms	Neonatal, infancy, childhood
Postsynaptic	CNTNAP2	CNTNAP2	Cell adhesion	Focal, tonic	Infancy, childhood
	IQSEC2	IQSEC2	Guanine nucleotide exchange factor	Atypical absence, GTCs	Infancy, childhood
	PCDH19	PCDH19	Cell adhesion	GTC, tonic, absence, atonic, partial, myoclonic	Infancy
	SHANK3	SHANK3	Scaffolding	GTC, partial, absence, tonic, myoclonic, atonic	Infancy, childhood
	SYNGAP1	SynGAP	GTP-ase activating	GTC, atonic, absence with eyelid myoclonia, myoclonic	Childhood
	STXBP1	STXBF1	Vesicle trafficking	Infantile spasms, myoclonic, GTC, atonic, absence, partial	Neonatal, infancy

Table 4
Defects in intracellular pathways/organelles and associated epilepsy syndromes/seizure types

	Gene	Protein	Function	Epilepsy Syndromes/Seizure Types	Seizure Onset
mTOR pathway	*TSC1, TSC2*	TSC1, TSC2	Cell growth	Tuberous sclerosis	Infancy, childhood, adolescence, adulthood
	MTOR	mTOR	Cell growth	Focal cortical dysplasia	Variable age of onset
	RHEB	RHEB	Cell growth	Focal cortical dysplasia	Variable age of onset
	DEPDC5	DEPDC5	Cell growth	Focal cortical dysplasia	Neonatal, infancy, childhood
	NPRL2, NPRL3	NPRL2, NPRL3	Cell growth	Nocturnal frontal lobe epilepsy, frontal lobe epilepsy, temporal lobe epilepsy	Infancy, childhood
	AKT3	AKT3	Cell growth	Infantile spasm	Infancy
Mitochondria	*POLG*	POLG	mtDNA integrity	Alpers-Huttenlocher syndrome	Childhood
	MT-TK	tRNA-lysine	Mitochondrial protein synthesis	Myoclonic epilepsy with red ragged fibers	Childhood, adolescence, adulthood
	PDHA1	PDHA1	Pyruvate dehydrogenase complex	Infantile spasm, myoclonic absence, atypical absence, West syndrome, Lennox-Gastaut	Neonatal, infancy
	PDHB	PDHB	Pyruvate dehydrogenase complex	Infantile spasm, myoclonic absence, atypical absence, West syndrome, Lennox-Gastaut	Neonatal, infancy
Lysosome	*SCARB2*	LIMP-2	Lysosomal enzyme transport	AMRF	Adolescence, adulthood
	CLN1–CLN8, CLN10–CLN14	Lysosomal enzymes, lysosome-interacting proteins	Breakdown of metabolites in the lysosome	Myoclonic epilepsy, atypical absence	Variable age of onset depending on specific *CLN* gene defect
	NEU1	NEU1	Cleavage of sialic acid from glycoproteins/glycolipids	Progressive myoclonic epilepsy, GTC	Adolescence, adulthood

Abbreviations: AMRF, action myoclonus–renal failure; progressive myoclonic epilepsy; mtDNA, mitochondrial DNA; mTOR, mechanistic target of rapamycin; PDHB, pyruvate dehydrogenase complex E1-beta; tRNA, transfer RNA.

Table 5
Metabolic defects and associated epilepsy syndromes/seizure types

	Gene	Protein	Function	Epilepsy Syndromes/Seizure Types	Seizure Onset
Pyridoxine	ALDH7A1	Antiquitin	Lysine metabolism	Focal, GTC, infantile spasm, myoclonic	Neonatal, infancy, childhood
	PNPO	Peridoxine-5'-phosphate oxidase	Pyridoxine to pyridoxal 5' phosphate	GTC, tonic, clonic, myoclonic, focal	Neonatal
Biotin	BTD	Biotinidase	Biotin recycling	GTC, myoclonic, infantile spasm, Ohtahara syndrome	Neonatal, infancy
Folic acid	FOLR1	FOLR$_\alpha$	CNS folate transport	Myoclonic-astatic, myoclonic, GTC	Childhood
Glycine	GLDC	Glycine decarboxylase	Glycine metabolism	Nonketotic hyperglycinemia	Neonatal
	AMT	Aminomethyltransferase	Glycine metabolism	Nonketotic hyperglycinemia	Neonatal
Glutamate	SLC2A1	GLUT1	CNS glutamate transport	Focal, absence, myoclonic-astatic	Infancy
Uridine	CAD	CPSase/ATCase/DHOas	De novo pyrimidine biosynthesis	GTC, focal	Infancy

Abbreviation: CNS, central nervous system.

Mutations in other VGSC genes of the α subunit (*SCN2A*, *SCN3A*, *SCN8A*, *SCN9A*) and β subunit (*SCN1B*) occur less frequently but are also associated with seizures. Interestingly, seizures in patients with *SCN2A* mutations often disappear by about 18 months of age, possibly because of reduced Nav1.2 expression and compensatory expression of functional Nav1.6.[13] Gain-of-function[14] and loss-of-function[15] mutations have been identified in the *SCN3A* gene of patients with epileptic encephalopathy. Gain-of-function variants of the *SCN8A* gene, which codes for the Nav1.6 α subunit, have similarly been associated with epileptic encephalopathy[16–18] and mostly result from de novo mutations. Mutations in the *SCN9A* gene, which codes for Nav1.7, may have causal overlap with DS epilepsy as a potential modifier.[19] Of the 4 β subunit genes (encoding β1, β1b, β2, β3, and β4 proteins), the *SCN1B* gene has been linked to various forms of epilepsy.[20–24] A mutation in the *SCN1B* gene was identified in a patient with idiopathic epilepsy.[25]

Potassium Channels

Potassium channels regulate neuronal excitability by limiting the frequency, amplitude, and duration of action potentials.[26–28] Impairment of the repolarizing functions of potassium channels can lead to hyperexcitable and synchronous neuronal firing. Mutations of potassium channel genes in epilepsy have been identified, including *KCNA2*, *KCNB1*, *KCND2*, *KCNQ2*, *KCNQ3*, *KCNQ5*, *KCNH1*, *KCNH5*, *KCNJ10*, *KCNMA1*, and *KCNT1* (see **Table 1**). Voltage-gated potassium channels (VGPCs) are composed of 4 small α subunits coded separately by more than 40 genes[29,30] and can also bind modulatory β subunits that regulate localization and channel opening/closing.[31]

Variants of the *KCNA2* gene that encode for *Kv1.2* can cause epileptic encephalopathy with ataxia and tremors.[32–34] Gain-of-function or loss-of-function mutations of *KCNA2* that have differential effects on *Kv1.2* channel properties were also distinctly associated with focal and generalized seizures, respectively.[35] *KCNB1* encodes the *Kv2.1* α subunit and has been associated with infantile epilepsy.[36,37] A mutation affecting the potassium ion selectivity filter of Kv2.1 was revealed in a patient with intractable multifocal seizures that started at age 13 months.[38] The *KCND2* gene encodes for *Kv4.2*, which is highly expressed in the central nervous system (CNS).[39,40] A truncating mutation of the *KCND2* gene was identified in a patient with temporal lobe epilepsy.[41] A different *KCND2* gene variant was found in identical twins exhibiting seizures.[42] Mutations in *Kv7.2* channels encoded by *KCNQ2* are associated with benign familial neonatal seizures (BFNSs) and KCNQ2 developmental and epileptic encephalopathy.[43,44] Seizures may start during the first week of life but often disappear by 12 months of age in BFNS.[45,46] The Kv7.3 subunit encoded by the *KCNQ3* gene can form a heteromeric potassium channel with Kv7.2. Mutations of *KCNQ3* are less frequently linked to epilepsy, but variants in either *KCNQ2* or *KCNQ3* that affect their heteromerization can result in early-onset seizures.[47] Gain-of-function and loss-of-function mutations have also been described in *KCNQ5* (Kv7.5) in epileptic encephalopathy.[48] *KCNH1* encodes Kv10.1 channels, and mutations cause Temple-Baraitser syndrome, a neurodevelopmental disorder with severe intellectual disability and epilepsy.[49–52] Less is known about Kv10.2, which is encoded by the *KCNH5* gene; however, epileptic variants of *KCNH5* have been documented.[53]

The *KCNMA1* gene encodes the voltage-sensitive and calcium-sensitive $K_{Ca1.1}$ channel, which is part of the BK (big potassium) subgroup of VGPCs, which are highly expressed in excitatory neurons of the brain and produce a powerful hyperpolarizing potassium ion conductance.[54] Because of calcium sensitivity, $K_{Ca1.1}$ channels can modulate calcium-induced neurotransmitter release at the synapse. Case reports include patients with *KCNMA1* mutations with paroxysmal dyskinesia and epilepsy.[55,56]

Potassium channels that are non–voltage dependent but contribute to neuronal membrane excitability during action potential generation have been linked to epilepsy. These channels include the sequence like A calcium activated K+ channel (SLACK or $K_{Ca}4.1$ subunit) and the ATP-sensitive inward rectifier potassium channel 10 (Kir4.1). *KCNT1* encodes the SLACK or $K_{Ca}4.1$ subunit and *KCNT1* mutations have been identified in malignant migrating focal seizures of infancy (MMFSI) and autosomal dominant nocturnal frontal lobe epilepsy (ADNFLE), which is characterized by hypermotor seizures during sleep.[57]

The *KCNJ10* gene encodes the ATP-sensitive Kir4.1 inward rectifying potassium channels.[58,59] Mutations in *KCNJ10* have been identified in patients with genetic generalized epilepsies[60] and epilepsy, ataxia, sensorineural deafness, and tubulopathy (EAST) syndrome.[61,62]

Chloride Channels

Voltage-gated chloride channels control chloride homeostasis and thereby have effects on gamma-aminobutyric acid (GABA) A receptors. Variants of the *CLCN1* and *CLCN2* genes, which encode the voltage-gated chloride channels CLC-1 and CLC-2, respectively, have been identified in families with idiopathic epilepsy[63–68] (see **Table 1**). Rare *CLCN2* variants were associated with SCN1A mutations in patients with DS and early infantile epileptic encephalopathy, suggesting a possible role of *CLCN2* as a gene modifier.[69]

Potassium-Chloride Cotransporter

In mature CNS neurons, low intracellular chloride concentrations are imperative for the function of GABAergic neurotransmission in mediating inhibitory postsynaptic currents (IPSCs). The neuron-specific cotransporter K+/Cl− type-2 (KCC2), encoded by the *SLC12A5* gene, is expressed on the somatodendritic membrane and extrudes chloride using the potassium electrochemical force produced by the Na+/K+ATPase.[70] Early infancy epileptic encephalopathy with focal migrating seizures has been documented in families with biallelic *SLC12A5* loss-of-function mutations,[71–73] and idiopathic generalized epilepsy has been reported in patients with compound heterozygous *SLC12A5* mutations[74] (see **Table 1**). An Australian family with a history of early childhood–onset febrile seizures was reported to harbor a missense variant of the *SLC12A5* gene.[75]

Calcium Channels

Voltage-gated calcium channels (VGCCs) conduct an inward calcium current and contribute to neuronal excitability. VGCCs are generally categorized into low voltage–activated (LVA) and high voltage–activated (HVA) calcium channels, and mutations associated with epilepsy have been described (see **Table 1**). LVA, or T-type channels, are monomeric channels composed of a $Ca_V\alpha1$ subunit and function at voltages near the resting membrane potential.[76] Mutation of *CACNA1H* encoding the T-type Cav3.2 has been associated with idiopathic generalized epilepsy.[77] The HVA VGCCs (L, N, R, P, and Q types) are heteromeric channels composed of the principal pore-forming α1 subunit and ancillary subunits (β, α2, δ, and γ). HVA channels require much larger depolarization potentials to activate. In the CNS, the P/Q type Cav2.1 channel encoded by the *CACNA1A* gene mediates fast synaptic transmission at the presynaptic membrane.[76] Mutations in *CACNA1A* can lead to devastating early-life ischemic strokes and intractable epilepsy[78] as well as early-onset epileptic encephalopathy, widespread CNS atrophy, and reduced lifespan.[79] Variants of the *CACNA1A* gene leading to impaired Cav2.1 function are also associated with absence seizures and episodic ataxia[80] and may increase the frequency of absence seizures in a subset of patients with DS.[81] Mutations affecting the VGCC ancillary subunit β4 have been reported in patients with myoclonic epilepsy[82] and severe neurodevelopmental disorders with focal or tonic seizures.[83]

RECEPTORS/BINDING PROTEINS/SYNAPTIC PROTEINS
Gamma-aminobutyric Acid Receptors

GABA receptors are a major pharmacologic target in epilepsy.[84] GABA-A receptors are ligand-gated chloride channels that conduct IPSCs in the mature nervous system and are generally composed of 2 α subunits, 2 β subunits, and 1 γ subunit, which are each encoded by 6 α, 3 β, and 3 γ genes.[85] Genes encoding GABA receptor subunits with mutations linked to epilepsy include *GABRA1*, *GABRB3*, *GABRG2*, and *GABRD* (see **Table 2**), which can affect surface expression and receptor open time, or alter protein folding and oligomerization.[86] The *GABRA1* gene codes for GABA-A receptor α1 subunit. Mutations in *GABRA1* have been identified in patients with absence seizures, febrile seizures, generalized seizures, and epileptic encephalopathy.[87–90] Variants of the *GABRB3* gene, which codes for the GABA-A receptor β3 subunit, have been identified in young patients with childhood absence seizures and early-onset/infantile epileptic encephalopathy,[91–93] and may also underlie a subset of *SCN1A*-negative DS cases.[94] The *GABRG2* gene codes for GABA-A receptor subunit γ2. Variants of *GABRG2* are also strongly linked to epileptic encephalopathies and are a risk for absence, febrile, and generalized seizures.[95–97] Rare variants of the *GABRE* gene coding for the ε subunit have recently been found in patients with epilepsy.[98]

Nicotinic Acetylcholine Receptors

Nicotinic acetylcholine receptors (nAChRs) are ligand-gated ion channels encoded in humans by 16 genes and are assembled from 5 subunits into heteromeric or homomeric channels.[99–101] nAChRs are broadly distributed in the brain and modulate neuronal response to many neurotransmitter systems. The first discovery of a genetic mutation causing epilepsy was that of the nAChR subunit gene *CHRNA4*, associated with ADNFLE (now known as autosomal dominant sleep-related hypermotor epilepsy [ADSHE]) in 1995.[102] Since then, mutations have been discovered in *CHRNA2*, *CHRNA4*, and *CHRNB2* that code for the α2, α4, and β2 subunits, respectively, which are implicated in ADNFLE/ADSHE[103–108] (see **Table 2**). Although *CHRNA2* mutations are not strongly suspected in ADNFLE,[109] variants of *CHRNA2* may be a contributing component of benign familial infantile epilepsy.[110]

Glutamate Receptors

Glutamate receptors are a family of ligand-gated ion channels and metabotropic receptors and mediate most of the excitatory neurotransmission in the CNS.[111,112] The *N*-methyl-D-aspartate receptor (NMDAR) is an ion channel that conducts a slow but long inward calcium current on 2 simultaneous synaptic events: postsynaptic membrane depolarization and glutamate binding.[113] Genes coding for NMDAR subunits implicated in epilepsy include *GRIN1*, *GRIN2A*, and *GRIN2B*[114] (see **Table 2**). Mutations in *GRIN1* encoding for the ubiquitous NMDAR subunit GluN1 were identified in patients showing profound developmental delay, severe intellectual disability, and severe seizures.[115] Mutations in *GRIN2A* encoding the GluN2A subunit have been found in patients showing developmental delay and diverse seizure types, including absence, tonic, myoclonic, and syndromic epilepsy, such as childhood focal epilepsy, rolandic epilepsy, and epileptic encephalopathy,[116–119] and the epilepsy-aphasia disorders, including Landau-Kleffner syndrome (LKS).[117,120] Autosomal dominant inherited GRIN2B gene variants have been detected in patients with intellectual disability, schizophrenia, autism spectrum disorder, and with epileptic spasms, focal epilepsy, and epileptic encephalopathies.[121,122] Loss-of-function and gain-of-function mutations in the GRIN2B gene have been documented.[123] The discovery of GRIN2D mutations linked to severe epileptic encephalopathy has increased.[124–127]

SYNGAP1 and STXBP1

Mutations in genes encoding proteins critical for synapse formation, maintenance, and function are emerging as an important cause of epilepsy. The proteins encoded by such genes are found both in the presynaptic and postsynaptic space. SYNGAP1 (postsynaptic) and STXBP1 (presynaptic) (see **Table 3**) are two now well-established epilepsy genes that encode synaptic proteins.

SYNGAP1 encodes the synaptic GTP-ase activating protein (SynGAP), a major constituent of the postsynaptic density of excitatory synapses.[128,129] The first report of patients with SYNGAP1 mutations was in 2009 in individuals with nonsyndromic intellectual disability.[130] Epilepsy was discovered soon after to be a common phenotype in individuals with SYNGAP1 loss-of-function mutations.[131] With the larger cohorts of patients recently published, it is now clear that greater than 90% of individuals with SYNGAP1 loss-of-function mutations have epilepsy.[132,133] The most common seizure type in individuals with SYNGAP1 mutations are myoclonic absences, at times subtle and brief, that can be induced by chewing.[133,134] Other seizure types also occur in these patients, including atonic, myoclonic, and generalized tonic clonic seizures. The combination of atonic and myoclonic absences frequently leads to a diagnosis of Doose syndrome.

In contrast with SYNGAP1, mutations in STXBP1 often present with a severe, early-onset encephalopathy that often leads to clinical diagnoses of Ohtahara syndrome or West syndrome. The first mutations in STXBP1 were described in Ohtahara syndrome, a neonatal encephalopathy.[135] Some of those initial neonates progressed to West syndrome. Subsequent cohorts of patients with pathogenic STXBP1 mutations have broadened the spectrum of epilepsy to include later onset. At present, 85% of individuals with pathogenic mutations in STXBP1 are diagnosed with epilepsy, with most having onset in the first year of life.[136] Mutations in additional synaptic protein–encoding genes lead to epileptic encephalopathies (see **Table 3**).

mTORopathies

Mechanistic target of rapamycin (mTOR) is a serine/threonine kinase known as a master regulator of cell growth, migration, proliferation, and metabolism. mTOR associates with 2 distinct groups of proteins to form mTOR complex 1 (mTORC1) or mTOR complex 2 (mTORC2). Dysregulation of the mTOR pathway has been identified in cancer[137,138] and in the brain is associated with malformations of cortical development[139,140] (see **Table 4**).

Tuberous Sclerosis Complex

TSC is the prototypical mTORopathy, showing upregulation of mTOR activity caused by mutations in the TSC1 or TSC2 genes, which encode for the regulators hamartin and tuberin, respectively,[141,142] in the mTORC1 pathway. TSC is characterized by the formation of benign tumors affecting skin, heart, lungs, kidneys, brain, and other systems. Brain abnormalities in TSC include subependymal nodules and subependymal giant cell astrocytomas (SEGA).[143–145] From 80% to 90% of patients with TSC show early-onset seizures, often with infantile spasms (ISs) that evolve to multiple described seizure types associated with cortical tubers.[146–149] Identification of a cortical tuber as an epileptogenic focus and subsequent surgical resection may lead to reduced seizure frequency and may improve developmental delay.[147,150,151] Cortical tubers are characterized by dyslamination and are composed of a heterogenous group of malformed neuronal and glial cells.[152,153]

Other mTORopathies

Epilepsy may also be associated with upregulation of the mTOR pathway because of mutations in other upstream regulator genes.[154–156] Focal cortical dysplasia type II (FCDII) presents with cortical dyslamination, and cytomegalic and dysmorphic neurons.[157,158] Patients with FCDII often present with intractable epilepsy and mutations in mTOR pathway regulators, and variants of the *MTOR* gene itself have been reported in some.[140,159,160] In addition, mutations in genes coding for mTOR regulatory proteins such as DEPDC5, encoded by the *DEPDC5* gene,[161,162] and NPRL2/NPRL3, encoded by the *NPRL2/NPRL3* genes,[163] were revealed in patients with epilepsy and upregulation of mTORC1. Mutations in the upstream regulator *PTEN* in humans are not typically associated with epilepsy[164] but case reports do exist in some patients with Cowden syndrome that also experience seizures.[165–167] Parker and colleagues[168] described a rare infantile-onset epilepsy in the Old Order Mennonite population with associated cognitive impairment/delay, craniofacial dysmorphisms, and malformations of cortical development associated with deletion mutation in the *LYK5/STRADA* gene encoding the pseudokinase, STRADA, which is an upstream inhibitor in the mTOR pathway. The described deletion mutation in this gene renders the mTOR pathway upregulated, and treatment with rapamycin reduced seizure frequency and improved language development in these patients,[168] thereby proving it to be disease modifying. Mutations in genes for the mTOR upstream regulators *PIK3CA* and *AKT3* may also result in increased mTOR activation, and variants have been described in patients with seizures ranging from mild to severe.[139,169–172] Furthermore, in TSC and other malformations of cortical development associated with epilepsy, germline and brain somatic mutations in the mTOR and associated regulatory growth pathways have been described.[154,173]

INBORN ERRORS IN METABOLISM

Epilepsy caused by inborn errors in metabolism (IEM) is rare, but, when IEM are present, seizures and epilepsy are frequent aspects of the phenotype. Comorbidities of developmental delay and regression, intellectual disability, and behavioral impairments are common. These disorders often occur because of an inherited enzyme or cofactor deficiency that affects specific metabolic and biochemical pathways (see **Table 5**). Because some of the IEM are responsive to specific therapies, early diagnosis is critical. Although the IEM may present throughout life, there are several that present early in the neonatal/infancy period that involve vitamin or cofactor deficiencies that are amenable to treatment.

Pyridoxine

Pyridoxine-dependent epilepsy (PDE) is a rare, autosomal recessive epilepsy caused by mutations in the antiquitin gene (*ALDH7A1*)[174] causing deficiency of alpha-aminoadipic semialdehyde dehydrogenase (antiquitin), which leads to altered lysine metabolism, ultimately causing piperideine-6-carboxylate to accumulate and inactivate pyridoxal phosphate, which is the activated form of pyridoxine. Pyridoxine phosphate is a cofactor for glutamic acid decarboxylase (GAD), which is involved in GABA synthesis. Thus, this IEM is presumed to affect GABA inhibitory neurotransmission and thereby increase excitability in the CNS.[175–177] Presentation is newborn period through 3 years of age, diagnosis suspected based on pyridoxine challenge with electroencephalogram (EEG) monitoring and confirmed with genetic testing, and treatment is pyridoxine supplementation. Long-term neurodevelopmental impairments are variable and not directly associated with seizure control.[176,178,179]

Mutations in the pyridoxine 5′-phosphate oxidase (PNPO) gene result in nonfunctional PNPO and affect pyridoxine signaling, leading to low levels of pyridoxal 5′-phosphate (PLP), which is a cofactor for enzymes including GAD. Clinical presentation is different than for PDE, with premature birth and seizures (may occur in utero), hypoglycemia, lactic acidosis, and encephalopathy. Treatment is with PLP, the activated form of pyridoxine.[176]

Biotin

Mutations in the *BTD* gene result in biotinidase deficiency, which is involved in recycling biotin, an enzyme required for biotin-dependent carboxylase metabolism. The phenotype in biotin deficiency includes seizures, marked developmental delay, cognitive impairment, ataxia, skin rash, alopecia, hearing and vision impairment, and fungal infections. Biotin deficiency is identified as part of newborn screening and treatment is with biotin oral replacement therapy.[176,180]

Folinic Acid

Mutations of the *FOLR1* gene encoding the folate receptor alpha, a folate transporter, are associated with folinic acid–responsive seizures (FARS) caused by disruption of folate transport into the CNS. Treatment is with folinic acid but there are reported links to PDE suggesting that outcome may improve with both pyridoxine and folinic acid supplementation.[181] Presentation is in early childhood with seizures, developmental delay, and hypotonia.[176,182] FARS may have an autoimmune cause with similar but earlier presentation.

Glycine

Mutations in genes encoding the glycine cleavage enzyme system, including *GLDC* and *AMT*, are associated with nonketotic hyperglycinemia (NKH), which is an autosomal recessive disorder of glycine metabolism. These mutations cause glycine accumulation in the body with increases measured in plasma and cerebrospinal fluid (CSF). Presentation occurs in the neonatal period with encephalopathy, hypotonia, myoclonus with suppression burst EEG pattern, and subsequent development of drug-resistant epilepsy with severe intellectual disability.[183–185] Intervention is supportive (anticonvulsant treatment avoiding valproic acid because it may increase glycine levels) and targeted at decreasing glycine levels with sodium benzoate, but, in neonatal-onset NKH, developmental outcome is not altered, whereas seizure severity and frequency may be affected. Late-onset variants are considered attenuated forms of NKH with a less severe phenotype and are more responsive to therapy with sodium benzoate and dextromethorphan (*N*-methyl-D-aspartate receptor antagonism).[186]

Glutamate

Mutations in the SLC2A1 gene encoding the cerebral glucose transporter (GLUT1) lead to the GLUT1 deficiency syndrome, resulting in impaired glucose transport into the brain. Glut-1 deficiency may be via autosomal dominant inheritance or sporadic haploinsufficiency. GLUT1 deficiency syndrome classically presents with infantile-onset drug-resistant seizures, developmental delay, acquired microcephaly, abnormal tone, and movement disorder.[187,188] However, there is a broad clinical spectrum that includes developmental delay, epilepsy, paroxysmal exercise-induced dyskinesias, and cognitive impairments. Focal motor seizures are seen in infancy and, later, the predominant seizure type is generalized, including early-onset absence and myoclonic-astatic. Seizures may increase before meals or with fasting. Low CSF glucose levels (with blood glucose levels performed immediately before lumber puncture) support the diagnosis but may be normal in some GLUT1-deficient patients, so genetic testing for mutations in the *SLC2A1* gene is critical. The ketogenic diet is an effective therapy or the modified Atkins diet in milder cases. Medications that impair GLUT1 function, including phenobarbital and diazepam, should be avoided.[186]

Mitochondrial Disorders

Mitochondria consist of 37 genes[189] and the proximity of the mitochondrial DNA (mtDNA) to the ATP-producing machinery makes them particularly vulnerable to oxidative damage by reactive oxygen species (ROS). Various forms of epilepsy have been linked to mitochondrial defects that increase ROS production,[190–192] and studies suggest antioxidant therapy may be neuroprotective[192,193] (see **Table 4**). Mutations in mitochondrial genes may be associated with epilepsy.[194,195] Alpers-Huttenlocher syndrome is a rare and severe mitochondrial disease characterized by intractable seizures. Alpers-Huttenlocher syndrome is caused by mutations in the mitochondrial gene *POLG* encoding polymerase gamma, which maintains mtDNA integrity.[196] Alpers-Huttenlocher syndrome affects multiple organs with a variety of symptoms, including epilepsy with onset between 2 and 4 years and death occurring within 4 years after onset. Pathologic changes in the cortex include spongiosis, neuronal apoptosis, and astrogliosis, which may result from progressive loss of mitochondria. Myoclonic epilepsy with ragged red fibers (MERFF) is a rare and severe multisystem disorder characterized by epilepsy, ataxia, and dementia.[197] MERFF is caused by mutations in the mitochondrial genes for transfer RNA (tRNA), with more than 80% of cases caused by mutations in the *MT-TK* gene, which codes for tRNA lysine[197] and results in diminished synthesis of mitochondrial proteins.[198] The function of mitochondrial energetics depends on the coordination of nuclear-encoded and mitochondrial-encoded proteins.[189,199] Mutations in the nuclear genes *PHA1* (pyruvate dehydrogenase complex E1-alpha polypeptide) and *PDHB* (pyruvate dehydrogenase complex E1-beta) encoding components of the multienzyme pyruvate dehydrogenase complex (PDHc) lead to PDHc deficiency and epilepsy.[200]

Lysosomal Storage Diseases

Lysosomal storage diseases are a heterogenous groups of disorders and mutations in genes that affect lysosomal function and have also been reported to be associated with epilepsy (see **Table 4**). For example, mutations in the *SCARB2* gene, which codes for lysosomal integral membrane protein-2 (LIMP-2), are seen in action myoclonus–renal failure (AMRF) syndrome.[201,202] Some patients with AMRF experience seizures before renal dysfunction,[201] whereas others can show ataxia and epilepsy in the absence of renal failure.[203–205] Examination of postmortem histologic brain samples from patients with *SCARB2* mutations and a history of progressive myoclonic epilepsy reveal signs of neurodegeneration with excessive neuronal loss, gliosis, and granule deposition within astrocytes.[206] Neuronal ceroid lipofuscinoses (NCL [or Batten disease]) is a group of lysosomal storage disorders caused by mutations in *CLN* genes.[207,208] Mutations in *CLN1* to *CLN8* and *CLN10* to *CLN14* genes that code for a series of lysosomal or lysosomal-interacting proteins have been associated with severe epilepsy.[207,209] Similar to *SCARB2* variant–associated epilepsy, NCL neurologic disorder is characterized by neurodegeneration and the deposition of granular lipopigments.[210] The *NEU1* gene codes for neuraminidase 1, a lysosomal protein that catalyzes removal of sialic acid from glycoproteins, glycolipids, and oligosaccharides.[211] Mutations of the *NEU1* gene lead to sialidosis, a rare metabolic disorder and lysosomal storage disease.[212] Sialidosis type 1 is associated with ataxia and seizures[213,214] and presents with vacuolations and deposition of lipofuscinlike pigment in neurons of the neocortex, basal ganglia, thalamus, and brain stem.[212]

Epilepsy may constitute a major part of the phenotype in other genetic IEM. An example is uridine-responsive epileptic encephalopathy caused by mutation in the gene encoding CPSase/ATCase/DHOas (CAD), which is involved in de novo pyrimidine biosynthesis (see **Table 5**). Mutations in CAD were identified in children with neurodegeneration associated with developmental delay, epileptic encephalopathy, and anemia with anisopoikilocytosis. Uridine supplementation halted seizures, improved development, and reversed the anemia.[215] Urea cycle defects, organic acidemias, and aminoacidopathies also may be associated with epileptic encephalopathies presenting in the neonatal period or in milder cases later associated with infection or stress.[186] There are many other IEM disorders with seizures and epilepsy as a part of the phenotype, but it is beyond the scope of this article to describe them all.

Inheritance Epilepsy

The unveiling of a growing list of candidate genes in epilepsy reflects the underlying complexity and underscores the challenges in treatment. Twin studies and linkage analysis on extended families established a genetic basis and determined mendelian inheritance in monogenic epilepsies; however, many more forms of epilepsy show a complex pattern of heritability, suggesting interactions with susceptibility genes and environmental factors.[216,217] Mutations in the *SCN1A* gene provide a model of a monogenic epilepsy with complex expressivity possibly caused by gene modifiers.[218] Similarly, although there may be intrafamilial sharing of *TSC* gene variants, disease severity of TSC may differ between family members, including between twins.[219–222] Therefore, defining more precisely the genetic landscape against which a pathogenic variant is expressed may be informative to disease variability.

Genetic Evaluation

Neurologic examination, EEG, neuroimaging, and metabolic testing are part of a routine diagnostic work-up that can inform the proper therapy and genetic evaluation (**Fig. 1**). Genetic epilepsies often do not present with overt anatomic signs of a lesion or a delineated hyperexcitable focus. Furthermore, many forms of epilepsy are not part of a typical semiology and require more in-depth examination. If a conclusive cause cannot be identified after epilepsy is established, genetic testing is warranted. Lumbar puncture for CSF neurotransmitter studies and CSF and serum glucose levels may be considered. In some cases, single-gene testing may be considered based on semiology and course of seizures or family history. Genomic testing by next-generation sequencing is increasingly becoming a standardized part of the diagnostic protocol.[223] Gene panels narrow down the genetic analysis to commonly known epilepsy-associated genes. Commercially available panels can be customized to include a small number of suspected genes or hundreds of genes with established links to syndromic and nonsyndromic epilepsies. Moreover, genetic panels include the mitochondrial genome for diagnosing rarer forms of epilepsy.[195] If an epilepsy

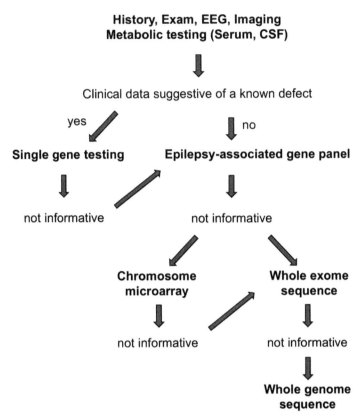

Fig. 1. Proposed algorithm for genetic evaluation in epilepsy. Routine diagnostic work-up and characterization of the seizure types can inform genetic work-up. Based on this information, the proposed algorithm for genetic testing is outlined. Of note is that, if all testing is negative but a genetic cause is strongly suspected, repeat genetic analysis is recommended every 1 to 2 years.

gene panel is not informative, array comparative genomic hybridization (aCGH) or whole exome sequencing (WES) can be used to evaluate for copy number variants and single nucleotide variants, respectively. In addition, if none of these provide an answer, whole genome sequencing is emerging as a diagnostic test. The results of genetic testing may guide treatment and modify or improve clinical management of patients with established seizure intractability.[223–225] Several studies have examined the diagnostic yield of genetic testing using WES or multigene panels in epilepsy and show a clear benefit, particularly in the pediatric population.[8,226–229] Parental testing can considerably expand the utility of patient genetic screening in cases with inconclusive results.[226] In cases of idiopathic epilepsy when a genetic cause is strongly suspected but state-of-the-art genetic testing described here shows no abnormalities, repeated genetic analysis is recommended every 1 to 2 years. Genetic counseling is recommended when genetic abnormalities are identified.

Therapeutic Considerations

Therapeutic intervention has traditionally been guided by clinical data related to seizure type and EEG data, particularly given that additional testing such as genetic is often not obtained until after imaging results and the response to initial therapeutics are known. Thus, therapies first follow those outlined for specific seizure types and epilepsy syndromes outlined in Akshat Katyayan and Gloria Diaz-Medina's article, "Epilepsy: Epileptic Syndromes and Treatment," elsewhere in this issue. As genetic testing is done more routinely and earlier in the course of epilepsy, therapeutics are guided by these results. For example, gain-of-function mutations of GABA-A receptors that result in suppressed inhibitory tone may not respond well to treatment with a GABA receptor agonist and instead exacerbate seizure frequency.[230] In DS, the use of traditional sodium channel blockers worsen seizures when used chronically.[231,232] Some first-line AEDs disrupt mitochondrial function and therefore are contraindicated in mitochondrial disease epilepsies.[233] Other genetic factors can influence the response to AEDs. For example, polymorphisms in genes for drug metabolizing enzymes such as the cytochrome P450 superfamily or the drug efflux transporter P-glycoprotein 1 (P-gp1) can alter the bioavailability of AEDs and may be associated with multidrug resistance.[234,235]

Immunomodulators

Immunomodulation is used in some specific forms of epilepsy, including autoimmune epilepsies, IS, electrographic status epilepticus of sleep, and LKS. Specifically related to genetic epilepsies is a case report of a patient with LKS related to a GRIN2A mutation who responded to immunomodulatory therapy.[236]

Cannabidiol

Cannabidiol (CBD) is approved for use in DS and Lennox-Gastaut syndrome.[237,238] There are reports that CBD may be effective in other genetic disorders associated with epilepsy such as TSC.[239]

Mechanistic Target of Rapamycin Modulation

Seizures associated with mTORopathies are frequently resistant to traditional AEDs. mTOR inhibitors initially used as antitumor agents are crossing over as potential treatment of epilepsy-related mTORopathies.[240,241] The naturally occurring mTOR inhibitor rapamycin (sirolimus) has shown significant usefulness in reducing the size of SEGAs and other tumors in TSC.[242–247] Small clinical studies showed moderate success in reducing seizure frequency in patients with TSC[248–251]; however, because of its immunosuppressant effects and gastric toxicity, treatment must be closely monitored.[252] Rapamycin analogues, such as everolimus, were designed to increase solubility and bioavailabilty.[253] Everolimus (Afinitor) effectively reduces tumor volume in TSC[254] and decreases partial-onset seizures in patients with TSC more than 2 years old,[255–258] although adverse events are still a concern.[259,260] Clinical studies have tentatively established the safe use of everolimus in patients with TSC less than 2 years old,[261] which, coupled with earlier diagnosis, opens up the prospect of long-term disease-modifying effects.

Therapies Targeting Genetic Mechanisms

There are preclinical studies to support a focus on genetic mechanisms involved in the regulation of excitability.[262] Other groups have focused gene approaches on specific gene mutations underlying epilepsy syndromes using traditional gene therapy with viral vectors and CRISPR (clustered regularly interspaced short palindromic repeats) technology. Recent preclinical studies in human cell lines and a mouse model of DS have used antisense oligonucleotides to increase expression of productive *Scn1a* transcripts with promising results in DS mice.[263] Preclinical studies targeting specific gene defects underlying epilepsy such as these will serve as the foundation to translate to humans.

Other Therapeutics

When the epilepsy evaluation indicates focal seizure onset or for specific seizure types/syndromes, evaluation for surgical intervention is indicated. Surgical interventions include resection, laser interstitial thermal therapy, and implantation of neurostimulation devices. Dietary therapy with the ketogenic diet may be considered for genetic epilepsies depending on the underlying gene defect and epilepsy syndrome. One specific disorder responsive to ketogenic diet is GLUT1 deficiency syndrome. Similarly, additional therapies will be guided by the specific gene mutations, such as the PDE, as described earlier.

Additional Considerations

Several inherited ion channelopathies have been implicated in sudden unexpected death in epilepsy (SUDEP) through molecular diagnostics and case reports.[17,264–266] As expected, defects in the Na^+ and K^+ channels known to cause cardiac arrhythmias account for a significant portion of the identified genetic causes of SUDEP. Mutations in *SCN1A*, *SCN8A*, and *KCNQ2*, along with a mutation in mTOR signaling (*DEPDC5*), have been observed in human patients with SUDEP to date.[264] It is hoped that ongoing registries and increased awareness will shed light on additional genetic and acquired causes for SUDEP.

DISCUSSION

Genetic evaluation for patients with refractory epilepsy, particularly with associated cognitive and behavioral impairments, is critical for focusing therapeutics as well as counseling the family and patient. This article describes many of the known gene mutations identified thus far in epilepsy as well as disorders with epilepsy as a prominent feature of the phenotype. Efforts at describing, for example, IEM associated with epilepsy have focused specifically on patients with known early treatments to modify the course of the disease. Because of the impact of early intervention, some of these disorders are included in newborn screening panels.

Much progress has been made in the several decades since the first identified gene mutation in epilepsy. Gene discovery in epilepsy and neurologic disease in general have driven the emphasis toward using this information not just for anticipatory guidance/counseling and prognosis but, importantly, to guide therapy and to focus on innovative therapeutics with disease-modifying effects. With epilepsy gene discovery, precision medicine is possible focused on correction of a specific gene defect or downstream effects. Disorders such as GLUT1 deficiency syndrome with highest treatment efficacy using the ketogenic diet highlight precision medicine in epilepsy.[267]

SUMMARY

Epilepsy gene panels and next-generation sequencing combined with routine diagnostic evaluation in epilepsy have facilitated the recognition of many gene defects associated with epilepsy. Ultimately, gene discovery will facilitate precision medicine in epilepsy and serve as the foundation for disease modification.

CLINICS CARE POINTS

- Genetic testing should be considered in any child with unexplained epilepsy.
- Repeat analysis or new genetic testing should be considered in the child with medically refractory epilepsy where previous genetic testing has not been informative because of continuous discovery of new genetic epilepsies.
- The chronic use of sodium channel inhibitors should be avoided in individuals with SCN1A mutations.
- Ketogenic diet should be considered in individuals with GLUT1 mutations.
- In infants or young children with medically refractory epilepsy, a pyridoxine challenge should be considered to diagnose PDE.
- CSF amino acids should be measured in infants or young children with medically refractory epilepsy to measure glycine levels for NKH, which can respond to sodium benzoate or dextromethorphan therapy.
- mTOR modulation with rapalogs should be considered in individuals with TSC and potentially other epilepsy syndromes associated with mutations involving hyperactive mTOR signaling.
- Immune modulation can be efficacious in a subset of genetic epilepsies, such as IS and LKS, that are resistant to other antiepileptic medications.
- In genetic epilepsies associated with ion channel mutations, and particularly with DS, families should be counseled on increased risk for SUDEP.

ACKNOWLEDGMENTS

This work was supported by grant 2017063 from the Doris Duke Charitable Foundation and the Joan and Stanford Alexander Endowed Chair for Neuropsychiatric Research (J.L. Holder), Foundation for Angelman Syndrome Therapeutics, and NIH (NS104665 [A. Anderson], 5T32NS043124 [L.A. Martinez]).

DISCLOSURE

No disclosures.

REFERENCES

1. Berkovic SF, Mulley JC, Scheffer IF, et al. Human epilepsies: interaction of genetic and acquired factors. Trends Neurosci 2006;29(7):391–7.
2. Coppola G. Malignant migrating partial seizures in infancy: an epilepsy syndrome of unknown etiology. Epilepsia 2009;50(Suppl 5):49–51.
3. Burgess R, Wang S, McTague A, et al. The Genetic Landscape of Epilepsy of Infancy with Migrating Focal Seizures. Ann Neurol 2019;86(6):821–31.
4. Møller RS, Dahl HA, Helbig I. The contribution of next generation sequencing to epilepsy genetics. Expert Rev Mol Diagn 2015;15(12):1531–8.
5. Møller RS, Hammer TB, Rubboli G, et al. From next-generation sequencing to targeted treatment of non-acquired epilepsies. Expert Rev Mol Diagn 2019; 19(3):217–28.
6. Hoelz H, Herdl C, Gerstl L, et al. Impact on Clinical Decision Making of Next-Generation Sequencing in Pediatric Epilepsy in a Tertiary Epilepsy Referral Center. Clin EEG Neurosci 2020;51(1):61–9.

7. Lemke JR, Riesch E, Scheurenbrand T, et al. Targeted next generation sequencing as a diagnostic tool in epileptic disorders. Epilepsia 2012;53(8): 1387–98.

8. Lindy AS, Stosser MB, Butler E, et al. Diagnostic outcomes for genetic testing of 70 genes in 8565 patients with epilepsy and neurodevelopmental disorders. Epilepsia 2018;59(5):1062–71.

9. Parrini E, Marini C, Mei D, et al. Diagnostic targeted resequencing in 349 patients with drug-resistant pediatric epilepsies identifies causative mutations in 30 different genes. Hum Mutat 2017;38(2):216–25.

10. Catterall WA. Voltage-gated sodium channels at 60: structure, function and pathophysiology. J Physiol 2012;590(11):2577–89.

11. Namadurai S, Yereddi NR, Cusdin FS, et al. A new look at sodium channel β subunits. Open Biol 2015;5(1):140192.

12. O'Malley HA, Isom LL. Sodium channel β subunits: emerging targets in channelopathies. Annu Rev Physiol 2015;77:481–504.

13. Liao Y, Deprez L, Maljevic S, et al. Molecular correlates of age-dependent seizures in an inherited neonatal-infantile epilepsy. Brain 2010;133(Pt 5):1403–14.

14. Zaman T, Helbig I, Božović IB, et al. Mutations in SCN3A cause early infantile epileptic encephalopathy. Ann Neurol 2018;83(4):703–17.

15. Lamar T, Vanoye CG, Calhoun J, et al. SCN3A deficiency associated with increased seizure susceptibility. Neurobiol Dis 2017;102:38–48.

16. Estacion M, O'Brien JE, Conravey A, et al. A novel de novo mutation of SCN8A (Nav1.6) with enhanced channel activation in a child with epileptic encephalopathy. Neurobiol Dis 2014;69:117–23.

17. Veeramah KR, O'Brien JE, Meisler MH, et al. De novo pathogenic SCN8A mutation identified by whole-genome sequencing of a family quartet affected by infantile epileptic encephalopathy and SUDEP. Am J Hum Genet 2012;90(3): 502–10.

18. Wagnon JL, Barker BS, Hounshell JA, et al. Pathogenic mechanism of recurrent mutations of SCN8A in epileptic encephalopathy. Ann Clin Transl Neurol 2016; 3(2):114–23.

19. Singh NA, Pappas C, Dahle EJ, et al. A role of SCN9A in human epilepsies, as a cause of febrile seizures and as a potential modifier of Dravet syndrome. Plos Genet 2009;5(9):e1000649.

20. Aeby A, Sculier C, Bouza AA, et al. SCN1B-linked early infantile developmental and epileptic encephalopathy. Ann Clin Transl Neurol 2019;6(12):2354–67.

21. Scheffer IE, Harkin LA, Grinton BE, et al. Temporal lobe epilepsy and GEFS+ phenotypes associated with SCN1B mutations. Brain 2007;130(Pt 1):100–9.

22. Wallace RH, Scheffer IE, Parasivam G, et al. Generalized epilepsy with febrile seizures plus: mutation of the sodium channel subunit SCN1B. Neurology 2002;58(9):1426–9.

23. Wallace RH, Wang DW, Singh R, et al. Febrile seizures and generalized epilepsy associated with a mutation in the Na+-channel beta1 subunit gene SCN1B. Nat Genet 1998;19(4):366–70.

24. Audenaert D, Claes L, Ceulemans B, et al. A deletion in SCN1B is associated with febrile seizures and early-onset absence epilepsy. Neurology 2003;61(6): 854–6.

25. Patino GA, Brackenbury WJ, Bao Y, et al. Voltage-gated Na+ channel β1B: a secreted cell adhesion molecule involved in human epilepsy. J Neurosci 2011;31(41):14577–91.

26. Jan LY, Jan YN. Voltage-gated potassium channels and the diversity of electrical signalling. J Physiol 2012;590(11):2591–9.

27. Johnston J, Forsythe ID, Kopp-Scheinpflug C. Going native: voltage-gated potassium channels controlling neuronal excitability. J Physiol 2010;588(Pt 17): 3187–200.

28. Mitterdorfer J, Bean BP. Potassium currents during the action potential of hippocampal CA3 neurons. J Neurosci 2002;22(23):10106–15.

29. Kim DM, Nimigean CM. Voltage-gated potassium channels: a structural examination of selectivity and gating. Cold Spring Harb Perspect Biol 2016;8(5): a029231.

30. Kuang Q, Purhonen P, Hebert H. Structure of potassium channels. Cell Mol Life Sci 2015;72(19):3677–93.

31. Sun X, Zaydman MA, Cui J. Regulation of Voltage-Activated K(+) channel gating by transmembrane β subunits. Front Pharmacol 2012;3:63.

32. Corbett MA, Bellows ST, Li M, et al. Dominant KCNA2 mutation causes episodic ataxia and pharmacoresponsive epilepsy. Neurology 2016;87(19):1975–84.

33. Sachdev M, Gaínza-Lein M, Tchapyjnikov D, et al. Novel clinical manifestations in patients with KCNA2 mutations. Seizure 2017;51:74–6.

34. Syrbe S, Hedrich UBS, Riesch E, et al. De novo loss- or gain-of-function mutations in KCNA2 cause epileptic encephalopathy. Nat Genet 2015;47(4):393–9.

35. Masnada S, Hedrich UBS, Gardella E, et al. Clinical spectrum and genotype-phenotype associations of KCNA2-related encephalopathies. Brain 2017; 140(9):2337–54.

36. Marini C, Romoli M, Parrini E, et al. Clinical features and outcome of 6 new patients carrying de novo KCNB1 gene mutations. Neurol Genet 2017;3(6):e206.

37. Saitsu H, Akita T, Tohyama J, et al. De novo KCNB1 mutations in infantile epilepsy inhibit repetitive neuronal firing. Sci Rep 2015;5:15199.

38. Thiffault I, Speca DJ, Austin DC, et al. A novel epileptic encephalopathy mutation in KCNB1 disrupts Kv2.1 ion selectivity, expression, and localization. J Gen Physiol 2015;146(5):399–410.

39. Birnbaum SG, Varga AW, Yuan LL, et al. Structure and function of Kv4-family transient potassium channels. Physiol Rev 2004;84(3):803–33.

40. Serôdio P, Rudy B. Differential expression of Kv4 K+ channel subunits mediating subthreshold transient K+ (A-type) currents in rat brain. J Neurophysiol 1998;79(2):1081–91.

41. Singh B, Ogiwara I, Kaneda M, et al. A Kv4.2 truncation mutation in a patient with temporal lobe epilepsy. Neurobiol Dis 2006;24(2):245–53.

42. Lee H, Lin MC, Kornblum HI, et al. Exome sequencing identifies de novo gain of function missense mutation in KCND2 in identical twins with autism and seizures that slows potassium channel inactivation. Hum Mol Genet 2014;23(13):3481–9.

43. Goto A, Ishii A, Shibata M, et al. Characteristics of KCNQ2 variants causing either benign neonatal epilepsy or developmental and epileptic encephalopathy. Epilepsia 2019;60(9):1870–80.

44. Weckhuysen S, Mandelstam S, Suls A, et al. KCNQ2 encephalopathy: emerging phenotype of a neonatal epileptic encephalopathy. Ann Neurol 2012;71(1): 15–25.

45. Coppola G, Castaldo P, Miraglia del Giudice E, et al. A novel KCNQ2 K+ channel mutation in benign neonatal convulsions and centrotemporal spikes. Neurology 2003;61(1):131–4.

46. Singh NA, Westenskow P, Charlier C, et al. KCNQ2 and KCNQ3 potassium channel genes in benign familial neonatal convulsions: expansion of the functional and mutation spectrum. Brain 2003;126(Pt 12):2726–37.

47. Bassi MT, Balottin U, Panzeri C, et al. Functional analysis of novel KCNQ2 and KCNQ3 gene variants found in a large pedigree with benign familial neonatal convulsions (BFNC). Neurogenetics 2005;6(4):185–93.

48. Lehman A, Thouta S, Mancini GMS, et al. Loss-of-Function and Gain-of-Function Mutations in KCNQ5 Cause Intellectual Disability or Epileptic Encephalopathy. Am J Hum Genet 2017;101(1):65–74.

49. Fukai R, Saitsu H, Tsurusaki Y, et al. De novo KCNH1 mutations in four patients with syndromic developmental delay, hypotonia and seizures. J Hum Genet 2016;61(5):381–7.

50. Mastrangelo M, Scheffer IE, Bramswig NC, et al. Epilepsy in KCNH1-related syndromes. Epileptic Disord 2016;18(2):123–36.

51. Simons C, Rash LD, Crawford J, et al. Mutations in the voltage-gated potassium channel gene KCNH1 cause Temple-Baraitser syndrome and epilepsy. Nat Genet 2015;47(1):73–7.

52. von Wrede R, Jeub M, Ariöz I, et al. Novel KCNH1 Mutations Associated with Epilepsy: Broadening the Phenotypic Spectrum of KCNH1-Associated Diseases. Genes (Basel). 2021;12(2):132.

53. Veeramah KR, Johnstone L, Karafet TM, et al. Exome sequencing reveals new causal mutations in children with epileptic encephalopathies. Epilepsia 2013;54(7):1270–81.

54. Contet C, Goulding SP, Kuljis DA, et al. BK Channels in the Central Nervous System. Int Rev Neurobiol 2016;128:281–342.

55. Wang J, Yu S, Zhang Q, et al. KCNMA1 mutation in children with paroxysmal dyskinesia and epilepsy: Case report and literature review. Translational Sci Rare Dis 2017;2:165–73.

56. Yeşil G, Aralaşmak A, Akyüz E, et al. Expanding the phenotype of homozygous KCNMA1 mutations; dyskinesia, epilepsy, intellectual disability, cerebellar and corticospinal tract atrophy. Balkan Med J 2018;35(4):336–9.

57. Lim CX, Ricos MG, Dibbens LM, et al. KCNT1 mutations in seizure disorders: the phenotypic spectrum and functional effects. J Med Genet 2016;53(4):217–25.

58. Hibino H, Inanobe A, Furutani K, et al. Inwardly rectifying potassium channels: their structure, function, and physiological roles. Physiol Rev 2010;90(1):291–366.

59. Kinboshi M, Ikeda A, Ohno Y. Role of astrocytic inwardly rectifying potassium (Kir) 4.1 channels in epileptogenesis. Front Neurol 2020;11:626658.

60. Guo Y, Yan KP, Qu Q, et al. Common variants of KCNJ10 are associated with susceptibility and anti-epileptic drug resistance in Chinese genetic generalized epilepsies. PLoS One 2015;10(4):e0124896.

61. Mir A, Chaudhary M, Alkhaldi H, et al. Epilepsy in patients with EAST syndrome caused by mutation in the KCNJ10. Brain Dev 2019;41(8):706–15.

62. Zhang H, Zhu L, Wang F, et al. Novel KCNJ10 Compound Heterozygous Mutations Causing EAST/SeSAME-Like Syndrome Compromise Potassium Channel Function. Front Genet 2019;10:912.

63. Bertelli M, Cecchin S, Lapucci C, et al. Quantification of chloride channel 2 (CLCN2) gene isoforms in normal versus lesion- and epilepsy-associated brain tissue. Biochim Biophys Acta 2007;1772(1):15–20.

64. Chen TT, Klassen TL, Goldman AM, et al. Novel brain expression of ClC-1 chloride channels and enrichment of CLCN1 variants in epilepsy. Neurology 2013; 80(12):1078–85.
65. D'Agostino D, Bertelli M, Gallo S, et al. Mutations and polymorphisms of the CLCN2 gene in idiopathic epilepsy. Neurology 2004;63(8):1500–2.
66. Everett K, Chioza B, Aicardi J, et al. Linkage and mutational analysis of CLCN2 in childhood absence epilepsy. Epilepsy Res 2007;75(2–3):145–53.
67. Saint-Martin C, Gauvain G, Teodorescu G, et al. Two novel CLCN2 mutations accelerating chloride channel deactivation are associated with idiopathic generalized epilepsy. Hum Mutat 2009;30(3):397–405.
68. Stogmann E, Lichtner P, Baumgartner C, et al. Mutations in the CLCN2 gene are a rare cause of idiopathic generalized epilepsy syndromes. Neurogenetics 2006;7(4):265–8.
69. Fernández-Marmiesse A, Roca I, Díaz-Flores F, et al. Rare Variants in 48 Genes Account for 42% of Cases of Epilepsy With or Without Neurodevelopmental Delay in 246 Pediatric Patients. Front Neurosci 2019;13:1135.
70. Blaesse P, Airaksinen MS, Rivera C, et al. Cation-chloride cotransporters and neuronal function. Neuron 2009;61(6):820–38.
71. Saito T, Ishii A, Sugai K, et al. A de novo missense mutation in SLC12A5 found in a compound heterozygote patient with epilepsy of infancy with migrating focal seizures. Clin Genet 2017;92(6):654–8.
72. Saitsu H, Watanabe M, Akita T, et al. Impaired neuronal KCC2 function by biallelic SLC12A5 mutations in migrating focal seizures and severe developmental delay. Sci Rep 2016;6:30072.
73. Stödberg T, McTague A, Ruiz AJ, et al. Mutations in SLC12A5 in epilepsy of infancy with migrating focal seizures. Nat Commun 2015;6:8038.
74. Kahle KT, Merner ND, Friedel P, et al. Genetically encoded impairment of neuronal KCC2 cotransporter function in human idiopathic generalized epilepsy. EMBO Rep 2014;15(7):766–74.
75. Puskarjov M, Seja P, Heron SE, et al. A variant of KCC2 from patients with febrile seizures impairs neuronal Cl- extrusion and dendritic spine formation. EMBO Rep 2014;15(6):723–9.
76. Simms BA, Zamponi GW. Neuronal voltage-gated calcium channels: structure, function, and dysfunction. Neuron 2014;82(1):24–45.
77. Eckle VS, Shcheglovitov A, Vitko I, et al. Mechanisms by which a CACNA1H mutation in epilepsy patients increases seizure susceptibility. J Physiol 2014; 592(4):795–809.
78. Gudenkauf FJ, Azamian MS, Hunter JV, et al. A novel CACNA1A variant in a child with early stroke and intractable epilepsy. Mol Genet Genomic Med 2020;8(10):e1383.
79. Reinson K, Õiglane-Shlik E, Talvik I, et al. Biallelic CACNA1A mutations cause early onset epileptic encephalopathy with progressive cerebral, cerebellar, and optic nerve atrophy. Am J Med Genet A 2016;170(8):2173–6.
80. Imbrici P, Jaffe SL, Eunson LH, et al. Dysfunction of the brain calcium channel CaV2.1 in absence epilepsy and episodic ataxia. Brain 2004;127(Pt 12): 2682–92.
81. Ohmori I, Ouchida M, Kobayashi K, et al. CACNA1A variants may modify the epileptic phenotype of Dravet syndrome. Neurobiol Dis 2013;50:209–17.
82. Escayg A, De Waard M, Lee DD, et al. Coding and noncoding variation of the human calcium-channel beta4-subunit gene CACNB4 in patients with idiopathic generalized epilepsy and episodic ataxia. Am J Hum Genet 2000;66(5):1531–9.

83. Coste de Bagneaux P, von Elsner L, Bierhals T, et al. A homozygous missense variant in CACNB4 encoding the auxiliary calcium channel beta4 subunit causes a severe neurodevelopmental disorder and impairs channel and non-channel functions. Plos Genet 2020;16(3):e1008625.

84. Greenfield LJ Jr. Molecular mechanisms of antiseizure drug activity at GABAA receptors. Seizure 2013;22(8):589–600.

85. Sigel E, Steinmann ME. Structure, function, and modulation of GABA(A) receptors. J Biol Chem 2012;287(48):40224–31.

86. Macdonald RL, Kang JQ, Gallagher MJ. Mutations in GABAA receptor subunits associated with genetic epilepsies. J Physiol 2010;588(Pt 11):1861–9.

87. Bai YF, Chiu M, Chan ES, et al. Pathophysiology of and therapeutic options for a GABRA1 variant linked to epileptic encephalopathy. Mol Brain 2019;12(1):92.

88. Cossette P, Liu L, Brisebois K, et al. Mutation of GABRA1 in an autosomal dominant form of juvenile myoclonic epilepsy. Nat Genet 2002;31(2):184–9.

89. Kapoor A, Vijai J, Ravishankar HM, et al. Absence of GABRA1 Ala322Asp mutation in juvenile myoclonic epilepsy families from India. J Genet 2003;82(1–2): 17–21.

90. Lachance-Touchette P, Brown P, Meloche C, et al. Novel α1 and γ2 GABAA receptor subunit mutations in families with idiopathic generalized epilepsy. Eur J Neurosci 2011;34(2):237–49.

91. Papandreou A, McTague A, Trump N, et al. GABRB3 mutations: a new and emerging cause of early infantile epileptic encephalopathy. Dev Med Child Neurol 2016;58(4):416–20.

92. Tanaka M, Olsen RW, Medina MT, et al. Hyperglycosylation and reduced GABA currents of mutated GABRB3 polypeptide in remitting childhood absence epilepsy. Am J Hum Genet 2008;82(6):1249–61.

93. Zhang Y, Lian Y, Xie N. Early onset epileptic encephalopathy with a novel GABRB3 mutation treated effectively with clonazepam: A case report. Medicine (Baltimore) 2017;96(50):e9273.

94. Le SV, Le PHT, Le TKV, et al. A mutation in GABRB3 associated with Dravet syndrome. Am J Med Genet A 2017;173(8):2126–31.

95. Haerian BS, Baum L. GABRG2 rs211037 polymorphism and epilepsy: a systematic review and meta-analysis. Seizure 2013;22(1):53–8.

96. Pedersen M, Kowalczyk M, Omidvarnia A, et al. Human GABRG2 generalized epilepsy: Increased somatosensory and striatothalamic connectivity. Neurol Genet 2019;5(4):e340.

97. Shen D, Hernandez CC, Shen W, et al. De novo GABRG2 mutations associated with epileptic encephalopathies. Brain 2017;140(1):49–67.

98. Markus F, Angelini C, Trimouille A, et al. Rare variants in the GABA(A) receptor subunit ε identified in patients with a wide spectrum of epileptic phenotypes. Mol Genet Genomic Med 2020;8(9):e1388.

99. Albuquerque EX, Pereira EF, Alkondon M, et al. Mammalian nicotinic acetylcholine receptors: from structure to function. Physiol Rev 2009;89(1):73–120.

100. Dani JA, Bertrand D. Nicotinic acetylcholine receptors and nicotinic cholinergic mechanisms of the central nervous system. Annu Rev Pharmacol Toxicol 2007; 47:699–729.

101. Hogg RC, Raggenbass M, Bertrand D. Nicotinic acetylcholine receptors: from structure to brain function. Rev Physiol Biochem Pharmacol 2003;147:1–46.

102. Steinlein OK, Mulley JC, Propping P, et al. A missense mutation in the neuronal nicotinic acetylcholine receptor alpha 4 subunit is associated with autosomal dominant nocturnal frontal lobe epilepsy. Nat Genet 1995;11(2):201–3.

103. Cadieux-Dion M, Meneghini S, Villa C, et al. Variants in CHRNB2 and CHRNA4 Identified in Patients with Insular Epilepsy. Can J Neurol Sci 2020;47(6):800–9.

104. Chen Y, Wu L, Fang Y, et al. A novel mutation of the nicotinic acetylcholine receptor gene CHRNA4 in sporadic nocturnal frontal lobe epilepsy. Epilepsy Res 2009;83(2–3):152–6.

105. Langenbruch L, Biskup S, Young P, et al. Two mutations in the nicotinic acetylcholine receptor subunit A4 (CHRNA4) in a family with autosomal dominant sleep-related hypermotor epilepsy. Epileptic Disord 2020;22(1):116–9.

106. Rozycka A, Skorupska E, Kostyrko A, et al. Evidence for S284L mutation of the CHRNA4 in a white family with autosomal dominant nocturnal frontal lobe epilepsy. Epilepsia 2003;44(8):1113–7.

107. Steinlein OK, Magnusson A, Stoodt J, et al. An insertion mutation of the CHRNA4 gene in a family with autosomal dominant nocturnal frontal lobe epilepsy. Hum Mol Genet 1997;6(6):943–7.

108. Villa C, Colombo G, Meneghini S, et al. CHRNA2 and nocturnal frontal lobe epilepsy: identification and characterization of a novel loss of function mutation. Front Mol Neurosci 2019;12:17.

109. Gu W, Bertrand D, Steinlein OK. A major role of the nicotinic acetylcholine receptor gene CHRNA2 in autosomal dominant nocturnal frontal lobe epilepsy (ADNFLE) is unlikely. Neurosci Lett 2007;422(1):74–6.

110. Trivisano M, Terracciano A, Milano T, et al. Mutation of CHRNA2 in a family with benign familial infantile seizures: Potential role of nicotinic acetylcholine receptor in various phenotypes of epilepsy. Epilepsia 2015;56(5):e53–7.

111. Nakanishi S. Molecular diversity of glutamate receptors and implications for brain function. Science 1992;258(5082):597–603.

112. Ozawa S, Kamiya H, Tsuzuki K. Glutamate receptors in the mammalian central nervous system. Prog Neurobiol 1998;54(5):581–618.

113. McBain CJ, Mayer ML. N-methyl-D-aspartic acid receptor structure and function. Physiol Rev 1994;74(3):723–60.

114. Xu XX, Luo JH. Mutations of N-Methyl-D-Aspartate Receptor Subunits in Epilepsy. Neurosci Bull 2018;34(3):549–65.

115. Lemke JR, Geider K, Helbig KL, et al. Delineating the GRIN1 phenotypic spectrum: A distinct genetic NMDA receptor encephalopathy. Neurology 2016; 86(23):2171–8.

116. Chen W, Tankovic A, Burger PB, et al. Functional Evaluation of a De Novo GRIN2A mutation identified in a patient with profound global developmental delay and refractory epilepsy. Mol Pharmacol 2017;91(4):317–30.

117. Gao K, Tankovic A, Zhang Y, et al. A de novo loss-of-function GRIN2A mutation associated with childhood focal epilepsy and acquired epileptic aphasia. PLoS One 2017;12(2):e0170818.

118. Yuan H, Hansen KB, Zhang J, et al. Functional analysis of a de novo GRIN2A missense mutation associated with early-onset epileptic encephalopathy. Nat Commun 2014;5:3251.

119. Xu XX, Liu XR, Fan CY, et al. Functional Investigation of a GRIN2A Variant Associated with Rolandic Epilepsy. Neurosci Bull 2018;34(2):237–46.

120. Yang X, Qian P, Xu X, et al. GRIN2A mutations in epilepsy-aphasia spectrum disorders. Brain Dev 2018;40(3):205–10.

121. Lemke JR, Hendrickx R, Geider K, et al. GRIN2B mutations in West syndrome and intellectual disability with focal epilepsy. Ann Neurol 2014;75(1):147–54.

122. Smigiel R, Kostrzewa G, Kosinska J, et al. Further evidence for GRIN2B mutation as the cause of severe epileptic encephalopathy. Am J Med Genet A 2016;170(12):3265–70.

123. Mullier B, Wolff C, Sands ZA, et al. GRIN2B gain of function mutations are sensitive to radiprodil, a negative allosteric modulator of GluN2B-containing NMDA receptors. Neuropharmacology 2017;123:322–31.

124. Camp CR, Yuan H. GRIN2D/GluN2D NMDA receptor: Unique features and its contribution to pediatric developmental and epileptic encephalopathy. Eur J Paediatr Neurol 2020;24:89–99.

125. Jiao J, Li L, Sun M, et al. Identification of a novel GRIN2D variant in a neonate with intractable epileptic encephalopathy-a case report. BMC Pediatr 2021; 21(1):5.

126. Tsuchida N, Hamada K, Shiina M, et al. GRIN2D variants in three cases of developmental and epileptic encephalopathy. Clin Genet 2018;94(6):538–47.

127. XiangWei W, Kannan V, Xu Y, et al. Heterogeneous clinical and functional features of GRIN2D-related developmental and epileptic encephalopathy. Brain 2019;142(10):3009–27.

128. Chen HJ, Rojas-Soto M, Oguni A, et al. A synaptic Ras-GTPase activating protein (p135 SynGAP) inhibited by CaM kinase II. Neuron 1998;20(5):895–904.

129. Kim JH, Liao D, Lau LF, et al. SynGAP: a synaptic RasGAP that associates with the PSD-95/SAP90 protein family. Neuron 1998;20(4):683–91.

130. Hamdan FF, Gauthier J, Spiegelman D, et al. Mutations in SYNGAP1 in autosomal nonsyndromic mental retardation. N Engl J Med 2009;360(6):599–605.

131. Berryer MH, Hamdan FF, Klitten LL, et al. Mutations in SYNGAP1 cause intellectual disability, autism, and a specific form of epilepsy by inducing haploinsufficiency. Hum Mutat 2013;34(2):385–94.

132. Jimenez-Gomez A, Niu S, Andujar-Perez F, et al. Phenotypic characterization of individuals with SYNGAP1 pathogenic variants reveals a potential correlation between posterior dominant rhythm and developmental progression. J Neurodev Disord 2019;11(1):18.

133. Vlaskamp DRM, Shaw BJ, Burgess R, et al. SYNGAP1 encephalopathy: A distinctive generalized developmental and epileptic encephalopathy. Neurology 2019;92(2):e96–107.

134. von Stülpnagel C, Hartlieb T, Borggräfe I, et al. Chewing induced reflex seizures ("eating epilepsy") and eye closure sensitivity as a common feature in pediatric patients with SYNGAP1 mutations: Review of literature and report of 8 cases. Seizure 2019;65:131–7.

135. Saitsu H, Kato M, Mizuguchi T, et al. De novo mutations in the gene encoding STXBP1 (MUNC18-1) cause early infantile epileptic encephalopathy. Nat Genet 2008;40(6):782–8.

136. Abramov D, Guiberson NGL, Burré J. STXBP1 encephalopathies: Clinical spectrum, disease mechanisms, and therapeutic strategies. J Neurochem 2020; 157(2):165–78.

137. Easton JB, Houghton PJ. mTOR and cancer therapy. Oncogene 2006;25(48): 6436–46.

138. Guertin DA, Sabatini DM. An expanding role for mTOR in cancer. Trends Mol Med 2005;11(8):353–61.

139. Jansen LA, Mirzaa GM, Ishak GE, et al. PI3K/AKT pathway mutations cause a spectrum of brain malformations from megalencephaly to focal cortical dysplasia. Brain 2015;138(Pt 6):1613–28.

140. Mirzaa GM, Campbell CD, Solovieff N, et al. Association of MTOR mutations with developmental brain disorders, including megalencephaly, focal cortical dysplasia, and pigmentary mosaicism. JAMA Neurol 2016;73(7):836–45.

141. Curatolo P. Mechanistic target of rapamycin (mTOR) in tuberous sclerosis complex-associated epilepsy. Pediatr Neurol 2015;52(3):281–9.

142. Orlova KA, Crino PB. The tuberous sclerosis complex. Ann N Y Acad Sci 2010; 1184:87–105.

143. Jóźwiak S, Nabbout R, Curatolo P. Management of subependymal giant cell astrocytoma (SEGA) associated with tuberous sclerosis complex (TSC): Clinical recommendations. Eur J Paediatr Neurol 2013;17(4):348–52.

144. Katz JS, Frankel H, Ma T, et al. Unique findings of subependymal giant cell astrocytoma within cortical tubers in patients with tuberous sclerosis complex: a histopathological evaluation. Childs Nerv Syst 2017;33(4):601–7.

145. Roth J, Roach ES, Bartels U, et al. Subependymal giant cell astrocytoma: diagnosis, screening, and treatment. Recommendations from the International Tuberous Sclerosis Complex Consensus Conference 2012. Pediatr Neurol 2013; 49(6):439–44.

146. Chu-Shore CJ, Major P, Camposano S, et al. The natural history of epilepsy in tuberous sclerosis complex. Epilepsia 2010;51(7):1236–41.

147. Jansen FE, Huiskamp G, van Huffelen AC, et al. Identification of the epileptogenic tuber in patients with tuberous sclerosis: a comparison of high-resolution EEG and MEG. Epilepsia 2006;47(1):108–14.

148. Thiele EA. Managing epilepsy in tuberous sclerosis complex. J Child Neurol 2004;19(9):680–6.

149. Weiner HL, Carlson C, Ridgway EB, et al. Epilepsy surgery in young children with tuberous sclerosis: results of a novel approach. Pediatrics 2006;117(5): 1494–502.

150. Arya R, Tenney JR, Horn PS, et al. Long-term outcomes of resective epilepsy surgery after invasive presurgical evaluation in children with tuberous sclerosis complex and bilateral multiple lesions. J Neurosurg Pediatr 2015;15(1):26–33.

151. Liang S, Zhang J, Yang Z, et al. Long-term outcomes of epilepsy surgery in tuberous sclerosis complex. J Neurol 2017;264(6):1146–54.

152. Mühlebner A, van Scheppingen J, Hulshof HM, et al. Novel histopathological patterns in cortical tubers of epilepsy surgery patients with tuberous sclerosis complex. PLoS One 2016;11(6):e0157396.

153. Talos DM, Kwiatkowski DJ, Cordero K, et al. Cell-specific alterations of glutamate receptor expression in tuberous sclerosis complex cortical tubers. Ann Neurol 2008;63(4):454–65.

154. Lim JS, Kim WI, Kang HC, et al. Brain somatic mutations in MTOR cause focal cortical dysplasia type II leading to intractable epilepsy. Nat Med 2015;21(4): 395–400.

155. Marsan E, Baulac S. Review: Mechanistic target of rapamycin (mTOR) pathway, focal cortical dysplasia and epilepsy. Neuropathol Appl Neurobiol 2018; 44(1):6–17.

156. Sisodiya SM, Fauser S, Cross JH, et al. Focal cortical dysplasia type II: biological features and clinical perspectives. Lancet Neurol 2009;8(9):830–43.

157. Lin YX, Lin K, Kang DZ, et al. Similar PDK1-AKT-mTOR pathway activation in balloon cells and dysmorphic neurons of type II focal cortical dysplasia with refractory epilepsy. Epilepsy Res 2015;112:137–49.

158. Patil VV, Guzman M, Carter AN, et al. Activation of extracellular regulated kinase and mechanistic target of rapamycin pathway in focal cortical dysplasia. Neuropathology 2016;36(2):146–56.

159. Liu J, Reeves C, Michalak Z, et al. Evidence for mTOR pathway activation in a spectrum of epilepsy-associated pathologies. Acta Neuropathol Commun 2014; 2:71.

160. Zhao S, Li Z, Zhang M, et al. A brain somatic RHEB doublet mutation causes focal cortical dysplasia type II. Exp Mol Med 2019;51(7):1–11.

161. Baulac S, Ishida S, Marsan E, et al. Familial focal epilepsy with focal cortical dysplasia due to DEPDC5 mutations. Ann Neurol 2015;77(4):675–83.

162. Ribierre T, Deleuze C, Bacq A, et al. Second-hit mosaic mutation in mTORC1 repressor DEPDC5 causes focal cortical dysplasia-associated epilepsy. J Clin Invest 2018;128(6):2452–8.

163. Ricos MG, Hodgson BL, Pippucci T, et al. Mutations in the mammalian target of rapamycin pathway regulators NPRL2 and NPRL3 cause focal epilepsy. Ann Neurol 2016;79(1):120–31.

164. Pilarski R. PTEN hamartoma tumor syndrome: a clinical overview. Cancers (Basel) 2019;11(6):844.

165. Adachi T, Takigawa H, Nomura T, et al. Cowden syndrome with a novel PTEN mutation presenting with partial epilepsy related to focal cortical dysplasia. Intern Med 2018;57(1):97–9.

166. Child ND, Cascino GD. Mystery case: Cowden syndrome presenting with partial epilepsy related to focal cortical dysplasia. Neurology 2013;81(13):e98–9.

167. Elia M, Amato C, Bottitta M, et al. An atypical patient with Cowden syndrome and PTEN gene mutation presenting with cortical malformation and focal epilepsy. Brain Dev 2012;34(10):873–6.

168. Parker WE, Orlova KA, Parker WH, et al. Rapamycin prevents seizures after depletion of STRADA in a rare neurodevelopmental disorder. Sci Transl Med 2013;5(182):182ra153.

169. Alcantara D, Timms AE, Gripp K, et al. Mutations of AKT3 are associated with a wide spectrum of developmental disorders including extreme megalencephaly. Brain 2017;140(10):2610–22.

170. Nellist M, Schot R, Hoogeveen-Westerveld M, et al. Germline activating AKT3 mutation associated with megalencephaly, polymicrogyria, epilepsy and hypoglycemia. Mol Genet Metab 2015;114(3):467–73.

171. Yeung KS, Tso WWY, Ip JJK, et al. Identification of mutations in the PI3K-AKT-mTOR signalling pathway in patients with macrocephaly and developmental delay and/or autism. Mol Autism 2017;8:66.

172. Loconte DC, Grossi V, Bozzao C, et al. Molecular and Functional Characterization of Three Different Postzygotic Mutations in PIK3CA-Related Overgrowth Spectrum (PROS) Patients: Effects on PI3K/AKT/mTOR Signaling and Sensitivity to PIK3 Inhibitors. PLoS One 2015;10(4):e0123092.

173. Møller RS, Weckhuysen S, Chipaux M, et al. Germline and somatic mutations in the MTOR gene in focal cortical dysplasia and epilepsy. Neurol Genet 2016; 2(6):e118.

174. Mills PB, Struys E, Jakobs C, et al. Mutations in antiquitin in individuals with pyridoxine-dependent seizures. Nat Med 2006;12(3):307–9.

175. Cirillo M, Venkatesan C, Millichap JJ, et al. Case report: intravenous and oral pyridoxine trial for diagnosis of pyridoxine-dependent epilepsy. Pediatrics 2015;136(1):e257–61.

176. Cosnahan AS, Campbell CT. Inborn errors of metabolism in pediatric epilepsy. J Pediatr Pharmacol Ther 2019;24(5):398–405.
177. Rahman S, Footitt EJ, Varadkar S, et al. Inborn errors of metabolism causing epilepsy. Dev Med Child Neurol 2013;55(1):23–36.
178. Basura GJ, Hagland SP, Wiltse AM, et al. Clinical features and the management of pyridoxine-dependent and pyridoxine-responsive seizures: review of 63 North American cases submitted to a patient registry. Eur J Pediatr 2009; 168(6):697–704.
179. Rankin PM, Harrison S, Chong WK, et al. Pyridoxine-dependent seizures: a family phenotype that leads to severe cognitive deficits, regardless of treatment regime. Dev Med Child Neurol 2007;49(4):300–5.
180. Wolf B. Worldwide survey of neonatal screening for biotinidase deficiency. J Inherit Metab Dis 1991;14(6):923–7.
181. Gallagher RC, Van Hove JL, Scharer G, et al. Folinic acid-responsive seizures are identical to pyridoxine-dependent epilepsy. Ann Neurol 2009;65(5):550–6.
182. Agadi S, Quach MM, Haneef Z. Vitamin-responsive epileptic encephalopathies in children. Epilepsy Res Treat 2013;2013:510529.
183. Dulac O. Epileptic encephalopathy with suppression-bursts and nonketotic hyperglycinemia. Handb Clin Neurol 2013;113:1785–97.
184. Iqbal M, Prasad M, Mordekar SR. Nonketotic hyperglycinemia case series. J Pediatr Neurosci 2015;10(4):355–8.
185. Kure S, Kato K, Dinopoulos A, et al. Comprehensive mutation analysis of GLDC, AMT, and GCSH in nonketotic hyperglycinemia. Hum Mutat 2006;27(4):343–52.
186. Sharma S, Prasad AN. Inborn errors of metabolism and epilepsy: current understanding, diagnosis, and treatment approaches. Int J Mol Sci 2017;18(7):1384.
187. Campistol J, Plecko B. Treatable newborn and infant seizures due to inborn errors of metabolism. Epileptic Disord 2015;17(3):229–42.
188. Papetti L, Parisi P, Leuzzi V, et al. Metabolic epilepsy: an update. Brain Dev 2013;35(9):827–41.
189. Taanman JW. The mitochondrial genome: structure, transcription, translation and replication. Biochim Biophys Acta 1999;1410(2):103–23.
190. Kovac S, Domijan AM, Walker MC, et al. Prolonged seizure activity impairs mitochondrial bioenergetics and induces cell death. J Cell Sci 2012;125(Pt 7): 1796–806.
191. Puttachary S, Sharma S, Stark S, et al. Seizure-induced oxidative stress in temporal lobe epilepsy. Biomed Res Int 2015;2015:745613.
192. Yang N, Guan QW, Chen FH, et al. Antioxidants targeting mitochondrial oxidative stress: promising neuroprotectants for epilepsy. Oxid Med Cell Longev 2020;2020:6687185.
193. Lin TK, Chen SD, Lin KJ, et al. Seizure-induced oxidative stress in status epilepticus: is antioxidant beneficial? Antioxidants (Basel) 2020;9(11):1029.
194. Lim A, Thomas RH. The mitochondrial epilepsies. Eur J Paediatr Neurol 2020; 24:47–52.
195. Saneto RP. Epilepsy and mitochondrial dysfunction: a single center's experience. J Inborn Errors Metab Screen 2017;5. 2326409817733012.
196. Saneto RP, Cohen BH, Copeland WC, et al. Alpers-Huttenlocher syndrome. Pediatr Neurol 2013;48(3):167–78.
197. Velez-Bartolomei F, Lee C, Enns G. MERRF. In: Adam MP, Ardinger HH, Pagon RA, et al, editors. GeneReviews(®). Seattle (WA): University of Washington, Seattle Copyright © 1993-2020, University of Washington, Seattle; 1993. Available at: https://www.ncbi.nlm.nih.gov/books/NBK1520/. GeneReviews is a

registered trademark of the University of Washington, Seattle. All rights reserved.

198. Shoffner JM, Lott MT, Lezza AM, et al. Myoclonic epilepsy and ragged-red fiber disease (MERRF) is associated with a mitochondrial DNA tRNA(Lys) mutation. Cell 1990;61(6):931–7.

199. Schon EA, DiMauro S, Hirano M. Human mitochondrial DNA: roles of inherited and somatic mutations. Nat Rev Genet 2012;13(12):878–90.

200. Prasad C, Rupar T, Prasad AN. Pyruvate dehydrogenase deficiency and epilepsy. Brain Dev 2011;33(10):856–65.

201. Badhwar A, Berkovic SF, Dowling JP, et al. Action myoclonus-renal failure syndrome: characterization of a unique cerebro-renal disorder. Brain 2004;127(Pt 10):2173–82.

202. Zeigler M, Meiner V, Newman JP, et al. A novel SCARB2 mutation in progressive myoclonus epilepsy indicated by reduced β-glucocerebrosidase activity. J Neurol Sci 2014;339(1–2):210–3.

203. Dibbens LM, Michelucci R, Gambardella A, et al. SCARB2 mutations in progressive myoclonus epilepsy (PME) without renal failure. Ann Neurol 2009;66(4): 532–6.

204. Rubboli G, Franceschetti S, Berkovic SF, et al. Clinical and neurophysiologic features of progressive myoclonus epilepsy without renal failure caused by SCARB2 mutations. Epilepsia 2011;52(12):2356–63.

205. Tian WT, Liu XL, Xu YQ, et al. Progressive myoclonus epilepsy without renal failure in a Chinese family with a novel mutation in SCARB2 gene and literature review. Seizure 2018;57:80–6.

206. Fu YJ, Aida I, Tada M, et al. Progressive myoclonus epilepsy: extraneuronal brown pigment deposition and system neurodegeneration in the brains of Japanese patients with novel SCARB2 mutations. Neuropathol Appl Neurobiol 2014;40(5):551–63.

207. Kohlschütter A, Schulz A, Denecke J. Epilepsy in neuronal ceroid lipofuscinoses. J Pediatr Epilepsy 2014;3:199–206.

208. Nita DA, Mole SE, Minassian BA. Neuronal ceroid lipofuscinoses. Epileptic Disord 2016;18(S2):73–88.

209. Canafoglia L, Gilioli I, Invernizzi F, et al. Electroclinical spectrum of the neuronal ceroid lipofuscinoses associated with CLN6 mutations. Neurology 2015;85(4): 316–24.

210. Radke J, Stenzel W, Goebel HH. Human NCL Neuropathology. Biochim Biophys Acta 2015;1852(10 Pt B):2262–6.

211. Maurice P, Baud S, Bocharova OV, et al. New insights into molecular organization of human neuraminidase-1: transmembrane topology and dimerization ability. Sci Rep 2016;6:38363.

212. Franceschetti S, Canafoglia L. Sialidoses. Epileptic Disord 2016;18(S2):89–93.

213. Aravindhan A, Veerapandiyan A, Earley C, et al. Child Neurology: Type 1 sialidosis due to a novel mutation in NEU1 gene. Neurology 2018;90(13):622–4.

214. Mohammad AN, Bruno KA, Hines S, et al. Type 1 sialidosis presenting with ataxia, seizures and myoclonus with no visual involvement. Mol Genet Metab Rep 2018;15:11–4.

215. Koch J, Mayr JA, Alhaddad B, et al. CAD mutations and uridine-responsive epileptic encephalopathy. Brain 2017;140(2):279–86.

216. Koeleman BPC. What do genetic studies tell us about the heritable basis of common epilepsy? Polygenic or complex epilepsy? Neurosci Lett 2018; 667:10–6.

217. Ottman R. Analysis of genetically complex epilepsies. Epilepsia 2005;46(Suppl 10):7–14.
218. de Lange IM, Mulder F, van 't Slot R, et al. Modifier genes in SCN1A-related epilepsy syndromes. Mol Genet Genomic Med 2020;8(4):e1103.
219. Humphrey A, Higgins JN, Yates JR, et al. Monozygotic twins with tuberous sclerosis discordant for the severity of developmental deficits. Neurology 2004; 62(5):795–8.
220. Jentarra GM, Rice SG, Olfers S, et al. Evidence for population variation in TSC1 and TSC2 gene expression. BMC Med Genet 2011;12:29.
221. Martin N, Zügge K, Brandt R, et al. Discordant clinical manifestations in monozygotic twins with the identical mutation in the TSC2 gene. Clin Genet 2003; 63(5):427–30.
222. Wang F, Xiong S, Wu L, et al. A novel TSC2 missense variant associated with a variable phenotype of tuberous sclerosis complex: case report of a Chinese family. BMC Med Genet 2018;19(1):90.
223. Thodeson DM, Park JY. Genomic testing in pediatric epilepsy. Cold Spring Harb Mol Case Stud 2019;5(4):a004135.
224. Demos M, Guella I, DeGuzman C, et al. Diagnostic yield and treatment impact of targeted exome sequencing in early-onset epilepsy. Front Neurol 2019;10:434.
225. Tsang MH, Leung GK, Ho AC, et al. Exome sequencing identifies molecular diagnosis in children with drug-resistant epilepsy. Epilepsia Open 2019;4(1): 63–72.
226. Balciuniene J, DeChene ET, Akgumus G, et al. Use of a dynamic genetic testing approach for childhood-onset epilepsy. JAMA Netw Open 2019;2(4):e192129.
227. Butler KM, da Silva C, Alexander JJ, et al. Diagnostic Yield From 339 Epilepsy Patients Screened on a Clinical Gene Panel. Pediatr Neurol 2017;77:61–6.
228. Kothur K, Holman K, Farnsworth E, et al. Diagnostic yield of targeted massively parallel sequencing in children with epileptic encephalopathy. Seizure 2018;59: 132–40.
229. Zhang L, Gao J, Liu H, et al. Pathogenic variants identified by whole-exome sequencing in 43 patients with epilepsy. Hum Genomics 2020;14(1):44.
230. Absalom NL, Liao VWY, Kothur K, et al. Gain-of-function GABRB3 variants identified in vigabatrin-hypersensitive epileptic encephalopathies. Brain Commun 2020;2(2):fcaa162.
231. Wirrell EC, Nabbout R. Recent advances in the drug treatment of dravet syndrome. CNS Drugs 2019;33(9):867–81.
232. Tai C, Abe Y, Westenbroek RE, et al. Impaired excitability of somatostatin- and parvalbumin-expressing cortical interneurons in a mouse model of Dravet syndrome. Proc Natl Acad Sci U S A 2014;111(30):E3139–48.
233. Finsterer J, Zarrouk-Mahjoub S. Management of epilepsy in MERRF syndrome. Seizure 2017;50:166–70.
234. Klotz U. The role of pharmacogenetics in the metabolism of antiepileptic drugs: pharmacokinetic and therapeutic implications. Clin Pharmacokinet 2007;46(4): 271–9.
235. López-García MA, Feria-Romero IA, Serrano H, et al. Influence of genetic variants of CYP2D6, CYP2C9, CYP2C19 and CYP3A4 on antiepileptic drug metabolism in pediatric patients with refractory epilepsy. Pharmacol Rep 2017; 69(3):504–11.
236. Fainberg N, Harper A, Tchapyjnikov D, et al. Response to immunotherapy in a patient with Landau-Kleffner syndrome and GRIN2A mutation. Epileptic Disord 2016;18(1):97–100.

237. Devinsky O, Cross JH, Laux L, et al. Trial of cannabidiol for drug-resistant seizures in the dravet syndrome. N Engl J Med 2017;376(21):2011–20.

238. Perucca E. Cannabinoids in the treatment of epilepsy: hard evidence at last? J Epilepsy Res 2017;7(2):61–76.

239. Hess EJ, Moody KA, Geffrey AL, et al. Cannabidiol as a new treatment for drug-resistant epilepsy in tuberous sclerosis complex. Epilepsia 2016;57(10): 1617–24.

240. Griffith JL, Wong M. The mTOR pathway in treatment of epilepsy: a clinical update. Future Neurol 2018;13(2):49–58.

241. Wong M. A critical review of mTOR inhibitors and epilepsy: from basic science to clinical trials. Expert Rev Neurother 2013;13(6):657–69.

242. Birca A, Mercier C, Major P. Rapamycin as an alternative to surgical treatment of subependymal giant cell astrocytomas in a patient with tuberous sclerosis complex. J Neurosurg Pediatr 2010;6(4):381–4.

243. Davies DM, de Vries PJ, Johnson SR, et al. Sirolimus therapy for angiomyolipoma in tuberous sclerosis and sporadic lymphangioleiomyomatosis: a phase 2 trial. Clin Cancer Res 2011;17(12):4071–81.

244. Franz DN, Leonard J, Tudor C, et al. Rapamycin causes regression of astrocytomas in tuberous sclerosis complex. Ann Neurol 2006;59(3):490–8.

245. He W, Chen J, Wang YY, et al. Sirolimus improves seizure control in pediatric patients with tuberous sclerosis: A prospective cohort study. Seizure 2020; 79:20–6.

246. Lucchesi M, Chiappa E, Giordano F, et al. Sirolimus in infants with multiple cardiac rhabdomyomas associated with tuberous sclerosis complex. Case Rep Oncol 2018;11(2):425–30.

247. Peces R, Peces C, Cuesta-López E, et al. Low-dose rapamycin reduces kidney volume angiomyolipomas and prevents the loss of renal function in a patient with tuberous sclerosis complex. Nephrol Dial Transpl 2010;25(11):3787–91.

248. Canpolat M, Gumus H, Kumandas S, et al. The use of rapamycin in patients with tuberous sclerosis complex: Long-term results. Epilepsy Behav 2018;88: 357–64.

249. Canpolat M, Per H, Gumus H, et al. Rapamycin has a beneficial effect on controlling epilepsy in children with tuberous sclerosis complex: results of 7 children from a cohort of 86. Childs Nerv Syst 2014;30(2):227–40.

250. Cardamone M, Flanagan D, Mowat D, et al. Mammalian target of rapamycin inhibitors for intractable epilepsy and subependymal giant cell astrocytomas in tuberous sclerosis complex. J Pediatr 2014;164(5):1195–200.

251. Overwater IE, Bindels-de Heus K, Rietman AB, et al. Epilepsy in children with tuberous sclerosis complex: Chance of remission and response to antiepileptic drugs. Epilepsia 2015;56(8):1239–45.

252. Li M, Zhou Y, Chen C, et al. Efficacy and safety of mTOR inhibitors (rapamycin and its analogues) for tuberous sclerosis complex: a meta-analysis. Orphanet J Rare Dis 2019;14(1):39.

253. Yuan R, Kay A, Berg WJ, et al. Targeting tumorigenesis: development and use of mTOR inhibitors in cancer therapy. J Hematol Oncol 2009;2:45.

254. Franz DN, Belousova E, Sparagana S, et al. Long-term use of everolimus in patients with tuberous sclerosis complex: final results from the EXIST-1 study. PLoS One 2016;11(6):e0158476.

255. Franz DN, Lawson JA, Yapici Z, et al. Everolimus for treatment-refractory seizures in TSC: Extension of a randomized controlled trial. Neurol Clin Pract 2018;8(5):412–20.

256. French JA, Lawson JA, Yapici Z, et al. Adjunctive everolimus therapy for treatment-resistant focal-onset seizures associated with tuberous sclerosis (EXIST-3): a phase 3, randomised, double-blind, placebo-controlled study. Lancet 2016;388(10056):2153–63.

257. Krueger DA, Wilfong AA, Holland-Bouley K, et al. Everolimus treatment of refractory epilepsy in tuberous sclerosis complex. Ann Neurol 2013;74(5):679–87.

258. Samueli S, Abraham K, Dressler A, et al. Efficacy and safety of Everolimus in children with TSC - associated epilepsy - Pilot data from an open single-center prospective study. Orphanet J Rare Dis 2016;11(1):145.

259. Davies M, Saxena A, Kingswood JC. Management of everolimus-associated adverse events in patients with tuberous sclerosis complex: a practical guide. Orphanet J Rare Dis 2017;12(1):35.

260. Krueger DA, Capal JK, Curatolo P, et al. Short-term safety of mTOR inhibitors in infants and very young children with tuberous sclerosis complex (TSC): Multicentre clinical experience. Eur J Paediatr Neurol 2018;22(6):1066–73.

261. Saffari A, Brösse I, Wiemer-Kruel A, et al. Safety and efficacy of mTOR inhibitor treatment in patients with tuberous sclerosis complex under 2 years of age - a multicenter retrospective study. Orphanet J Rare Dis 2019;14(1):96.

262. Mesraoua B, Deleu D, Kullmann DM, et al. Novel therapies for epilepsy in the pipeline. Epilepsy Behav 2019;97:282–90.

263. Han Z, Chen C, Christiansen A, et al. Antisense oligonucleotides increase Scn1a expression and reduce seizures and SUDEP incidence in a mouse model of Dravet syndrome. Sci Transl Med 2020;12(558):eaaz6100.

264. Chahal CAA, Salloum MN, Alahdab F, et al. Systematic review of the genetics of sudden unexpected death in epilepsy: potential overlap with sudden cardiac death and arrhythmia-related genes. J Am Heart Assoc 2020;9(1):e012264.

265. Goldman AM, Behr ER, Semsarian C, et al. Sudden unexpected death in epilepsy genetics: Molecular diagnostics and prevention. Epilepsia 2016; 57(Suppl 1):17–25.

266. Shmuely S, Sisodiya SM, Gunning WB, et al. Mortality in dravet syndrome: a review. Epilepsy Behav 2016;64(Pt A):69–74.

267. Klepper J, Akman C, Armeno M, et al. Glut1 Deficiency Syndrome (Glut1DS): State of the art in 2020 and recommendations of the international Glut1DS study group. Epilepsia Open 2020;5(3):354–65.

Epilepsy
Epileptic Syndromes and Treatment

Akshat Katyayan, MD[a,b,]*, Gloria Diaz-Medina, MD[a,b]

KEYWORDS

- Epilepsy • Epilepsy syndrome • Infantile spasms • Lennox-Gastaut syndrome
- Childhood absence epilepsy • Juvenile myoclonic epilepsy
- Childhood epilepsy with centrotemporal spikes • Dravet syndrome

KEY POINTS

- An epilepsy syndrome is a specific set of seizure types and EEG and imaging features that tend to have age-dependent features, triggers, and often prognosis.
- Epilepsy syndromes may be classified based on age of presentation and outcomes.
- Characterization of epilepsy syndromes may help guide choice and duration of treatment and predict outcomes.
- Common pediatric epilepsy syndromes include West syndrome, Lennox-Gastaut syndrome, Dravet syndrome, Panayiotopoulos syndrome, childhood epilepsy with centrotemporal spikes, childhood absence epilepsy, juvenile myoclonic epilepsy.

BACKGROUND

Epilepsy has traditionally been defined as a disorder of the brain characterized by predisposition to have recurrent unprovoked seizures, widely accepted as 2 or more seizures at least 24 hours apart. In 2014, The International League Against Epilepsy (ILAE) proposed a practical definition of epilepsy[1] as a disease of the brain defined by any of the following conditions:

1. At least 2 unprovoked (or reflex) seizures occurring more than 24 hours apart.
2. One unprovoked (or reflex) seizure and a probability of further seizures similar to the general recurrence risk (at least 60%) after 2 unprovoked seizures, occurring over the next 10 years.
3. Diagnosis of an epilepsy syndrome.

In 2017, ILAE updated the classification of seizures and epilepsy with an emphasis on etiologic classification[2,3]; this represents a significant change from the last classification in 1989. There are 3 levels of diagnosis in the new classification:

---

[a] Department of Pediatrics, Baylor College of Medicine, Texas Children's Hospital, 6701, Fannin Street, Suite 1250, Houston, TX 77030, USA; [b] Department of Neurology, Baylor College of Medicine, Texas Children's Hospital, 6701, Fannin Street, Suite 1250, Houston, TX 77030, USA
* Corresponding author. 6701, Fannin Street, Suite 1250, Houston, TX 77030.
E-mail address: AKSHAT.KATYAYAN@BCM.EDU

Neurol Clin 39 (2021) 779–795
https://doi.org/10.1016/j.ncl.2021.04.002
0733-8619/21/© 2021 Elsevier Inc. All rights reserved.

1. Seizure type: focal onset, generalized onset, unknown onset (**Fig. 1**)
2. Epilepsy type: focal, generalized, combined focal and generalized, unknown (**Fig. 2**)
3. Epilepsy syndrome

ILAE recommends an attempt to determine the cause of patient's epilepsy at all 3 levels of diagnosis.

There are 6 etiologic groups identified: structural, genetic, infectious, metabolic, immune, and unknown. It is possible to have more than one cause in a patient.

CONCEPT OF EPILEPSY SYNDROME

An epilepsy syndrome is the third and final level of epilepsy diagnosis. An epilepsy syndrome is a specific set of seizure types and elecroencephalographic (EEG) and imaging features that tend to have age-dependent features, triggers, and often prognosis.[3]

NEED FOR A SYNDROMIC DIAGNOSIS (WHEN POSSIBLE)

1. Initiation of antiseizure medications (ASMs) and choice of ASM: Many age-dependent epilepsy syndromes have specific treatment implications. For example, many cases of benign epilepsy with centrotemporal spikes (BECTS) may not need treatment with ASMs. Childhood absence epilepsy (CAE) is typically treated with ethosuximide or valproic acid. Sodium channel blockers are contraindicated in Dravet syndrome (DS).

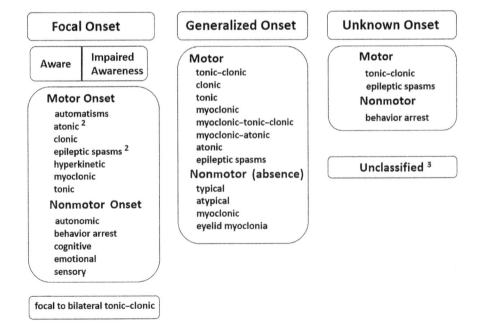

Fig. 1. ILAE classification of seizures (1).1- Definitions, other seizure types and descriptors are listed in the accompanying ILAE paper (2). 2- Degree of awareness usually is not specified. 3- Due to inadequate information or inability to place in other categories.

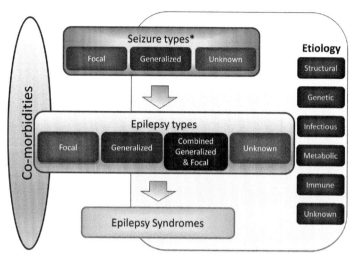

Fig. 2. ILAE classification of epilepsies.*Denotes onset of seizure.

2. Duration of treatment: Some epilepsy syndromes have age-dependent resolution, and hence its identification can guide duration of treatment. Most cases of CAE achieve seizure resolution by adolescence. Patients with juvenile myoclonic epilepsy (JME) typically need treatment for a long duration, many times lifelong.
3. Prognosis: Identification of an epilepsy syndrome may have prognostic implications. The outcomes of BECTS and PS are generally considered favorable, although neuropsychological comorbidities have been increasingly identified in typical patients. The outcomes for West syndrome and Lennox-Gastaut syndrome (LGS) are generally poor, with most patients experiencing developmental delay and refractory epilepsy.

CLASSIFICATION OF EPILEPSY SYNDROMES

There is no formal classification for epilepsy syndromes by ILAE. However, informal methods of classification have been suggested, mainly by age.

1. By age: ILAE educational Web site www.epilepsydiagnosis.org classifies epilepsy syndromes based on age[4] (**Table 1**)
2. By outcomes:
   - Self-limited, previously called benign, typically refers to epilepsy syndromes that often show spontaneous resolution. The term pharmacoresponsive is used for epilepsy syndromes that are well controlled on appropriately chosen ASMs. Examples include BECTS, CAE, and PS. The term benign is not recommended anymore given the concomitant cognitive abnormalities associated with these syndromes
   - Pharmacoresistant, previously called catastrophic or malignant. The term pharmacoresistant is not officially recognized by ILAE, but it is a logical opposite to the term pharmacoresponsive. These epilepsy syndromes typically do not show spontaneous resolution and often meet criteria for refractory epilepsy, with many associated with poor developmental outcomes (epileptic and developmental encephalopathy). Examples include West syndrome and LGS.

Table 1
Epilepsy syndrome classification based on age

Neonatal/Infantile Onset	Childhood Onset	Adolescent/Adult Onset	Any Age
Self-limited neonatal seizures and self-limited familial neonatal epilepsy	Epilepsy with myoclonic atonic seizures	Juvenile absence epilepsy	Familial focal epilepsy with variable foci
Self-limited familial and nonfamilial infantile epilepsy	Epilepsy with eyelid myoclonia	Juvenile myoclonic epilepsy	Reflex epilepsies
Early myoclonic encephalopathy	Lennox-Gastaut syndrome	Epilepsy with generalized tonic-clonic seizures alone	Progressive myoclonic epilepsies
Ohtahara syndrome	Childhood absence epilepsy	Autosomal dominant epilepsy with auditory features	
West syndrome	Epilepsy with myoclonic absences	Other familial temporal lobe epilepsies	
Dravet syndrome	Panayiotopoulos syndrome		
Myoclonic epilepsy in infancy	Childhood occipital epilepsy		
Epilepsy of infancy with migrating focal seizures	Photosensitive occipital lobe epilepsy		
Myoclonic encephalopathy in nonprogressive disorders	Childhood epilepsy with centrotemporal spikes		
Febrile seizures plus, genetic epilepsy with febrile seizures plus	Atypical childhood epilepsy with centrotemporal spikes		
	Epileptic encephalopathy with continuous spike and wave during sleep		
	Landau-Kleffner syndrome		
	Autosomal dominant nocturnal frontal lobe epilepsy		

KEY FEATURES OF EPILEPSY SYNDROMES COMMONLY SEEN IN GENERAL NEUROLOGY PRACTICE

In the following sections, we describe salient features of common pediatric epilepsy syndromes. Description of all epilepsy syndromes is beyond the scope of this article.

WEST SYNDROME

Introduction: West syndrome is described as a triad of epileptic spasms (ES), hypsarrhythmia on EEG, and psychomotor regression. The term ES is now interchangeably used with infantile spasms because whereas more than 85% of patients have onset in infancy, some have onsets after infancy. It is rare to have onset of ES beyond 2 years of age. West syndrome is not rare, and the incidence is 2 to 4 per 1000 live births.[5]

Clinical features: The main seizure type in West syndrome is ES. These seizures are clinically seen as brief, flexor, extensor, or mixed axial jerks typically occurring in clusters on awakening from sleep. The child may cry typically after the spasm but occasionally before. In early and/or treated cases, ES can be subtle and can just consist of a head nod or eye roll.

EEG features: The interictal EEG feature of West syndrome in most patients is hypsarrhythmia. There is no consensus definition for hypsarrhythmia, but cardinal features agreed upon by most neurophysiologists include a high-voltage background slowing (typically >200 μV), frequent or abundant multifocal spikes, and disorganization of the background (**Fig. 3**). The last parameter is highly subjective and leads to poor inter-rater reliability in diagnosis.[6] The ictal patterns with ES can be variable but classically seen as a slow wave of medium to high amplitude followed by diffuse flattening; an electrodecrement, considered the most important feature; and fast activity (**Fig. 4**). The "x" denotes when the mother reported the spasm.

An initial 24-hour study capturing extended sleep is recommended in most patients suspected of having ES to capture ictal events and to look at extended sleep samples, as hypsarrhythmia may only be present in certain sleep segments.[5]

Diagnosis: The diagnostic approach to a patient with West syndrome starts with understanding the different etiologies. Broadly, patients can be subdivided into

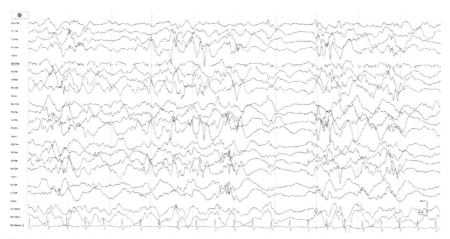

Fig. 3. Hypsarrhythmia EEG showing high-voltage, disorganized background with multifocal spikes.

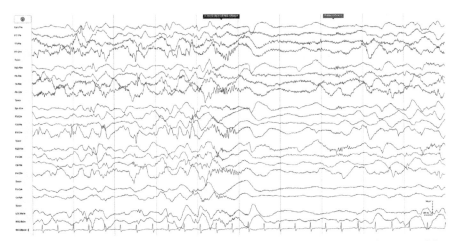

Fig. 4. Epileptic spasm ictal EEG with high-voltage slow wave, followed by flattening (electrodecrement). The "x" denotes when the mother reported the spasm.

symptomatic (with known etiology, 60%–70% of cases) or cryptogenic (without known etiology, 10%–40% of cases). In the symptomatic group, structural central nervous system abnormalities are the most common followed by genetic and metabolic.

After a thorough history and physical examination, an MRI of the brain is the highest yield study, followed by a genetic workup usually in the form of an epilepsy genetic panel with a chromosomal microarray. Depending on the clinical suspicion and outcome of initial workup, other studies, including spinal tap, metabolic studies, and further genetic work can be considered.

Management: Treatment of ES falls under 2 broad categories: hormonal (injectable or oral steroids) and vigabatrin. Vigabatrin is the preferred treatment in patients with tuberous sclerosis complex. For most other patients, hormonal therapy is the preferred initial method, especially in cryptogenic patients, in whom the outcomes have been shown to be better with hormonal treatment.[7] It should be noted that short-term outcomes (cessation of spasms at 2–6 weeks) is better with hormonal treatment[8] but long-term outcomes (at 2 years of age) are the same.[7]

For reference, the protocol used at Texas Children's Hospital is attached (**Fig. 5**A). A follow-up EEG (preferably an overnight study) is recommended at 2 weeks to assess response. Response is graded as an all-or-none phenomenon, with complete cessation of ES and resolution of hypsarrhythmia.[5]

Although adrenocorticotropic hormone has been the preferred hormonal treatment, studies have now shown comparable efficacy of high-dose oral steroids in treatment of ES[9]; this has been added as an option to our treatment protocol (**Fig. 5**B).

More recently, data have suggested combination therapy (hormonal treatment with vigabatrin) to be superior, at least to short-term to individual therapy alone, albeit with more risks for side effects.[10]

Early epilepsy surgery may be curative in patients who are good surgical candidates. Standard ASMs are generally not effective, although ketogenic diet may be of more benefit.

Prognosis: The prognosis of West syndrome is guarded and depends on the underlying cause. A significant majority (80% or more) of patients with West syndrome will have intellectual disability[5] and even more will have active epilepsy, although ES usually cease by 3 to 5 years and many evolve into LGS.

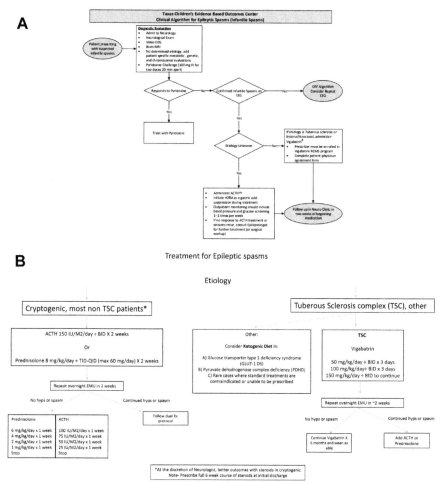

Fig. 5. (*A*) Clinical algorithm for epileptic spasms at Texas Children's Hospital. (*B*) Treatment algorithm for epileptic spasms at Texas Children's Hospital.[a] Dose per table 5b, [b] can also consider prednisolone.

LENNOX-GASTAUT SYNDROME

Introduction: LGS is also classified as an epileptic and developmental encephalopathy. The classic triad of LGS is multiple seizure types, including tonic, atonic, myoclonic, atypical absence seizures; interictal findings of slow spike wave complexes; and associated intellectual disability. Age of onset is typically between 3 and 5 years, and many cases evolve from a prior diagnosis of West syndrome.

Clinical features: Tonic seizures are the most common and characteristic seizure type of LGS. These seizures are seen as sustained axial or appendicular muscle contractions that may last for a few seconds to a few minutes. These seizures are often subtle and frequent in sleep. Atonic seizures (drop attacks) can be seen in up to 50% of patients. Atypical absence seizures, usually seen as alteration of awareness that has a gradual onset and termination (thereby distinguishing from typical absence seizures), are also frequent and may result in nonconvulsive status epilepticus (NCSE).[11] Myoclonic seizures, generalized tonic-clonic seizures (GTCSs), and focal seizures are also seen.

EEG features: The hallmark interictal finding in LGS are slow spike wave complexes, seen typically as bilaterally synchronous 1- to 2-Hz diffuse spike wave complexes, often occurring in prolonged runs and may be associated with atypical absence seizures and NCSE (**Fig. 6**). Bursts of paroxysmal fast rhythms in the 10 to 20 Hz range (typically generalized, hence called generalized paroxysmal fast activity) are seen in sleep and are also the ictal signature of tonic seizures (**Fig. 7**). The notation indicates that the eyes are open wide and deviated. Most experts believe the presence of paroxysmal fast activity during sleep, which may or may not be associated with tonic seizures, to be present to establish a diagnosis of LGS.

Diagnosis: Diagnosis typically requires overnight video-EEG monitoring to characterize ictal and interictal patterns. MRI of the brain and genetic testing will result in diagnostic yield in most patients.

Management: A 2013 Cochrane review for treatment of LGS concluded that the optimal treatment of LGS is uncertain and no study to date has shown any one drug to be highly efficacious; lamotrigine, rufinamide, topiramate, and felbamate may be helpful as add-on therapy.[12] Expert opinions identify valproic acid as one of the most commonly used agent for LGS, although it is not specifically licensed for its use. Clobazam is considered highly effective for atonic seizures. Felbamate is considered to be one of the most effective medications for treatment of seizures in LGS, but use is reserved for refractory patients owing to increased risk for aplastic anemia and liver failure.[13] More recently, cannabidiol has been approved for the treatment of seizures in LGS and is an increasingly popular choice. Ketogenic diet remains an effective nonpharmacologic option. Vagus nerve stimulator and corpus callosotomy (for atonic seizures) are effective surgical options in refractory cases. Focal resective surgery, especially in the presence of a single or unilateral lesion, should be considered, at times on a palliative basis, even if no convincing lateralizing ictal or interictal features are found.[14]

Prognosis: Most patients with LGS continue to have refractory seizures and intellectual disability into adulthood, although many evolve from a generalized to a focal epilepsy syndrome.

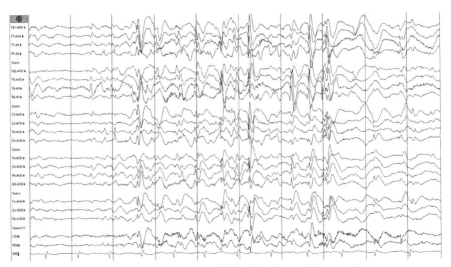

Fig. 6. Lennox-Gastaut syndrome, interictal EEG with "slow spike-wave".

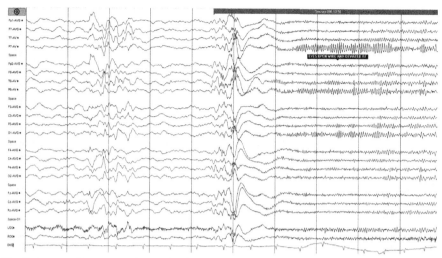

Fig. 7. Lennox-Gastaut syndrome, ictal EEG, with electrodecrement and fast activity. Notation of eyes open wide and deviated to right.

DRAVET SYNDROME

Introduction: DS (previously known as severe myoclonic epilepsy of infancy) is an early-onset medically intractable epilepsy syndrome that typically presents during the first year of life and causes an epileptic encephalopathy. The incidence of DS is estimated at 1 per 22,000 to 40,000, and it affects males twice as often as females.[15] The clinical diagnosis is supported by the presence of abnormalities in the sodium channel gene SCN1A (found in 70%–80% of cases).[16]

Clinical features: This syndrome is characterized by onset of seizures typically around 6 months of age. The seizure type consists of prolonged, febrile, and afebrile hemiclonic or generalized clonic seizures in a previously healthy child, often resulting in status epilepticus. Seizures are often provoked by fever or immunizations. Over the subsequent months, affected individuals experience recurrent febrile and afebrile seizures that often affect alternate sides of the body. Between 1 and 4 years of age, other seizure types develop, including myoclonic and atypical absences, focal seizures, and GTCS. In some individuals, myoclonic seizures do not develop and other seizure types, particularly focal or multifocal seizures, are the predominant seizure types.

Seizures tend to become less frequent and less severe in adolescence and adulthood. The most common seizure type in adulthood is generalized tonic-clonic, which may be focal in onset and occurs mainly during sleep.[17]

Head size and neurologic examination are usually normal initially; over time ataxia (60%), pyramidal signs (20%), uncoordinated movements, and interictal myoclonus may develop.[18] Neurodevelopment is typically normal in the first year of life followed by decline later on.

EEG features: EEG is typically normal during the first year of life. Subsequently, the EEG background may be slow. Generalized spike and polyspike wave and multifocal spikes usually develop by the second to fifth years of life. A photoparoxysmal response may be seen.

Diagnosis: DS is a clinical diagnosis that should be suspected in an infant younger than 1 year with repeated and prolonged febrile and afebrile seizures.[18] The presence of SCN1A mutation provides a strong argument, as well as other genetic abnormalities (PCDH19, GABRG2, SCN1B, and SCN2A) that may cause a similar phenotype as DS.

Neuroimaging is usually normal at onset.

Management: Goal of treatment is to significantly reduce seizure frequency, particularly of prolonged seizures, because a greater degree of cognitive and behavioral impairment has been linked to a higher frequency of both convulsive and nonconvulsive seizures.

With regard to emergency rescue, a benzodiazepine would be first line for home including intranasal midazolam or intranasal or rectal diazepam. In patients with DS, it is reasonable to indicate use of emergency medication immediately rather than wait a customary period of time. Subsequent second-line medication may depend on previous response of an individual to such medication, as well as local protocols.

For chronic treatment, first-line ASMs are valproic acid and clobazam. However, most children will require addition of a second-line agent. At present, most epileptologists consider stiripentol, topiramate, or the ketogenic diet as the best second-line options for patients who continue to experience poor seizure control despite valproic acid and clobazam.[19] Cannabidiol and fenfluramine are recently approved and are being increasingly used as second-line agents.[6] Third-line agents include addition of an antiepileptic drug, such as clonazepam, levetiracetam, zonisamide, ethosuximide (for atypical absence seizures), and phenobarbital, or consideration of vagus nerve stimulator.[20] Sodium channel blockers such as lamotrigine, carbamazepine, oxcarbazepine, and phenytoin may worsen seizures.

Prognosis: Children with DS have high mortality, and death may be due to status epilepticus, sudden unexpected death in epilepsy (up to approximately 15-fold higher than in those with other childhood epilepsies), or accidental death, and it may also be related to seizures associated with drowning or injury.[15] Most patients with DS will have moderate to severe delay into adulthood.

PANAYIOTOPOULOS SYNDROME

Introduction: Panayiotopoulos syndrome (PS) is an early childhood epilepsy with focal autonomic seizures that are often prolonged with EEG that shows shifting and/or multiple foci, often with occipital predominance.[21,22] Onset is between 3 and 6 years of age.[23] The prevalence of PS is 13% among early-onset epilepsies and 6% in children between 1 and 15 years.[23]

Clinical features: Autonomic seizures and autonomic status epilepticus are hallmark of the disease, in a normally developing child. These usually present with a full triad of nausea, retching, and vomiting that occurs in 80% of patients.[24] Other autonomic features include pupillary (especially mydriasis), circulatory (pallor, cyanosis), thermoregulatory, and cardiorespiratory changes. Most seizures start in sleep. Seizures are often prolonged (minutes to hours), constituting NCSE (lasting more than 30 minutes). However, the child recovers without residual neurologic or cognitive deficit. As the seizure evolves, other more conventional epilepsy manifestations appear, such as loss of responsiveness and head and eye deviation, and hemiclonic activity may develop.

Seizures are infrequent in most patients, with 25% having a single seizure and 50% having 6 seizures or less. Seizures usually resolve by age 11 to 13 years.

EEG features: The background EEG is normal. The interictal EEG is characterized by sleep-potentiated multifocal high-voltage, repetitive spikes and sharp waves in 90% of patients, with occipital spikes seen in 60% of patients (**Fig. 8**).

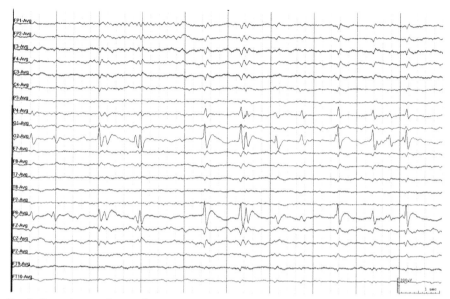

Fig. 8. Panayiotopoulos syndrome EEG with high-amplitude, occipital spikes.

Diagnosis: PS is a clinical diagnosis, supported by EEG findings. Neuroimaging is typically normal.

Management: Prophylactic treatment with ASM may not be needed for most patients because of infrequent seizures. Most neurologists treat recurrent seizures with ASMs such as carbamazepine, oxcarbazepine or levetiracetam.

Prognosis: PS has a good prognosis. Remission often occurs within 1 to 2 years of onset.

CHILDHOOD EPILEPSY WITH CENTROTEMPORAL SPIKES

Introduction: Childhood epilepsy with centrotemporal spikes, also referred to as BECTS or Rolandic epilepsy is the most common childhood epilepsy syndrome accounting for 15% to 20% of all epilepsies in children. Mean age of onset is between 6 and 9 years.

Clinical features: Presentation is with nocturnal focal aware seizures corresponding to the origin in the Rolandic (centrotemporal) cortex, manifesting as hemifacial sensorimotor seizures with associated gurgling and hypersalivation and speech arrest. Focal to bilateral tonic-clonic seizures may occur in up to 50% of patients.[25] The term benign is not preferred now because of association with cognitive dysfunction in most patients, including attention and memory impairment and learning difficulties,[26] and is not necessarily related to seizure control.

Atypical evolutions may be seen in a significant minority of patients (9%–50%, depending on the criteria used). These evolutions may vary from status epilepticus, Landau-Kleffner syndrome, electrical status epilepticus in sleep (ESES), epileptic encephalopathy with continuous spike and wave during sleep, and atypical benign childhood focal epilepsy.[27] The classic atypical variant was first described in 1982[28] and evolves from a typical focal epilepsy presentation into a generalized epilepsy syndrome, with atypical absence and atonic and negative myoclonic seizures.

EEG features: The classic interictal epileptiform abnormality is a biphasic discharge characterized by a prominent, negative sharp wave with a relatively rounded peak, at times preceded by a short-duration positive prespike and followed by a prominent positive sharp wave (amplitude up to 50% of the preceding negative sharp wave).[29] The later negative slow wave is often subtle and lower in amplitude than the preceding negative sharp wave. Location is in the centrotemporal region with a positivity in the frontal region, commonly referred to as a tangential dipole. Discharges can be unilateral or bilateral, independent or bilateral synchronous, and sleep potentiated as a rule (**Fig. 9**).

Diagnosis: A careful history and classic EEG findings are sufficient for diagnosis in most patients. Neuroimaging is generally not indicated, unless there are atypical features on history and examination or on EEG, such as focal slowing.

Management: Many patients do not need ASMs, which are indicated if seizures are frequent or have multiple convulsive seizures. Carbamazepine, levetiracetam, and oxcarbazepine are the most commonly used ASMs. However, in patients with atypical evolution, carbamazepine and phenobarbital may precipitate ESES and/or generalized seizures[30] and hence broad-spectrum ASMs such as valproic acid and benzodiazepines are preferred.

Prognosis: This is considered a self-limited epilepsy with most patients experiencing remission within 2 to 4 years of onset, almost always after puberty.

CHILDHOOD ABSENCE EPILEPSY

Introduction: CAE is the second most common pediatric epilepsy syndrome after BECTS. CAE is an idiopathic/genetic generalized epilepsy syndrome characterized mainly by typical absence seizures. Age of onset is between 4 and 10 years, and children usually have normal development. However, cognitive abnormalities are commonly found in these patients.

Clinical features: The prototypical seizure in CAE is a typical absence seizure, characterized by a brief (usually 5–10 seconds), sudden impairment of awareness, often

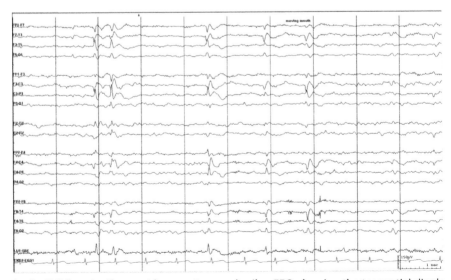

Fig. 9. Childhood epilepsy with centrotemporal spikes EEG, showing the tangential dipole.

noticed by caregivers as a staring episode from which the child is not distractible. Oral automatisms and eye movements are common. Seizures happen multiple times a day. Seizures can be easily provoked by hyperventilation, leading to a provisional diagnosis in many patients at the office visit.

Presence of other seizure types during the active stages of absence seizures is considered exclusionary for CAE. However, a significant minority (12%) of patients with CAE may develop generalized tonic-clonic seizures later during the course,[31] often after remission from absence seizures. Diagnostic criteria for CAE have been proposed by Panayiotopoulos[23] and are widely accepted.

Children with CAE commonly have significant attention issues,[32] anxiety, behavioral dyscontrol, and cognitive, emotional, and language problems. These deficits can persist despite adequate seizure control by ASMs.

EEG features: Classic ictal EEG findings with absence seizures are 3-Hz generalized spike waves, although they may vary in frequency from 2.5 to 3.5 Hz (usually faster at onset and slower at termination) (**Fig. 10**). The figure indicates that the eyelids are fluttering. Interictal background is normal, and occipital intermittent rhythmic delta activity may be seen (**Fig. 11**). NCS refers to no clinical signs.

Diagnosis: History and EEG are usually sufficient for diagnosis. Neuroimaging is not needed in typical cases. Testing for glucose transporter-1 (GLUT-1) should be considered in early-onset absence seizures, even in the absence of other typical clinical features of GLUT-1.

Management: The drug of choice for CAE is ethosuximide followed by valproic acid and lamotrigine.[33] Ethosuximide and valproic acid have comparable efficacy, but ethosuximide has a better side effect profile and a lower risk for attention issues. Other medications such as levetiracitam, topiramate, acetazolamide have been studied but are generally considered less effective. Ketogenic diet therapies have good efficacy

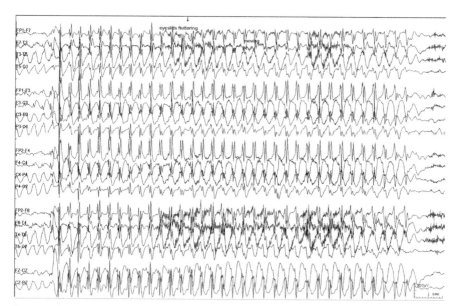

Fig. 10. Childhood absence epilepsy ictal EEG showing 3-Hz spike-and-wave seizure, with notation of eyelids fluttering.

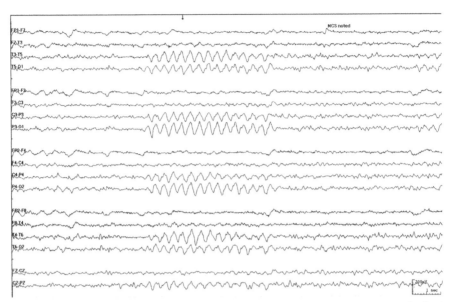

Fig. 11. Childhood absence epilepsy interictal EEG showing occipital intermittent rhythmic delta activity. The notation NCS refers to no clinical signs.

and should be considered in refractory cases after combination therapy with first-line agents has failed.

Prognosis: Seizure remission often occurs by puberty, but some patients may develop GTCS in adolescence. Behavioral problems may persist despite remission of absence seizures.

JUVENILE MYOCLONIC EPILEPSY

Introduction: JME is one of the most common genetic/idiopathic generalized epilepsies (IGEs).[3] JME is characterized by myoclonic seizures (97% of patients), GTCSs (58%), absence seizures (9%), or all 3 seizure types (21%).[34] Onset is typically around puberty. Prevalence is 8% to 10% among adult and adolescent patients with epilepsies.[23]

Clinical features: Presentation is with myoclonic seizures and GTCSs shortly after awakening from sleep in a normally developing adolescent. Myoclonic seizures can be subtle or severe, and the patient may drop objects or fall. These usually occur in clusters and often with an accelerating frequency and severity may precede a GTCS, as the so-called myoclonic-tonic-clonic generalized seizure.[35] Sleep deprivation and fatigue, particularly after excessive alcohol intake, are precipitants of myoclonic jerks and GTCSs.

EEG features: The background is normal. The interictal EEG is characterized by sleep-potentiated fast generalized spike and polyspike wave discharge, usually at 3.5 to 6 Hz (**Fig. 12**). The figure shows a fast spike and wave and polyspikes. The typical EEG discharge of myoclonic jerk is a single generalized burst of polyspike and wave discharges. Absence seizures are associated with regular fast (3.5–6 Hz) generalized spike and polyspike wave discharges. In one-third of cases, a photoparoxysmal response to intermittent photic stimulation is seen. Hyperventilation may

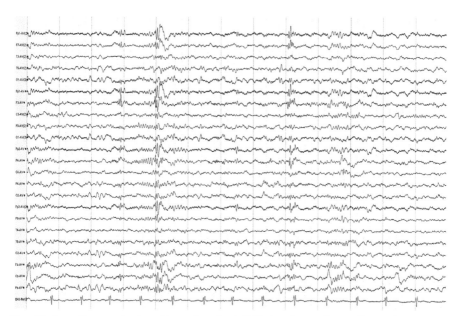

Fig. 12. Juvenile myoclonic epilepsy interictal EEG showing a fast spike and wave and polyspikes.

augment epileptiform discharges, although less reliably than in CAE or juvenile absence epilepsy.

Diagnosis: JME is a clinical diagnosis, supported by EEG findings. Neuroimaging is typically normal.

Management: Valproic acid is still considered the first-choice treatment, which is effective in 80% of the cases.[36] Levetiracetam and lamotrigine are alternative first choices in women of child-bearing age. Lamotrigine may exacerbate myoclonus, which may be prevented by the addition of clonazepam. Other add-on treatments if the first-line treatment fail are topiramate, zonisamide, clobazam, and acetazolamide. Vagal nerve stimulation may be considered as a last resort in pharmacoresistant cases.[36]

Several ASMs are contraindicated in JME including phenytoin, carbamazepine, oxcarbazepine, gabapentin, pregabalin, tiagabine, and vigabatrin because they can exacerbate myoclonic jerks in JME.

Prognosis: Most patients can achieve complete seizure control through a combination of ASM and adequate sleep. JME is considered a lifelong condition in which taper of ASMs should not be considered.

DISCLOSURE

The authors have nothing to disclose.

REFERENCES

1. Fisher RF, Acevedo C, Arzimanoglou A, et al. ILAE official report: a practical clinical definition of epilepsy. Epilepsia 2014;55(4):475–82.

2. Fisher RF, Cross JH, French JA, et al. Operational classification of seizure types by the International League Against Epilepsy: Position Paper of the ILAE Commission for Classification and Terminology. Epilepsia 2017;58(4):522–30.

3. Scheffer IE, Berkovic S, Capovilla G, et al. ILAE classification of the epilepsies: position paper of the ILAE Commission for Classification and Terminology. Epilepsia 2017;58(4):512–21.

4. Epilepsy syndromes. Available at: www.epilpesydiagnosis.org. Accessed October 28, 2020.

5. Pellock JM, Hrachovy R, Shinnar S, et al. Infantile spasms: A U.S. consensus report. Epilepsia 2010;51(10):2175–89.

6. Hussain SA, Kwong G, Millichap JJ, et al. Hypsarrhythmia assessment exhibits poor interrater reliability: a threat to clinical trial validity. Epilepsia 2015;56:77–81.

7. Lux AL, Edwards SW, Hancock E, et al. The United Kingdom Infantile Spasms Study (UKISS) comparing hormone treatment with vigabatrin on developmental and epilepsy outcomes to age 14 months: a multicentre randomised trial. Lancet Neurol 2005;4:712–7.

8. Lux AL, Edwards SW, Hancock E, et al. The United Kingdom Infantile Spasms Study comparing vigabatrin with prednisolone or tetracosactide at 14 days: a multicentre, randomised controlled trial. Lancet 2004;364:1773–8.

9. Wanigasinghe J, Arambepola C, Sri Ranganathan S, et al. Randomized,single-blind, parallel clinical trial on efficacy of oral prednisolone versus intramuscular corticotropin on immediate and continued spasm control in west syndrome. Pediatr Neurol 2015;53:193–9.

10. O'Callaghan FJK, Edwards SW, Alber FD, et al. Safety and effectiveness of hormonal treatment versus hormonal treatment with vigabatrin for infantile spasms (ICISS): a randomised, multicentre, open label trial. Lancet Neurol 2017;16:33–42.

11. Arzimanoglou A, French J, Blume WT, et al. Lennox Gastaut Syndrome: a consensus approach on diagnosis, assessment, management and trial methodology. Lancet Neurol 2009;8:82–93.

12. Hancock EC, Cross JH. Treatment of Lennox-Gastaut syndrome. Cochrane Database Syst Rev 2013;(2):CD003277.

13. Vanstraten AF, Ng YT. Update on the management of Lennox-Gastaut syndrome. Pediatr Neurol 2012;3:153–61.

14. Kang JW, Eom S, Hong W, et al. Long-term outcome of resective epilepsy surgery in patients with Lennox-Gastaut syndrome. Pediatrics 2018;142(4):e20180449.

15. Connolly MB. Dravet syndrome: diagnosis and long-term course. Can J Neurol Sci 2016;43:S3–8.

16. Claes L, Del-Favero J, Ceulemanns B, et al. De novo mutations in sodium channel SCN1A cause severe myoclonic epilepsy of infancy. Am J Hum Genet 2001;68:1327–32.

17. Genton P, Velizarova R, Dravet C. Dravet syndrome: the long-term outcome. Epilepsia 2011;52(Suppl 2):44–9.

18. Dravet C. The core Dravet syndrome phenotype. Epilepsia 2011;52(Suppl. 2):3–9.

19. Wirrell EC. The treatment of Dravet syndrome. Can J Neurol Sci 2016;43:S13–8.

20. Cross JH, Caraballo RH, Nabbout R, et al. Dravet syndrome: treatment options and management of prolonged seizures. Epilepsia 2019;60(S3):S39–48.

21. Ferrie C, Caraballo R, Covanis A, et al. Panayiotopoulos syndrome: a consensus view. Dev Med Child Neurol 2006;48:236–40.

22. Covanis A. Panayiotopoulos syndrome: a benign childhood autonomic epilepsy frequently imitating encephalitis, syncope, migraine, sleep disorder, or gastroenteritis. Pediatrics 2006;118:1237–43.
23. Panayiotopolous CP. Idiopathic generalized epilepsies. In: A clinical guide to epileptic syndromes and their management. 2nd edition. Springer Healthcare; 2010. p. 347–56, 384, 394–401.
24. Graziosi A, Pellegrino N, Stefano VD, et al. Misdiagnosis and pitfalls in Panayiotopoulos syndrome. Epilepsy Behav 2019;98:124–8.
25. Panayiotopolous CP. Benign childhood focal seizures and related epilepsy syndromes. In: A clinical guide to epileptic syndromes and their management. 2nd edition. Springer Healthcare; 2010. p. 341–2.
26. Garcia-Ramos C, Jackson DC, Lin JJ, et al. Cognition and brain development in children with benign epilepsy with central temporal spikes. Epilepsia 2015; 56(10):1615–22.
27. Kramer U. Atypical presentations of benign childhood epilepsy with central temporal spikes: a review. J Child Neurol 2008;23:785–90.
28. Aicardi J, Chevrie JJ. Atypical benign partial epilepsy of childhood. Dev Med Child Neurol 1982;24:281–92.
29. Pan A, Lüders HO. Epileptiform discharges in benign focal epilepsy of childhood. Epileptic Disord 2001;2(4):29–36.
30. Fejerman N. Atypical rolandic epilepsy. Epilepsia 2009;50(Suppl. 7):9–12.
31. Shinnar S, Cnaan A, Hu F, et al. Long-term outcomes of generalized tonic-clonic seizures in a childhood absence epilepsy trial. Neurology 2015;85(13):1108–14.
32. Masur D, Shinnar S, Cnaan A, et al. Pretreatment cognitive deficits and treatment effects on attention in childhood absence epilepsy. Neurology 2013;81:1572–80.
33. Glauser TA, Cnaan A, Shinnar S, et al. Ethosuximide, valproic acid and lamotrigine in childhood absence epilepsy. N Engl J Med 2010;362(9):790–9.
34. Panayiotopoulos CP, Obeid T, Tahan AR. Juvenile myoclonic epilepsy: a 5-year prospective study. Epilepsia 1994;35:285–96.
35. Delgado-Escueta AV, Enrile-Bacsal F. Juvenile myoclonic epilepsy of Janz. Neurology 1984;34:285–94.
36. Brodie MJ. Modern management of juvenile myoclonic epilepsy. Expert Rev Neurother 2016;16(6):681–8.

Neuromodulation in Pediatric Epilepsy

Irfan Ali, MD*, Kim Houck, MD

KEYWORDS

- Epilepsy • Refractory epilepsy • Neurostimulation • Neuromodulation • RNS • VNS
- DBS • TMS

KEY POINTS

- Neuromodulation with vagus nerve stimulation (VNS), closed-loop responsive neurostimulation (RNS), and deep brain stimulation (DBS) are effective treatments of drug-resistant epilepsy.
- Sustained and continued seizure reduction over 10 years in patients with VNS ($P<.01$).
- Quality of life improvement independent of seizure control with VNS.
- Median seizure reduction of 75% at 9 years with RNS.
- Statistically significant improvement in naming ($P<.001$) and memory ($P = .03$) after 2 years of RNS treatment in patients with temporal lobe epilepsy.

INTRODUCTION

Epilepsy is one of the most common neurologic disorders, affecting 1.2% of the world's population. There are 3 million adults and 470,000 children with epilepsy in the United States.[1] In an analysis of 1098 patients, 35% did not become seizure-free after 3 antiseizure medications.[2] Despite more than 30 available antiseizure medications, dietary treatments, and targeted epilepsy surgeries, many patients continue to have seizures.[3] An epileptogenic focus in the eloquent cortex, multiple seizure foci, primary generalized epilepsy, or patients' unwillingness to undergo traditional surgery further limits surgical interventions. Therapeutic nervous system stimulation is another treatment option for such patients. Various techniques have been in use for decades to treat neurologic diseases that were not manageable with traditional medicines and/or therapies available in the past. Therapeutic neurostimulation has shown efficacy in treating pain, depression, movement disorders, and epilepsy, with either open-loop or closed-loop modalities. Most recently, the use of closed-loop responsive neurostimulation therapy has been increasing, including children of younger age groups. Despite

The authors I. Ali and K. Houck, confirm they have nothing to disclose for this article.
Texas Children's Hospital, 6701 Fannin Street, Suite 1250, Houston, TX 77030, USA
* Corresponding author.
E-mail address: ixali@texaschildrens.org

neurologic.theclinics.com

all the technological advances, the underlying mechanisms of neurostimulation and of epilepsy networks remain to be fully elucidated.

HISTORICAL BACKGROUND

Neuromodulation alters neuronal activity by delivering a targeted electrical stimulus to a specific neurologic site in the body. The first reported use of neurostimulation dates back to Hippocrates, who is said to have used an electric fish to cause numbness. In 15 AD, Scriboniusis specifically recommended Torpedo fish shock for the treatment of pain.[4] In the late nineteenth century, Horsley stimulated the human cortex for the first time in epilepsy patients.[5] At the beginning of the twentieth century, the development of Electreat skin stimulation devices for pain opened the doors for neurostimulation in modern medicine.[6] With time, scientists discovered the role of deep brain structures in epilepsy: the 3 Hz spike-wave activity could be initiated in the cortex or thalamus and propagate via widespread thalamocortical connections.[7] In the mid-twentieth century, Penfield and Jasper demonstrated that cortical stimulation could disrupt epileptiform activity.[8] In 1985, Zabara[9] hypothesized vagus nerve stimulation (VNS) antagonizes hypersynchronous states in laboratory animals. These and many other studies set the foundation for the development of implantable neurostimulation devices for epilepsy.

NEUROSTIMULATION MODALITIES

The various neuromodulation options in epilepsy are either open-loop or closed-loop neurostimulation.[10,11] Among the open-loop category, invasive VNS and deep brain stimulation (DBS) are approved by the US Food and Drug Administration (FDA) for epilepsy. The noninvasive techniques using transcutaneous VNS, transcranial magnetic stimulation (TMS), direct cortical stimulation, and trigeminal nerve stimulation are not approved by the FDA for the treatment of epilepsy. However, transcutaneous VNS is an approved treatment in Europe. The following sections describe these modalities in detail.

VAGUS NERVE STIMULATION
Device Background and Mechanism of Action

The VNS consists of an implantable pulse generator and lead wire. The device is implanted subcutaneously in the left upper chest, with the lead wire coiled around the left vagus nerve (**Fig. 1**). VNS exerts its antiepileptic effects via several purported mechanisms. Although the exact mechanisms are not fully understood, animal models indicate that the locus coeruleus (LC) is a crucial structure.[12] Noradrenergic neurons from the LC have connections to various brain regions, including the hippocampus, thalamus, hypothalamus, orbitofrontal cortex, and cerebellum. The diffuse noradrenergic projection system and other circuitries, including the reticular activating system, central autonomic network, and limbic system, are purported to be altered by vagal afferent activities, giving rise to the antiepileptic properties of this therapy.[13]

Indications

The VNS therapy system is indicated for use as adjunctive therapy in reducing the frequency of seizures in patients 4 years of age and older with focal onset seizures that are refractory to antiseizure medications.[14] Studies have also shown efficacy in individuals with primary generalized epilepsy.[15–17]

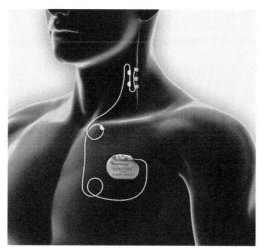

Fig. 1. VNS system. The generator is implanted in the left upper chest. The lead wire is tunneled subcutaneously and coiled around the vagus nerve within the carotid sheath. (*Courtesy of* LivaNova USA, Inc., Houston, TX.)

Application

In current commercial models, the VNS operates in 3 modes: "Normal," "Automatic Stimulation" (AutoStim), and "Magnet." These modalities are designed to prevent seizures, respond automatically to a seizure biomarker (tachycardia), and provide on-demand therapy to stop or shorten a seizure, respectively. In Normal mode, the generator is cycling for a specified time at the programmed settings. AutoStim is activated when the device detects a percentage increase in heart rate from baseline. Magnet mode is activated when a magnet is passed over the generator for 1 to 2 seconds and then removed from the area. There are 5 primary setting parameters: output current (milliamperes, mA), frequency (hertz, Hz), pulse width (microseconds, μSec), on-time (seconds, sec), and off-time (minutes, min). Initially, the goal is to titrate output current approximately once every 2 weeks, with adjustments in pulse width and frequency as needed to optimize efficacy and tolerability[18] (**Fig. 2**).[7] Adjustments by decreasing pulse width and frequency alone or together improve tolerability. Similarly, AutoStim mode allows various adjustments for sensitivity to tachycardia detection. Following the response to treatment further adjustments may be made in the duty cycle, defined as the percentage of time the device is stimulating. Increased duty cycle is associated with increased efficacy,[19] but also decreased generator battery longevity. AutoStim and Magnet use also affect battery longevity. On average, battery life ranges from 4.5 to 7.5 years.[14]

Complications/Concerns

Common adverse effects include hoarseness, cough, paresthesias, and shortness of breath.[14] These tend to improve over time.[20,21] In some cases, worsening of preexisting obstructive sleep apnea or new-onset obstructive sleep apnea may occur. Postoperative infection occurs in fewer than 3%, although children (4–11 years of age) may have a greater risk of infection compared with adolescent and adult patients (≥12 years of age). Children may also have a higher risk of lead fracture, lead extrusion, or generator migration. Otherwise, treatment-emergent adverse events in patients 4 to 11 year old are similar to patients ≥12 years.[14]

Phase 1: Output Current

Increase Output Current to therapeutic effect as tolerated by the patient

NORMAL MODE: 0.25 mA steps to therapeutic effect[12]

AUTOSTIM MODE: Normal Mode + 0.125 mA
AutoStim should be comfortable for patients

MAGNET MODE Normal Mode + 0.25 mA
Magnet Mode should be > than AutoStim Mode

Standard Protocol

		Visit	1	2	3	4	5	6	7
NORMAL	Output Current	mA	0.25	0.5	0.75	1.0	1.25	1.5	1.75
	Signal Frequency	Hz	20	20	20	20	20	20	20
	Pulse Width	µsec	250	250	250	250	250	250	250
	Signal ON Time	seconds	30	30	30	30	30	30	30
	Signal OFF Time	minutes	5	5	5	5	5	5	5
AUTOSTIM	Output Current	mA	0.375	0.625	0.875	1.125	1.375	1.625	1.875
	Pulse Width	µsec	250	250	250	250	250	250	250
	ON Time	seconds	60	60	60	60	60	60	60
MAGNET	Output Current	mA	0.5	0.75	1.0	1.25	1.5	1.75	2.0
	Pulse Width	µsec	500	500	500	500	500	500	500
	ON Time	seconds	60	60	60	60	60	60	60

> Suggested programming settings ≥ 2 wk post-op
> More frequent visits (1 - 2 wk) are suggested in Phase 1
> Multiple 0.25 mA increases may be made in a single visit to reach therapeutic range sooner; ensure patient tolerability before making additional adjustments

Fig. 2. Recommended dosing guidelines for Phase 1 of VNS programming. (*From* Sentiva Dosing Guide 2019. LivaNova USA, Inc. (C) 2019 https://vnstherapy.com/healthcare-professionals/sites/vnstherapy.com.healthcare-professionals/files/SenTiva_Dosing_Guide_2019-DIGITAL.PDF; with permission.)

Clinical Outcomes

Five clinical studies evaluating the efficacy of the VNS therapy system in reducing seizures have been reviewed.[22–26] Long-term data from uncontrolled follow-up have also been collected. For the acute phase studies, 454 patients, ages 3 to 63 years, were implanted. Patient exposure totaled 901 device-years, with a mean patient exposure of 24 months (range 8 days to 7.4 years). Long-term studies with open-label protocols have included follow-ups for up to 11 years.[14] Overall, these studies showed a responder rate, defined as ≥50% reduction in median seizure frequency, in half to two-thirds of patients.[23–27] One in 4 patients experienced a ≥90% seizure reduction.[23,27] In addition, the seizure-reducing effects appeared to improve over time.[14,22,23] A significant reduction in seizure duration and intensity, as well as improved postictal recovery, have also been demonstrated.[28,29] Significant decrease in sudden unexpected death in epilepsy (SUDEP) risk,[30] reduction in status epilepticus,[31,32] and improvement in quality of life[33] have been shown. Efficacy for children aged 4 to 11 years has also been demonstrated. After 12 months of treatment, there were no statistically significant differences in median percent reduction in seizures for patients 4 to 11 years of age compared with patients ≥12 years age, although median baseline seizure rate was higher (4–11 years old: 85.7 seizures/mo; 12–21 years old: 30.4 seizures/mo; >21 years old: 17.4 seizures/mo). Across the 5 clinical studies, Bayesian hierarchical models estimate a responder rate of 37% in children ages 4 to 11 years (95% credible interval: 26%, 48%).[14]

RESPONSIVE NEUROSTIMULATION
Device Background and Mechanism of Action

The RNS device is the only closed-loop neurostimulation system available to date to treat drug-resistant epilepsy. The system consists of 2 implantable leads, each having 4 contacts. These can be either depth electrodes for the deeper structures or surface electrodes effaced to the cerebral cortex. The leads are placed via burr holes, or stereotactic surgical techniques. Simultaneously, a metal housing is implanted in the skull, sacrificing the cranial bone's equivalent size, which harbors the neurostimulator device under the scalp. Currently, the available neurostimulation device has a battery life of 8 years. The RNS system provides a unique opportunity to record Electrocorticograpgy (ECoG) and deliver stimulation.[10] Lesser and colleagues[34] showed that if rhythmic during functional brain mapping, after discharges, could be disrupted with a train of pulse stimulation if delivered early at the onset. The stimulation of cortical neurons induces both immediate and long-term changes locally and at distant sites, affecting the epileptic network.[35] The slow structural changes in the neuronal cell membranes change the neuronal depolarization patterns. To maximize the therapeutic effects, identification, and engagement of the epileptogenic network are crucial. RNS delivers electric stimulation on the detection of specific predetermined epileptiform discharges in real-time.

Indications

The FDA approved the RNS system in 2013 to treat drug-resistant epilepsy with focal onset disabling seizures, with less than 2 epileptogenic foci, in patients 18 years of age or older. Device size is small (**Fig. 3**). Device placement requires a presurgical evaluation to identify a seizure onset zone for lead placement. A surgical procedure follows this by a trained neurosurgeon for precise placement of the intracranial leads and the device, requiring craniotomy (**Fig. 4**). There have been more than 3000 RNS system implantations since its approval in 2013. Tertiary care pediatric centers have implanted a total of 196 RNS systems in children to date.

Application

The RNS operates in detection only, detection and treatment, or MRI safety modes. The initial ECoG recording is in detection mode. Seizures are detected using line length, area, or bandpass, and time-domain analysis methods. An electrographic seizure detection, magnet swipe by the patient, and a preset specific time of the day are the most common ECoG recording triggers. The device can store 12 minutes of ECoG activity at a given time in divided epochs that range from 30 to 240 seconds each. Approximately 1 month after implantation, the patient usually follows up in the

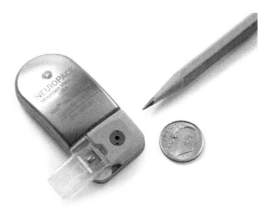

Fig. 3. Size comparison (device with dime and pencil). (All NeuroPace copyrighted images provided by Courtesy of NeuroPace.)

outpatient setting with an epileptologist trained to manage the device. After recording and reviewing the habitual seizures, the neurophysiologist/epileptologist determines the earliest seizure onset and specifies detection parameters as triggers for the neurostimulation. Stimulation parameters are also programmed. The device can be programmed to deliver stimulation to selected individual contacts within each electrode. Following a trigger, the device delivers 2 bursts of stimulation of the targeted contacts (**Fig. 5**). The initial stimulation is with a charge density of 0.5 micro coulombs per centimeter squared ($\mu C/cm^2$) at the contact point using a pulse width of 160 µs (frequency 200 Hz [1–333 Hz]) and a pulse duration of 100 ms (10–5000 ms). The patient is seen in the clinic every 3 months to assess the clinical response, review the recorded ECoG data, and adjust the charge density by 0.5 $\mu C/cm^2$ each visit to achieve a satisfactory response. The device can deliver a maximum charge density of 25 ($\mu C/cm^2$)[36]; however, clinical response is usually achieved with discharge density between 0.8 to 6 ($\mu C/cm^2$).[37] MRI safety mode is available and prevents the depletion of the device battery during MRI (**Fig. 6**).

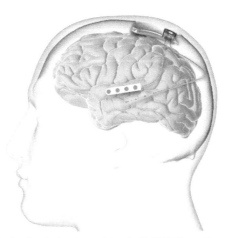

Fig. 4. Image of device/leads implanted in skull. (All NeuroPace copyrighted images provided by Courtesy of NeuroPace.)

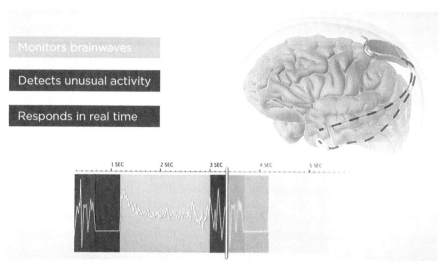

Fig. 5. The RNS device records real-time ECoG to detect seizures at their onset and delivers neurostimulation to disrupt seizure activity. (All NeuroPace copyrighted images provided by Courtesy of NeuroPace.)

Clinical Outcomes

Successful disruption of epileptiform activity was demonstrated by Kossoff and colleagues[38] using external neurostimulation during subdural monitoring, thus revealing promising results to suppress seizure activity. Subsequently, an FDA-approved, multicenter, randomized, double-blinded, placebo-controlled feasibility study,

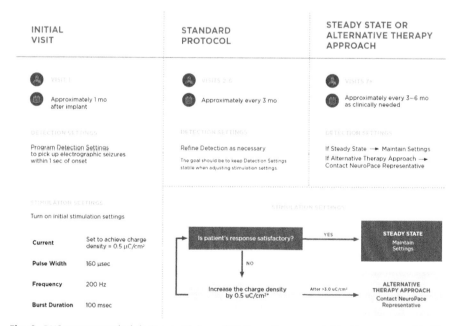

Fig. 6. RNS recommended dosing guidelines. (All NeuroPace copyrighted images provided by Courtesy of NeuroPace.) * indicates the increments should be equal or less than 0.5uC/cm2.

followed by the pivotal phase 3 study, demonstrated the safety and efficacy of closed-loop neurostimulation.[39] Morrell and colleagues[40] reported 191 patients with intracranial electrodes implanted at 1 or 2 foci after failing at least 2 medications and having at least 3 seizures per month. These patients were randomized 1:1 for stimulation versus sham groups, and physicians gathering outcome data were blinded entirely for the 12-week evaluation period. All the patients showed seizure reduction after the implantation of the device. The seizure frequency remained reduced in the stimulation group (41%) compared with sham (9.4%). Among the treatment group, 29% of participants showed a more than 50% reduction in frequency at the end of the blinded period, which increased to 46% at 2 years postimplant.[40] After 9 years of stimulation, a 2020 update on these patients showed a median seizure reduction of 75% and greater than 50% seizure reduction in 73% of participants. One-third of the participants achieved more than 90% seizure reduction in the most recent 6 months, and 28% had at least one period of greater than 6 months without seizures.[37] Loring and colleagues[41] found no cognitive adverse effects. There was no group decline on any of the 14 objective neuropsychological measures at baseline and after a blinded period of 1 and 2 years of neurostimulation in 175 patients.[41] Statistically significant improvements with naming (Boston naming test; $P < .001$) and verbal memory (Rey Auditory Verbal Learning Test; $P = .03$) were noted in patients with neocortical temporal and mesial temporal lobe epilepsy, respectively.[41]

In patients with temporal lobe epilepsy, long-term ambulatory ECoG monitoring revealed several significant findings. This long-term data changed the presumed unilateral or bilateral temporal lateralization in 20% of patients with bilateral temporal implantation. Notably, 7 (64%) of 11 patients with presumed unilateral temporal lobe epilepsy had bilateral electrographic seizures. Conversely, 7 (13%) of 71 patients with presumed bilateral temporal lobe epilepsy had unilateral electrographic seizures.[42] Hirsch and colleagues showed chronic ambulatory ECoG monitoring for presumed bilateral temporal epilepsy successfully identified candidates for surgical resection after a mean recording duration of 42 months. Of these patients, 25 (16%) of 157 had unilateral temporal lobe resection, and all remained seizure-free at 24 months follow-up.[43] Besides, chronic responsive neurostimulation improves the quality of life[44] and decreases SUDEP risk significantly from 6.1 (patients in the placebo arm of treatment-resistant epilepsy trials) to 2 per thousand patients/stimulation years ($P < .009$).[45]

Complications/Concerns

Responsive neurostimulation is a safe and well-tolerated treatment option with no chronic stimulation side effects.[46] Wu and colleagues[47] found relatively stable impedances at the electrode-neural interface of chronically implanted depth and subdural electrodes for 24 to 36 months. Responsive brain neurostimulation does not disturb sleep, as arousals precede neurostimulation on polysomnography.[48] The rate of serious adverse events is comparable to that of DBS devices.[49] There is a 2.7% intracranial hemorrhage rate with the implantation procedure, with no long-term sequelae.[40] For every neurostimulator implanted, there is an infection risk of 3.7% and an erosion risk of 0.8%.[50] Other procedures, such as electroconvulsive therapy, TMS, and diathermy procedures, are contraindicated in patients with RNS systems. Computed tomography scans are generally considered safe. It is always better to contact a physician familiar with the RNS system for proper guidance before any radiological procedure or extracorporeal shockwave lithotripsy.

DEEP BRAIN STIMULATION
Device Background and Mechanism of Action

DBS has been FDA-approved to treat drug-resistant focal epilepsy in patients 18 years of age and older. It has established efficacy in the treatment of movement disorders since the 1990s. Although there is long-standing safety data for DBS use in adults, further evaluation is needed to determine the safety and efficacy in pediatric epilepsy patients. The treatment system includes a depth electrode implanted stereotactically in the anterior nucleus of the thalamus and a pulse generator implanted in the chest or abdomen. A trained neurologist programs the pulse generator, which delivers neurostimulation to the thalamus. The central mechanisms of DBS result in increased transmission of both excitatory and inhibitory neurotransmitters within basal ganglia-thalamocortical circuitry. These include inhibition of action potential through sodium channel-mediated depolarization inhibition, direct distal axonal synaptic inhibition, depletion of neurotransmitters at distal terminals, and potentiating any of the preceding mechanisms via direct stimulation: the net therapeutic effect results from the contribution of these mechanisms to various extents.[51]

Clinical Outcomes

A review of Zangiabadi and colleagues[52] encompassed studies for neurostimulation between 1980 to 2018 in humans and animals, including stimulation of the anterior and centromedian nuclei of the thalamus, hippocampus, basal ganglia, cerebellum, and hypothalamus in drug-resistant epilepsy patients. It concluded that anterior thalamic nucleus stimulation could be recommended.[52] As demonstrated in animal models, high-frequency stimulation of the anterior nucleus of the thalamus increases seizure thresholds.[53] In a study of 5 patients with medically refractory epilepsy treated with DBS, Mojgan Hodaie and colleagues[54] reported a 54% mean reduction in seizure frequency at 15 months follow-up, with 2 patients experiencing $\geq$75% reduction. In the double-blinded, randomized, controlled Stimulation of the Anterior Nucleus of the Thalamus in Epilepsy (SANTE) Trial, Fisher and colleagues[55] reported a median seizure reduction 40.4% after 13 months in 110 patients. In a 5-year update of the SANTE trial, Salanova and colleagues[56] reported more than 50% reduction in seizures in 54% of the participants, a sustained and incremental beneficial effect. Quality of life improvement was also statistically significant.[56]

TRANSCRANIAL MAGNETIC STIMULATION
Background

TMS is a noninvasive procedure that uses magnetic fields to induce electric field changes, thereby inducing electrical currents that activate neurons in the brain cortex. The stimulation area is usually 2 to 3 cm deep from the brain surface, targeted using a hand-held magnetic coil, integrated with MRI-based stereotactic navigation software. Stereotactic localization of the stimulation coil is necessary to guide TMS therapy precisely over cortical areas of interest. Stimulation parameters include intensity, interstimulus interval, and rate. Single-pulse or repetitive pulse trains are also programmable.

Applications

The most common application for navigated TMS is for mapping of the motor cortex, using single-pulse stimulations while simultaneously recording electromyography (EMG) measurements. Repetitive TMS (rTMS) is used for the treatment of the major depressive disorder, as well as noninvasive mapping of the language cortex. With rTMS, underlying brain activity in a targeted region of cortex is inhibited by repeated magnetic pulses.[57] Although it is not currently FDA-approved for the treatment of epilepsy, rTMS has successfully been used to reduce epileptic seizures. In a study of 7 patients with a continuous form of a focal epileptic seizure, Epilepsia Partialis Continua (EPC), investigators were able to induce a 20 to 30-minute cessation of seizures in 43% of patients, and more than 1-day cessation of seizure in 29% of patients.[58] In another study of 7 patients with intractable extratemporal lobe epilepsy, rTMS induced a 19% decrease in seizure frequency.[59]

Complications/Concerns

TMS therapy is overall well-tolerated. Common adverse effects include headache, lightheadedness, scalp discomfort at the site of stimulation, and transient paresthesias of the face, or spasms of facial muscles. Rarely, TMS may induce seizures. Nonetheless, TMS is well-tolerated among patients with epilepsy. In one large-scale review of 28 independent studies of rTMS in epilepsy, which included a total of 287 human subjects, there were no reported cases of status epilepticus or life-threatening seizures. Approximately 10% of patients experienced a mild headache, and 1.4% (4 total patients) had a seizure during the rTMS treatment.[60] In children with epilepsy, several studies have also indicated that there is no increased risk of seizures from rTMS therapy.[58,61–63] Due to these potential adverse effects, especially regarding therapeutic outcomes, further studies are necessary to evaluate the efficacy and tolerability of rTMS for the treatment of epilepsy.

EXTERNAL TRIGEMINAL NERVE STIMULATION

A double-blinded, randomized, controlled trial of 50 patients evaluated the efficacy of external trigeminal nerve stimulation (e-TNS) in epilepsy treatment. Subjects were randomized to active stimulation, control stimulation, or sham groups. The treatment group experienced a significant reduction in seizure frequency after a 3-month blinded period ($P = .01$).[64] Follow-up of 35 of these patients at 1 year showed a sustained reduction in seizure frequency.[65] Although not approved for epilepsy treatment, e-TNS is in use for headaches and ADHD.

OTHER NEUROMODULATION MODALITIES

In addition to the neuromodulation modalities mentioned previously, transcranial Alternating Current Stimulation (t-ACS), transcranial Direct Current Stimulation (t-DCS), transcutaneous VNS (t-VNS), and Transcutaneous Electric Nerve Stimulation are other forms of neurostimulation that require further research for their efficacy in the treatment of epilepsy.

SUMMARY

Neuromodulation alters neuronal activity with electrical impulses delivered to targeted neurologic sites. Among several neuromodulation systems, VNS, RNS, and DBS are effective treatments for drug-resistant epilepsy. Other modalities, including TMS, e-TNS, and other external stimulation therapies, suggest benefits as well. The underlying neurophysiologic mechanisms by which these devices exert their antiepileptic effects are diverse, and require full elucidation; however, key components include the locus ceruleus (for VNS), cortex (for RNS), and anterior nucleus of the thalamus through the Papez circuit (for DBS). Neuromodulation via these modalities reduces seizure frequency, decreases SUDEP risk, and improves quality of life. RNS treatment improves naming and verbal memory in patients with temporal lobe epilepsy. Although the data in children are not as robust as in adults, there is growing evidence and experience in children with various neurostimulation devices. Further studies are needed to evaluate the safety and efficacy of neuromodulation for pediatric drug-resistant epilepsy.

CLINICS CARE POINTS

- On subsequent visits, if tolerated, multiple 0.25-mA increases can be made during VNS ramping.
- Magnet over VNS device will stop the device and deliver the treatment once moved away.
- More on-time than off-time can result in vagus nerve injury.
- If seizure worsen after current increment for RNS treatment, lower the current and may adjust the pulse width.
- Always test increased therapy in the office and make sure the changes are registered before the patient leave, it will take 1 to 2 minutes.

REFERENCES

1. Center for Disease Control and Prevention. Epilepsy Fast Facts 2015. Available at: https://www.cdc.gov/epilepsy/data/index.html. Accessed October 30, 2020.
2. Kwan P, Brodie MJ. Early identification of refractory epilepsy. N Engl J Med 2000; 342(5):314–9.
3. Jobst BC, Cascino GD. Resective epilepsy surgery for drug-resistant focal epilepsy: a review. JAMA 2015;313(3):285–93.
4. Tsoucalas G, Karamanou M, Lymperi M, et al. The "torpedo" effect in medicine. Int Marit Health 2014;65(2):65–7.
5. Isitan C, Yan Q, Spencer DD, et al. Brief history of electrical cortical stimulation: a journey in time from Volta to Penfield. Epilepsy Res 2020;166:106363.
6. Gildenberg PL. History of electrical neuromodulation for chronic pain. Pain Med 2006;7:S7–13.
7. Gholam K, Motamedi RPL, Miglioretti DL, et al. Optimizing parameters for terminating cortical afterdischarges with pulse stimulation. Epilepsia 2002;43(8): 836–46.
8. Jiruska P, de Curtis M, Jefferys JG, et al. Synchronization and desynchronization in epilepsy: controversies and hypotheses. J Physiol 2013;591(4):787–97.
9. Zabara J. Inhibition of experimental seizures in canines by repetitive vagal stimulation. Epilepsia 1992;33(6):1005–12.
10. Sun FT, Morrell MJ. Closed-loop neurostimulation: the clinical experience. Neurotherapeutics 2014;11(3):553–63.
11. Wu C, Sharan AD. Neurostimulation for the treatment of epilepsy: a review of current surgical interventions. Neuromodulation 2013;16(1):10–24 [discussion: 24].
12. Krahl SC, Kevin, Smith D, et al. Locus coeruleus lesions suppress the seizure-attenuating effects of vagus nerve stimulation. Epilepsia 1998;39(7):709–14.
13. Giorgi FSP, Chiara, Biagioni F, et al. The role of norepinephrine in epilepsy: from the bench to the bedside. Neurosci Biobehavioral Rev 2004;28(5):507–24.
14. Nova L. VNS Therapy® system. Epilepsy Physician's ManualVNS Therapy® System; 2020. Available at: file:///C:/Users/ixali/Downloads/VNS%20Therapy%20System%20Epilepsy%20Physician's%20Manual%20(US)%20(1).PDF.

15. Kostov HLP, Røste GK. Is vagus nerve stimulation a treatment option for patients with drug-resistant idiopathic generalized epilepsy? Acta Neurol Scand 2007; 115:55–8.

16. Sankaraneni RM, Patil A, Singh S. Outcome of Vagal Nerve Stimulation for The Treatment of Primary Generalized Epilepsy. Neurology 2020;84:2883.

17. Marti AS, Parrent A, McLachlan R, et al. BS16. VNS in generalized epilepsy: an assessment on the efficacy. Clin Neurophysiol 2018;129:219.

18. Liva Nova. VNS Therapy Sentiva Dosing Guidelines. 2019. Available at: https:// vnstherapy.com/healthcare-professionals/sites/vnstherapy.com.healthcare-professionals/files/SenTiva_Dosing_Guide_2019-DIGITAL.PDF.

19. DeGiorgio CM, Thompson J, Lewis P, et al. Vagus nerve stimulation: analysis of device parameters in 154 patients during the long-term XE5 study. Epilepsia 2001;42(8):1017–20.

20. Morris GLM 3rd, Mueller WM. Long-term treatment with vagus nerve stimulation in patients with refractory epilepsy. The Vagus Nerve Stimulation Study Group E01-E05. Neurology 1999;53(8):1731–5.

21. Ben-Menachem E. Vagus nerve stimulation, side effects, and long-term safety. J Clin Neurophysiol 2001;18(5):415–8.

22. Elliott RM, Morsi A, Tanweer O, et al. Efficacy of vagus nerve stimulation over time: review of 65 consecutive patients with treatment-resistant epilepsy treated with VNS > 10 years. Epilepsy Behav 2011;20(3):478–83.

23. Kawai K, Tanaka T, Baba H, et al. Outcome of vagus nerve stimulation for drug-resistant epilepsy: the first three years of a prospective Japanese registry. Epileptic Disord 2017;19(3):327–38.

24. Labar D. Vagus nerve stimulation for 1 year in 269 patients on unchanged antiepileptic drugs. Seizure 2004;13(6):392–8.

25. Vonck KT, Thadani V, Gilbert K, et al. Vagus nerve stimulation for refractory epilepsy: a transatlantic experience. J Clin Neurophysiol 2004;21:283–9.

26. De Herdt VB, Boon P, Ceulemans B, et al. Vagus nerve stimulation for refractory epilepsy. A Belgian multicenter study 2007;11(5):261–9.

27. Elliot RM, Morsi A, Kalhornalo S, et al. Vagus nerve stimulation in 436 consecutive patients with treatment-resistant epilepsy: Long-term outcomes and predictors of response. Epilepsy Behav 2011;20(1):57–63.

28. Boon PV, Vonck K, Rijckevorsel K, et al. A prospective, multicenter study of cardiac-based seizure detection to activate vagus nerve stimulation. Seizure 2015;32:52–61.

29. Orosz I, McCormick D, Zamponi N, et al. Vagus nerve stimulation for drug-resistant epilepsy: a European long-term study up to 24 months in 347 children. Epilepsia 2014;55(10):1576–84.

30. Ryvlin P, So EL, Gordon CM, et al. Long-term surveillance of SUDEP in drug-resistant epilepsy patients treated with VNS therapy. Epilepsia 2018;59(3): 562–72.

31. Helmers SD, Duh MS, Guérin A, et al. Clinical and economic impact of vagus nerve stimulation therapy in patients with drug-resistant epilepsy. Epilepsy Behav 2011;22(2):370–5.

32. Bernstein AL, Hess T. Vagus nerve stimulation therapy for pharmacoresistant epilepsy: effect on health care utilization. Epilepsy Behav 2007;10(1):134–7.

33. Englot DJ, Hassnain KH, Rolston JD, et al. Quality-of-life metrics with vagus nerve stimulation for epilepsy from provider survey data. Epilepsy Behav 2017;66:4–9.

34. Lesser RP, Kim SH, Beyderman L, et al. Brief bursts of pulse stimulation terminate afterdischarges caused by cortical stimulation. Neurology 1999;53(9):2073–81.

35. Stypulkowski PH, Stanslaski SR, Jensen RM, et al. Brain stimulation for epilepsy–local and remote modulation of network excitability. Brain Stimul 2014;7(3):350–8.

36. Fountas KN, Smith JR, Murro AM, et al. Implantation of a closed-loop stimulation in the management of medically refractory focal epilepsy: a technical note. Stereotact Funct Neurosurg 2005;83(4):153–8.

37. Nair DR, Laxer KD, Weber PB, et al. Nine-year prospective efficacy and safety of brain-responsive neurostimulation for focal epilepsy. Neurology 2020;95(9):e1244–56.

38. Kossoff EH, Ritzl EK, Politsky JM, et al. Effect of an external responsive neurostimulator on seizures and electrographic discharges during subdural electrode monitoring. Epilepsia 2004;45(12):1560–7.

39. Anderson WS, Kossoff EH, Bergey GK, et al. Implantation of a responsive neurostimulator device in patients with refractory epilepsy. Neurosurg Focus 2008;25(3):E12.

40. Morrell MJ, Group RNSSiES. Responsive cortical stimulation for the treatment of medically intractable partial epilepsy. Neurology 2011;77(13):1295–304.

41. Loring DW, Kapur R, Meador KJ, et al. Differential neuropsychological outcomes following targeted responsive neurostimulation for partial-onset epilepsy. Epilepsia 2015;56(11):1836–44.

42. King-Stephens D, Mirro E, Weber PB, et al. Lateralization of mesial temporal lobe epilepsy with chronic ambulatory electrocorticography. Epilepsia 2015;56(6):959–67.

43. Hirsch LJ, Mirro EA, Salanova V, et al. Mesial temporal resection following long-term ambulatory intracranial EEG monitoring with a direct brain-responsive neurostimulation system. Epilepsia 2020;61(3):408–20.

44. Meador KJ, Kapur R, Loring DW, et al. Quality of life and mood in patients with medically intractable epilepsy treated with targeted responsive neurostimulation. Epilepsy Behav 2015;45:242–7.

45. Devinsky O, Friedman D, Duckrow RB, et al. Sudden unexpected death in epilepsy in patients treated with brain-responsive neurostimulation. Epilepsia 2018;59(3):555–61.

46. Gregory K, Bergey MMJM, Mizrahi EM, et al. Long-term treatment with responsive brain stimulation in adults with refractory partial seizures. Neurology 2015;84(8):810–7.

47. Wu C, Evans JJ, Skidmore C, et al. Impedance variations over time for a closed-loop neurostimulation device: early experience with chronically implanted electrodes. Neuromodulation 2013;16(1):46–50 [discussion: 50].

48. Ruoff L, Jarosiewicz B, Zak R, et al. Sleep disruption is not observed with brain-responsive neurostimulation for epilepsy. Epilepsia Open 2020;5(2):155–65.

49. Martin AJ, Starr PA, Ostrem JL, et al. Hemorrhage detection and incidence during magnetic resonance-guided deep brain stimulator implantations. Stereotact Funct Neurosurg 2017;95(5):307–14.

50. Weber PB, Kapur R, Gwinn RP, et al. Infection and erosion rates in trials of a cranially implanted neurostimulator do not increase with subsequent neurostimulator placements. Stereotact Funct Neurosurg 2017;95(5):325–9.

51. Lee KHM, Elizabeth M, Bhala C. Neuromodulation. 2nd edition. London: Academic Press; 2018.

52. Zangiabadi N, Ladino LD, Sina F, et al. Deep brain stimulation and drug-resistant epilepsy: a review of the literature. Front Neurol 2019;10:601.

53. Wyckhuys T, Raedt R, Vonck K, et al. Comparison of hippocampal Deep Brain Stimulation with high (130Hz) and low frequency (5Hz) on afterdischarges in kindled rats. Epilepsy Res 2010;88(2–3):239–46.
54. Mojgan Hodaie RAW, Dostrovsky JO, Lozano AM. Chronic anterior thalamus stimulation for intractable epilepsy. epilepsia 2002;43(6):603–8.
55. Fisher R, Salanova V, Witt T, et al. Electrical stimulation of the anterior nucleus of thalamus for treatment of refractory epilepsy. Epilepsia 2010;51(5):899–908.
56. Vicenta Salanova MTW, Worth R, Henry TR, et al. Long-term efficacy and safety of thalamic stimulation for drug-resistant partial epilepsy. Neurology 2015;84: 1017–25.
57. Chen RCJ, Gerloff C, Celnik P, et al. Depression of motor cortex excitability by low-frequency transcranial magnetic stimulation. Neurology 1997;48(5): 1398–403.
58. Rotenberg A, Bae EH, Takeoka M, et al. Repetitive transcranial magnetic stimulation in the treatment of epilepsia partialis continua. Epilepsy Behav 2009; 14(1):253–7.
59. Kinoshita MIA, Begum T, Yamamoto J, et al. Low-frequency repetitive transcranial magnetic stimulation for seizure suppression in patients with extratemporal lobe epilepsy—A pilot study. Seizure 2005;14(6):387–92.
60. Bae EH, Schrader LM, Machii K, et al. Safety and tolerability of repetitive transcranial magnetic stimulation in patients with epilepsy: a review of the literature. Epilepsy Behav 2007;10(4):521–8.
61. Graff-Guerrero A, Gonzáles-Olvera J, Ruiz-García M, et al. rTMS reduces focal brain hyperperfusion in two patients with EPC. Acta Neurol Scand 2004;109(4): 290–6.
62. Morales OG, Henry ME, Nobler MS, et al. Electroconvulsive therapy and repetitive transcranial magnetic stimulation in children and adolescents: a review and report of two cases of epilepsia partialis continua. Child Adolesc Psychiatr Clin N Am 2005;14(1):193–210, viii–ix.
63. Sun W, Fu W, Mao W, et al. Low-frequency repetitive transcranial magnetic stimulation for the treatment of refractory partial epilepsy. Clin EEG Neurosci 2011; 42(1):40–4.
64. Christopher M, DeGiorgio MJS, Cook IA, et al. Randomized controlled trial of trigeminal nerve stimulation for drug-resistant epilepsy. neurology 2013;80(9): 786–91.
65. Soss J, Heck C, Murray D, et al. A prospective long-term study of external trigeminal nerve stimulation for drug-resistant epilepsy. Epilepsy Behav 2015;42:44–7.

Inflammatory Diseases of the Central Nervous System

Nikita Malani Shukla, MD[a],*, Timothy E. Lotze, MD[a], Eyal Muscal, MD[b]

KEYWORDS

- Pediatric neuroinflammatory diseases • Pediatric neuroimmunology
- Pediatric demyelinating disease • Pediatric autoimmune encephalitis

KEY POINTS

- Pediatric neuroinflammatory disorders encompass demyelinating diseases, immune-mediated epilepsies, rheumatologic conditions with neurologic manifestations, and certain genetic disorders with inflammatory pathophysiology.
- Each disorder has a distinct pathophysiology that guides treatment and determines prognosis.
- Neuroinflammatory diseases should be considered in any child that presents with encephalopathy, focal neurologic deficits, seizures, or movement disorders.

INTRODUCTION

Pediatric neuroinflammatory conditions are a complex group of immune-mediated disorders with a wide range of clinical presentations, including focal neurologic deficits, encephalopathy, seizures, movement disorders, and psychiatric manifestations. Initial evaluation often involves multiple disciplines, including neurology, rheumatology, and psychiatry, as well as extensive investigation including MRI of the brain and spine, serum and cerebrospinal fluid (CSF) studies, electroencephalography (EEG), ophthalmologic examination, and neuropsychological assessment.

Pediatric neuroinflammatory conditions can be classified according to clinical presentation, pathophysiologic mechanism (ie, antibody-mediated vs innate immunity-mediated) or imaging and laboratory findings. In this article, we group these conditions into acquired demyelinating diseases, immune-mediated epilepsies/encephalopathies, primary rheumatologic conditions with central nervous system (CNS) manifestations, CNS vasculitis, and neurodegenerative/genetic conditions with immune-mediated pathophysiology.

[a] Department of Neurology and Developmental Neuroscience, Texas Children's Hospital, Baylor College of Medicine, 6701 Fannin Street, Suite 1250, Houston, TX 77030, USA; [b] Department of Pediatrics, Texas Children's Hospital, Baylor College of Medicine, Co-appointment in Department of Neurology and Developmental Neuroscience, 6701 Fannin Street, 11th Floor, Houston, TX 77030, USA
* Corresponding author.
E-mail address: malani@bcm.edu

Neurol Clin 39 (2021) 811–828
https://doi.org/10.1016/j.ncl.2021.04.004
0733-8619/21/© 2021 Elsevier Inc. All rights reserved.

ACQUIRED DEMYELINATING CONDITIONS

There has been significant progress in understanding pediatric demyelinating diseases over the past 10 years, including elucidating pathophysiologic mechanisms, discovery of antibody markers, and development of targeted treatments depending on the specific demyelinating condition.[1] These disorders can be divided into monophasic and multiphasic diseases, although it can be difficult to predict the risk of further demyelinating events at first presentation.

MONOPHASIC DEMYELINATING DISEASE
Acute Disseminated Encephalomyelitis

Definition
Acute disseminated encephalomyelitis (ADEM) is defined as a first polyfocal CNS event with presumed inflammatory demyelinating cause. The presence of encephalopathy and MRI abnormalities consistent with demyelination are required to meet diagnostic criteria.

Epidemiology
ADEM is the most common demyelinating disease in children, and its incidence is estimated to be 0.3 to 0.6 per 100,000 per year. The median age of presentation is 5 to 8 years old and it occurs more frequently in male patients.[2]

Pathophysiology
ADEM typically occurs in the postinfectious period (2–3 weeks following a viral infection); however, a causal relationship has not been established. It is histopathologically characterized by macrophage and lymphocyte infiltration of the perivascular regions.[3]

Clinical presentation
Patients present with acute onset of encephalopathy and polyfocal neurologic deficits, which can include ataxia, dysarthria, focal weakness, vision loss due to optic neuritis (ON), and weakness or sensory changes due to spinal cord syndrome. Seizures occur more frequently in patients with ADEM compared with other acquired demyelinating diseases. These symptoms can be preceded by a prodromal phase of fever, headache, nausea, and vomiting. ADEM progresses rapidly, with a clinical nadir at approximately 2 to 5 days.[2]

Typically, ADEM is a monophasic event with no new disease activity after 3 months of disease onset; however multiphasic ADEM (MDEM) does occur and is defined as a second ADEM event more than 3 months after the initial event. ADEM also can be followed by ON (ADEM-ON) or be the first presentation of a neuromyelitis optica spectrum disorder (NMO-SD). In 2% to 3% of patients, ADEM can be followed by a non-ADEM event that then meets criteria for diagnosis of multiple sclerosis.[2]

Fulminant forms of ADEM can require admission to the intensive care unit (ICU), mechanical ventilation for airway protection, and invasive monitoring of intracranial pressure due to cerebral edema. A hemorrhagic form of ADEM, acute hemorrhagic leukoencephalopathy, has also been reported.

Diagnostic laboratory tests and imaging
Infectious workup, including herpes simplex virus polymerase chain reaction, should be initiated in cases of suspected ADEM. Other serum studies include complete blood count, erythrocyte sedimentation rate, C-reactive protein, anti-aquaporin-4 (AQP-4) antibodies, and anti-myelin oligodendrocyte protein (MOG) antibodies.

CSF is usually notable for an elevated white count with lymphocytic predominance and elevated protein levels. Elevated immunoglobulin (Ig)G Index has also been reported; however, CSF-specific oligoclonal bands (OCBs) are not typically found in patients with ADEM.[2]

MRI brain and spine demonstrate multiple T2 fluid-attenuated inversion recovery (FLAIR) lesions that are bilateral, asymmetric, and poorly marginated, involving both the gray and white matter. Spinal cord involvement is seen in around 30% of patients. Contrast-enhancing lesions are present in around 30% of patients (**Fig. 1**).[1,2]

Treatment

Treatment of acute attacks of demyelinating disease, including ADEM, is based on consensus guidelines and expert opinion and discussed in **Box 1**.[1,2] Longer-term treatments such as monthly high-dose steroids or monthly intravenous immunoglobulin (IVIg) can be used in patients with MDEM or ADEM-ON.

Outcome

Most children with monophasic ADEM are reported to have full recovery. There are, however, studies that show that even one demyelinating event leads to decreased white matter growth and long-term neurocognitive deficits such as learning difficulties and attention problems.[4]

Clinically Isolated Syndrome

Clinically isolated syndrome (CIS) is an umbrella term that is used for a first-time demyelinating event other than ADEM. Estimated incidence is 0.5 to 1.66 per 100,000 children.[5] Clinical phenotypes include ON, transverse myelitis, brainstem syndrome, and any other monofocal or multifocal first-time event (without associated

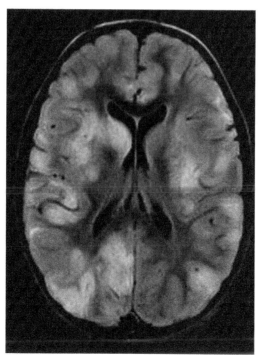

Fig. 1. T2 Axial FLAIR image showing extensive demyelinating lesions involving both the gray and white matter in ADEM.

> **Box 1**
> **Treatment of acute attacks of demyelinating disease**
>
> - High-dose corticosteroids (usually intravenous [IV] methylprednisolone 30 mg/kg/d) followed by oral steroid taper over 4 to 6 weeks.
> - IVIg in cases that do not fully respond to steroids.
> - Plasmapheresis in severe cases

encephalopathy). Studies have shown that approximately 80% of patients go on to have a second attack in a median time of 0.7 years (range between 0.3 and 2.2 years).[6]

Evaluation of patients presenting with CIS should include MRI of the brain and spine. Ophthalmologic examination should be performed, including optical coherence tomography, where available. Visual evoked potentials can be useful to identify subclinical ON in some patients. Serum studies include anti-MOG antibodies, AQP-4 antibodies, and vitamin D levels, as well as antinuclear antibody and antiphospholipid antibodies to evaluate for systemic autoimmune mimickers of demyelinating disease. Obtaining CSF is recommended, as the presence of OCBs can assist in making an earlier diagnosis of multiple sclerosis. **Box 2** lists predictors of progression to multiple sclerosis after CIS. Recent infection preceding the CIS event suggests lower risk of evolution into MS.[5,7]

Acute treatment of CIS is discussed in **Box 1**, although in patients with suspected NMO-SD or fulminate transverse myelitis, plasmapheresis should be initiated more promptly given improved outcomes in this subset of patients.[10]

MULTIPHASIC DEMYELINATING DISEASE
Multiple Sclerosis

Definition
Pediatric-onset multiple sclerosis (POMS) is defined as MS with onset before 18 years of age, using the 2017 McDonald Criteria. To meet criteria for diagnosis, patients must prove dissemination in space (DIS) and dissemination in time (DIT). DIS is proven by lesions in 2 or more of the MS-typical areas. DIT can be proven by more than 1 attack, new lesions on serial MRIs, presence of contrast-enhancing and non–contrast-enhancing lesions on one MRI, or presence of OCBs in CSF.[1]

> **Box 2**
> **Predictors of progression to multiple sclerosis after clinically isolated syndrome**
>
> - Female gender[6]
> - Age>10 y[1]
> - Postpubertal status in female patients[1]
> - Positive cerebrospinal fluid oligoclonal bands[6]
> - MRI brain lesions[6]
> - Multifocal/polyfocal symptoms at onset[6]
> - Low vitamin D levels[1]
> - Remote Epstein-Barr virus infection[1]

Epidemiology

Three percent to 5% of all MS cases have pediatric onset. Mean age of onset in POMS is 11 years; however, most patients are older than 15.[1] There is a known female predilection for MS, although not in the younger than 11 years age group.[3]

Pathophysiology

MS is an autoimmune disease in which T and B lymphocytes are activated and in turn activate the CNS microglia and astrocytes, creating an inflammatory environment.[1] The characteristic pathologic finding in MS is a confluent, sharply demarcated white matter lesion with demyelination, inflammation, and gliosis. In comparison with adult MS, POMS is found to be more inflammatory and cause more axonal damage.[3]

Clinical presentation

Patients with POMS present with a relapsing-remitting subtype of MS. In fact, the diagnosis of a progressive form of MS in the pediatric population should raise suspicion for a leukodystrophy or mitochondrial disease.

Patients can present with ON, transverse myelitis, cerebral attacks, and brainstem attacks affecting vision, strength, bowel/bladder control, extraocular movements, and sensation.

In addition to acute attacks, up to a third of patients with POMS report cognitive difficulties that interfere with their school performance, and depression and anxiety are prevalent in this patient population.[11]

Diagnostic laboratory tests and imaging

Pertinent laboratory tests and workup are the same as those for CIS.

Classic MS lesions on MRI are larger than 3 mm, ovoid, sharply demarcated, and homogeneous in signal intensity. Lesions should be asymmetric and present in the MS-typical areas: periventricular, cortical/juxtacortical, infratentorial, and spinal cord (**Fig. 2**).

Neuropsychological evaluation is important to assess any cognitive issues that may arise.

Treatment

Treatment of acute attacks in POMS is discussed in **Box 1**.

There has been tremendous development in the disease-modifying treatments (DMTs) for preventing disease progression in MS, which has led to a shift in treatment paradigm from a stepwise escalation approach to initiation of treatment with higher efficacy medications.[12]

Currently, only fingolimod, an oral sphingosine-1-phosphate immunomodulator, is approved by the Food and Drug Administration for use in patients with POMS; however, glatiramer acetate (injectable), dimethyl fumarate (oral), natalizumab (infusion), and rituximab (infusion) are commonly used in clinical practice. Decision on which DMT to start is based on patient and parent preference, availability of medications, tolerability of side effects, and disease severity. The goal of therapy is to achieve no evidence of disease activity (NEDA), which is defined as no relapses, no new MRI lesions, and no increase in disability.[13]

Outcome

Disability accrual in POMS is measured by the Expanded Disability Status Scale (EDSS). Although patients with POMS tend to recover from relapses better than their adult counterparts, their long disease duration and more active disease can lead to significant disability over time. Prognosis is worse in patients with highly active disease or in those who do not fully recover from relapses.[14]

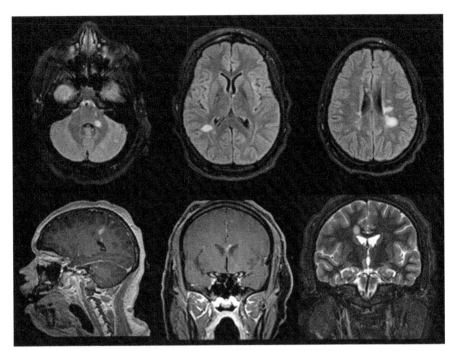

Fig. 2. Axial FLAIR (*top row*) and coronal FLAIR (*bottom row, right*) images from a patient with confirmed POMS show multiple ovoid, hyperintense lesions within the white matter. On the contrast-enhanced sequence (*bottom row*), several lesions show ill-defined contrast enhancement.

Neuromyelitis Optica Spectrum Disorder

Definition
NMO-SD is a spectrum of demyelinating disease with prominent features of ON and longitudinally extensive transverse myelitis (LETM). Diagnostic criteria (**Table 1**) for NMO-SD classify patients based on presence or absence of AQP-4 antibodies, with most patients being AQP-4 IgG positive.[1] Anti-MOG antibodies are also found in patients with NMO-SD with a reported frequency of approximately 10%. Dual seropositivity has not yet been reported. Approximately 15% of pediatric NMO-SD cases are seronegative for both antibodies.[15,16]

Epidemiology
Three percent to 5% of all NMO-SD cases have pediatric onset with a typical age of onset of 10 to 12 years. Girls are more likely to be affected than boys.[16]

Pathophysiology
Pathology shows demyelination due to AQP-4 antibodies activating the complement system after binding to the AQP-4 water channel on astrocyte foot processes. This autoimmune astrocytopathic picture is distinct from the inflammation seen in MS.[3]

Clinical presentation
Pediatric NMO-SD is a relapsing disease and common relapses include vision loss due to ON, weakness, sensory changes, or bowel/bladder issues due to LETM and intractable nausea/vomiting due to area postrema syndrome.

Table 1
Diagnostic criteria of Neuromyelitis Optica Spectrum Disorder

Antibody Status	Needed for Diagnosis
Aquaporin-4 positive	1 Core clinical characteristic, exclusion of alternative diagnosis
Aquaporin-4 negative	2 Core clinical characteristics with the following criteria: a One characteristic must be either ON, LETM, or area postrema syndrome b Dissemination in space of 2 core characteristics c Fulfillment of MRI criteria, which includes involvement of more than one-half of the optic nerve in ON, LETM extending of ≥3 segments, and additional requirements for area postrema and brainstem syndrome

Abbreviations: LETM, longitudinally extensive transverse myelitis; ON, optic neuritis.

Of note, patients with pediatric NMO-SD are more likely to have coexisting autoimmune conditions, such as autoimmune thyroid disease, systemic lupus erythematosus, and Sjogren's syndrome (**Fig. 3**).[1]

Diagnostic laboratory tests and imaging

Serum studies should include testing for AQP-4 antibodies and anti-MOG antibodies.

CSF testing shows lymphocytic pleocytosis, often with a higher white count (>50 cells) than seen in CIS or multiple sclerosis. Elevated IgG index and oligoclonal banding can be seen in up to 30% of patients.[1]

Treatment

Treatment of acute attacks is discussed in **Box 1**. Of note, plasmapheresis is often initiated before IVIg in children with NMO-SD, as early initiation has shown improved outcomes in severe attacks in adult NMO-SD.[10]

Azathioprine, mycophenolate mofetil, and rituximab are commonly used first-line DMTs in NMO-SD and all have been found to reduce the rate of relapse in children.[15,16] New monoclonal antibody treatments such as tocilizumab, satralizumab, and eculizumab have shown efficacy in adult patients with NMO-SD and are sometimes used off-label in pediatric patients.

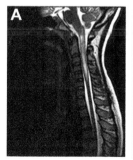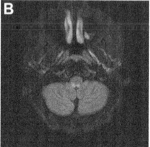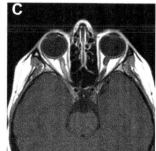

Fig. 3. Imaging from a patient with confirmed AQP-4 positive NMO-SD. (*A*) Sagittal FLAIR image shows LETM extending over greater than 3 segments in the cervical spinal cord. (*B*) Axial T2 FLAIR image shows a brainstem lesion associated with area postrema syndrome. (*C*) Sagittal T2 FLAIR image shows increased signal in the right optic nerve, consistent with ON.

Outcome

Pediatric NMO-SD is more active than POMS with a mean of 1.8 attacks in the first 2 years of disease and higher EDSS within 2 years of disease onset.[1]

MOG-RELATED DEMYELINATION

Anti-MOG antibodies are found in both monophasic and multiphasic demyelinating syndromes and commonly seen in patients with MDEM, ADEM-ON, relapsing ON, relapsing TM, and NMO-SD. Since anti-MOG testing has become available, positivity has been reported in 18% to 35% of children with acute demyelinating syndromes.[1,17]

The presence of anti-MOG antibodies suggests a non-MS disease course but otherwise offers limited insight into risk of relapse. Approximately 50% of patients found to have MOG antibodies follow a relapsing course and these relapses can occur within a few months or more than 10 years after the initial attack.[1]

Acute attacks are treated as discussed in **Box 1**.

Longer-term treatment in MOG-positive patients is typically initiated after the second attack or if patients meet criteria for NMO-SD. Treatment regimens include monthly IVIg, monthly high-dose steroids, mycophenolate mofetil, azathioprine, and rituximab. Optimal duration of treatment is unclear, however many centers suggest 2 years of treatment.[18]

IMMUNE-MEDIATED EPILEPSIES AND ENCEPHALOPATHIES

The link between epilepsy and neuroinflammation is one that has been studied for many years in the context of Rasmussen encephalitis (RE). More recently, epilepsy caused by antibody-mediated conditions (such as NMDA receptor encephalitis) and innate immunity-driven disorders such as FIRES has also been described. Of note, elevation in inflammatory markers has also been found in infantile spasms, suggesting that neuroinflammation plays some part in either the development or propagation of some epilepsy syndromes that were previously considered solely "genetic" in etiology.[19]

Autoimmune Encephalitis (Anti-NMDA Receptor Encephalitis)

Definition

Autoimmune encephalitis (AIE) is a group of disorders in which brain inflammation and dysfunction is caused by antibodies against neuronal receptors and cell surface proteins that are involved in neuronal excitability. Anti-NMDA receptor encephalitis is the most frequent form of AIE in the pediatric population and is the focus of this section.[20] AIE associated with other antibodies (such as anti-GAD and anti-VGKC) is exceedingly rare in the pediatric population and mostly found as a paraneoplastic disorder in adults.[20] Of note, Hashimoto encephalopathy, also known as steroid-responsive encephalopathy associated with autoimmune thyroiditis (SREAT), can have a similar clinical presentation and should be evaluated for in all suspected cases of AIE.[20]

Epidemiology

The California Encephalitis Project found that the frequency of anti-NMDA receptor encephalitis was greater than any single viral encephalitis, especially in younger patients, and more recent studies have confirmed a comparable prevalence to viral encephalitis.[21,22] Forty percent of all patients with anti-NMDA receptor encephalitis are younger than 18 years old.[9,20]

Pathophysiology
Anti-NMDA receptor antibodies are directed at the NR1 subunit of the NMDA receptor and cause selective crosslinking and internalization of NMDA receptors, leading to reduction in NMDA-mediated synaptic currents. In contrast to T-cell mediated processes, this does not lead to cell death and effects can be reversed once the antibody is no longer present.[8]

Clinical presentation
Clinical presentation varies based on the age of the patient. In older children, a prodromal phase of fever and headache is followed by onset of psychiatric and behavioral changes. This then progresses to decreased level of consciousness, seizures, movement disorders, and autonomic and vital sign instability. Children younger than 12 years tend to present with seizures, movement disorders, behavioral changes, and loss of speech or mutism.[20,23]

Anti-NMDA receptor encephalitis is associated with benign ovarian teratomas in up to 40% of young women. Testicular tumors are rarely found in male patients younger than 18 years. Anti-NMDA receptor encephalitis has also been reported to occur weeks or months after herpes simplex encephalitis.[24]

Diagnostic laboratory tests and imaging
Diagnosis is confirmed by demonstrating anti-NMDA receptor antibodies in the serum or CSF. MRI can be normal in 50% of patients. EEG typically shows diffuse background slowing and some may show prominent delta brush activity (faster frequencies admixed onto slower frequencies); the EEG can may also show electrographic seizures in approximately 60% of patients.[20]

Treatment
No definitive standard of treatment has been established, thus treatment is based on expert consensus. When teratoma is present, there is evidence that removal of the tumor and prompt immunotherapy leads to improved outcome. Children typically receive IV steroids and IVIg as first-line therapy with plasmapheresis reserved in most centers for cases with severe autonomic or vital sign instability. Increasingly, rituximab is being used after these treatments due to reports of efficacy and improved outcomes.[20,23]

Outcome
Patients with AIE often have prolonged hospital stays and need intensive inpatient rehabilitation. Eighty percent of patients are reported to have substantial or full recovery, although this recovery can take up to 2 years after initial presentation. Neurocognitive and psychiatric symptoms often linger, thus a multidisciplinary approach involving neurology, psychiatry, and cognitive rehabilitation is key to improving outcomes.

Clinical relapses occur in 12% of children and the efficacy of long-term immunosuppression in preventing relapses is not established.[20,25]

Challenge of seronegative autoimmune encephalitis
In patients with suspected AIE in whom no disease-causing antibody is found, the diagnosis of seronegative AIE can be made. Diagnostic criteria for seronegative AIE have been proposed and include presentation consistent with AIE, exclusion of other disorders, and evidence of CNS inflammation (ie, signal changes on MRI or CSF pleocytosis) (**Box 3**).[8,23]

> **Box 3**
> **Challenges of antibody testing in neuroinflammatory conditions[8]**
>
> The detection of specific antibodies has become more clinically relevant as more antibodies associated with neuroinflammatory conditions have been elucidated. However, it is equally important to be aware of the limitations of using the presence of an antibody to establish a definitive diagnosis. Anti-GAD antibodies, for example, can be found at lower titers in 1% of healthy people and up to 80% of those with type 1 diabetes. Only at high titers are anti-GAD antibodies associated with neurologic symptoms. Furthermore, the target antigens of these antibodies can have more than 1 subunit and antibodies against each of the subunits can have different clinical significance. For example, antibodies against the voltage-gated potassium channel complex (VGKC) itself are nonspecific and cannot be used to diagnose neuroinflammatory conditions. However, antibodies against 2 of its subunits, LGI and CASPR2 are pathogenic and associated with well-defined syndromes. Furthermore, patients can be dual seropositive for anti-NMDA receptor antibodies and either anti-myelin oligodendrocyte or anti-aquaporin-4 antibodies. Clinicians should be aware that overlapping demyelinating and autoimmune encephalitis syndromes can occur in these cases, and in patients with atypical features for either disease, one should consider evaluation for the other.[9]

Febrile Infection-Related Epilepsy Syndrome

Definition
Febrile infection-related epilepsy syndrome (FIRES) is a rare condition characterized by onset of refractory status epilepticus in a previously healthy child following a febrile illness.

Epidemiology
The estimated prevalence of FIRES is 1:1,000,000 and it occurs primarily in school-aged children with a median age of onset of 8 years.[26]

Clinical presentation
Children with FIRES have a routine febrile illness that is followed by new onset of seizures without any concomitant neurologic changes. The seizures evolve into status epilepticus, refractory to even anesthetic agents. Patients universally require ICU level care due to need for airway management secondary to status epilepticus and the large doses of anti-epileptics and sedatives that are used to treat the seizures. After this acute phase of refractory status epilepticus resolves, patients enter the chronic phase of FIRES, which is characterized by severe neurocognitive impairment and drug-resistant epilepsy.[26]

Pathophysiology
Given the close temporal relationship to febrile illness, FIRES is presumed to be an innate immune disorder triggered by infection. An intrathecal overproduction of proinflammatory and proconvulsant cytokines (such as interleukin-6) has been found in the CSF of children with FIRES, which likely elicits an explosive onset of epilepsy.[26,27]

Diagnostic laboratory tests and imaging
The diagnosis of FIRES is one of exclusion and initial workup should include infectious studies in both the serum and CSF, testing for autoimmune encephalitis including thyroid antibodies, metabolic studies, and consideration of whole-exome sequencing and mitochondrial next generation sequencing. CSF neopterin and cytokines can also be sent to aid in diagnosis, although their exact significant is unclear.[26]

Continuous EEG is used to guide therapeutic interventions, as well as to recognize nonconvulsive seizures.

MRI is often normal during the acute phase of FIRES but typically shows brain atrophy with hippocampal sclerosis within a month of seizure onset.[26]

Treatment
Following the failure of common anticonvulsants, IV pentobarbital and IV midazolam are used to obtain seizure control and often place patients in burst-suppression. The optimal length of burst-suppression is unknown and long periods of burst-suppression are associated with poorer neurocognitive outcomes (although this is likely also reflective of more severe disease).

Treatment with IV Steroids, IVIg, and plasmapheresis is often initiated due to concern for autoimmune encephalitis, although with limited response.[28]

Ketogenic diet has shown improved seizure control and improved neurocognitive outcomes in small groups of patients, thus is often initiated very quickly after the diagnosis of FIRES is suspected. Anakinra, an interleukin-1 receptor antagonist, has shown safety and efficacy in case reports and is being studied further in multicenter retrospective studies.[28]

Outcome
The acute phase of FIRES has a reported mortality rate of up to 60%. In reports of patients who did survive this acute phase, all were left with drug-resistant epilepsy and most with severe neurocognitive impairment. Ketogenic diet and potentially treatment with anakinra have shown some promise in improving neurocognitive outcomes.[26–28]

Rasmussen Encephalitis

Definition
RE is a progressive condition characterized by unihemispheric brain inflammation and eventual atrophy with resultant focal epilepsy, progressive hemiplegia, and cognitive decline.[29]

Epidemiology
RE is a rare condition with estimated incidence in studies ranging from 1.7 to 2.4 cases per 10 million people. The median age of onset is 6 years with no reported gender predominance.[29]

Pathophysiology
Histopathology in patients with RE shows unihemispheric cortical inflammation with neuronal loss and eventual gliosis. The trigger for the onset of inflammation has not been found despite extensive research into infectious agents and genetic changes that may predispose one to this type of immune response.[29]

Clinical presentation
Patients typically present with frequent focal seizures arising from one cerebral hemisphere and many have epilepsia partialis continua (EPC). If left untreated, children develop contralateral hemiparesis and cognitive decline within a year of onset of seizures. After this acute phase, there is a residual chronic phase of stable but severe motor and cognitive issues with refractory epilepsy.[29]

Diagnostic laboratory tests and imaging
No specific serum or CSF laboratory tests can make the diagnosis of RE; however, autoimmune encephalitis, CNS vasculitis, and neurologic manifestations of primary rheumatologic diseases should be ruled out to the best of the clinician's ability.

MRI is the mainstay for diagnosis of RE and typically within months of disease onset shows unilateral enlargement of the ventricular system with T2 FLAIR signal in the affected cortical or subcortical regions. Serial MRIs show progressive signal change and continued atrophy. Functional studies using fludeoxyglucose F-PET can show unilateral cerebral hypometabolism before MRI changes and can be helpful in making an early diagnosis.

EEG can show persistent high amplitude delta activity over the affected hemisphere within months of seizure onset. Epileptiform activity and seizures can be captured; however, EPC may not always have recognizable ictal EEG abnormalities.[29]

Treatment

Functional hemispherectomy remains the only curative option for the seizures associated with RE with studies showing improved cognitive outcomes with early intervention. Without surgical intervention, seizures, especially EPC, are refractory to medical management.

Case reports have shown positive outcomes with long-term corticosteroids, IVIg, tacrolimus, and rituximab; however, these treatments need to be studied in larger groups of patients to assess outcomes more effectively.[29]

Outcome

Outcome in RE depends on several factors, including severity of initial presentation, involvement of dominant versus nondominant hemisphere, and time to definitive treatment with surgical intervention.[29]

Opsoclonus Myoclonus Ataxia Syndrome

Definition

Opsoclonus myoclonus ataxia (OMA) is an immune-mediated encephalopathy with acute onset of neurologic deficits, often in the setting of neuroblastoma.

Epidemiology

In children, OMA typically develops in the first 2 years of life, with a mean age at presentation of 20 months.[30]

Pathophysiology

OMA is presumed to be an autoimmune condition due to rapid development of symptoms, findings of B-cell activation in the CSF, and response to immunotherapy, although no specific antibody has been found.[20] Fifty percent of pediatric patients with OMA have an underlying neural crest tumor, and it is postulated that there may be a common brain/neuroblastoma antigen that leads to CNS inflammation.[30]

Clinical presentation

Previously healthy, typically developing children present with new-onset ataxia, myoclonus, and opsoclonus, although presence of all 3 is not required for diagnosis. Children can develop gait failure and lose the ability to sit up due to ataxia. Speech regression and severe irritability with sleep disturbances are reported.[20,30]

Diagnostic laboratory tests and imaging

Although there is no specific marker for OMA, antibody panel testing for autoimmune encephalitis in the serum and CSF as well as routine CSF studies should be performed. In patients with suspected OMA, investigation for underlying neuroblastoma should include MRI of the chest/abdomen/pelvis, urinary catecholamine metabolites, and radiolabeled iodine scintigraphy (MIBG scan). If tumor is not identified at time of diagnosis, it is recommended to repeat testing for neuroblastoma in 6 months.[30]

Treatment and outcome

Early diagnosis and combination therapy with corticosteroid, IVIg, and rituximab has showed improvement in developmental outcome. Treatment often improves opsoclonus, myoclonus, and ataxia symptoms; however, patients can be left with residual cognitive, speech/language, and behavioral deficits, especially if treatment is delayed. Relapses are reported to occur in approximately 50% of patients, often in the setting of infections or tapering immunosuppression.[20,30,31]

CENTRAL NERVOUS SYSTEM MANIFESTATIONS OF RHEUMATOLOGIC DISEASE

Many primary rheumatologic diseases have associated neurologic complications, the most prevalent being systemic lupus erythematosus (SLE). SLE is an autoimmune condition that affects the joints, kidneys, skin, and bone marrow. Neuropsychiatric SLE syndromes (NPSLE) are reported in 20% to 95% of pediatric patients with SLE (15%–81% with neuropsychiatric manifestations at diagnosis) and are associated with higher morbidity and mortality.[32,33] Common neurologic issues include seizures, ischemic stroke, and psychosis. Subacute headaches, mood changes, and cognitive issues are also reported.[32] The pathophysiology of NPSLE involves small-vessel vasculopathy and thrombosis as well as parenchymal damage related to antineuronal antibodies and complement/cytokine mediated inflammation. Antiphospholipid antibodies (APL), which are found in most children with SLE, are associated with small-vessel vasculopathy, ischemic strokes, and focal CNS inflammation.[32] Treatment of pediatric NPSLE typically involves escalating immunosuppression for treatment of underlying SLE. Medications used include monthly cyclophosphamide for 6 months, rituximab, and oral steroids. Anticoagulation is added in cases complicated by thromboses.[33,34]

CNS infection and posterior reversible encephalopathy syndrome should also be considered in pediatric patients with SLE with neurologic dysfunction, given the use of immunosuppressive medications and chronic steroid use.[33,34]

Other less common pediatric rheumatologic conditions, such as Behcet syndrome, sarcoidosis, Sjogren syndrome, macrophage activation syndrome related to juvenile idiopathic arthritis, and monogenic autoinflammatory syndromes (such as periodic fever syndromes), also can present with neurologic complications and should be considered in patients with systemic symptoms, multi-organic involvement, and neurologic disease.

CENTRAL NERVOUS SYSTEM VASCULITIS

CNS vasculitis is an inflammatory disease involving the cerebral vasculature that can cause neurologic deficits and psychiatric disease in previously healthy children. CNS vasculitis can occur secondary to an underlying systemic illness, such as infection (mycobacterium tuberculosis, varicella zoster), rheumatologic disease (SLE, systemic vasculidities), or related to malignancy/radiation treatment of malignancy. CNS vasculitis in which no systemic illness or condition that can cause vasculitis is found is called childhood primary angiitis of the central nervous system (cPACNS).[35] Diagnostic criteria for primary angiitis were first proposed by Calabrese in adult patients and these have since been adapted for pediatric patients. cPACNS can be further classified into 3 subtypes, which are discussed in **Table 2**. There have been no large clinical trials to guide the care of children with cPACNS, thus treatment regimens are based on expert opinion (**Fig. 4**).[35–37]

Table 2
Classification of childhood primary angiitis of the central nervous system

Subtype/ Vessel Involvement	Clinical Presentation	Diagnostic Studies	Disease Course	Treatment
Nonprogressive large-medium vessel	Sudden-onset focal neurologic deficits Male>female	MRI with unilateral ischemic lesions in large vessel territories MRA with enhancement of vessels Angiography with unilateral stenoses, dilatations of the proximal segments of ACA, MCA, ICA	No progression/new vascular territory involvement after 3 mo (reclassified as progressive if this occurs)	Anti-thrombotic therapy-heparin X 3–6 mo followed by long-term aspirin Use of steroids is controversial
Progressive large-medium vessel	Focal and diffuse (headaches, cognitive dysfunction, mood changes) deficits Male > female	Increased inflammatory markers (ESR, CRP, WBC) MRI lesions in more than 1 vascular territory, some bilateral Anterior >posterior circulation involvement Angiography with stenoses, dilatations of the proximal segments of ACA, MCA, ICA	New stenoses on angiography beyond 3 mo of disease Patients typically have residual focal neurologic deficits	High-dose IV steroids × 3–5 d followed by oral steroids IV monthly cyclophosphamide pulses × 6 mo followed by mycophenolate mofetil or azathioprine
Small vessel	Seizures, movement disorders, diffuse neurologic and psychiatric deficits Female>male	Increased CSF cell count/protein MRI with inflammatory lesions (less commonly ischemic), leptomeningeal enhancement Normal MRA and angiography, brain biopsy with evidence of vascular inflammation often needed for diagnosis	Most with good recovery of neurologic deficits, can have continued seizures with need for long-term anti-epileptics	High-dose IV steroids × 3–5 d followed by oral steroids IV monthly cyclophosphamide pulses × 6 mo followed by mycophenolate mofetil or azathioprine

Abbreviations: ACA, anterior cerebral artery; CRP, C-reactive protein; CSF, cerebrospinal fluid; ESR, erythrocyte sedimentation rate; ICA, internal carotid artery; IV, intravenous; MCA, middle cerebral artery; WBC, white blood cells.

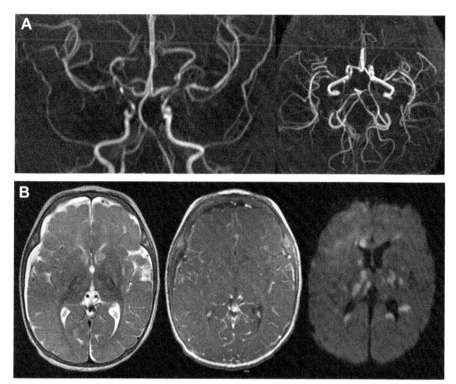

Fig. 4. (*A*) Coronal and axial MRA in a case of CNS vasculitis. A significant narrowing and irregularity is noted, affecting the distal internal carotid arteries bilaterally as well as the M1 and M2-segments of both middle cerebral arteries. (*B*) Axial T2 images show multi-focal, ill-defined T2-hyperintense lesions within the central gray matter, hemispheric white matter, and cortical gray matter bilaterally. Most of the T2-hyperintense lesions are more conspicuous on diffusion-weighted imaging (DWI) and reveal imaging character-istics compatible with cytotoxic edema (DWI-hyperintense). On the contrast-enhanced sequence, mild diffuse leptomeningeal enhancement is noted as well as an increased vessel enhancement.

GENETIC CONDITIONS WITH IMMUNE-MEDIATED PATHOPHYSIOLOGY

As the genetic basis of more neurologic disorders is found, many are found to have inflammatory pathophysiology with potential for treatment with immunomodulators. Aicardi-Goutieres, for example, is a monogenic type 1 interferonopathy with causative genetic mutations in the intracellular signaling machinery (TREX1 and RNASEH2A/2B/2C). This leads to overproduction of interferon, which in turn causes progressive en-cephalopathy characterized by intracranial calcifications, white matter disease, and CSF lymphocytosis. Systemic interferon overproduction causes skin lesions, glau-coma, hypothyroidism, and lupuslike disease. Patients can present with neurologic abnormalities at birth or in early childhood and severity of disease varies based on gene involvement, though phenotype can vary even within families.[38] JAK kinase in-hibitors are useful in blocking interferon activation in these patients and an open-label study with baricitinib showed decreased skin inflammation and improved devel-opmental abilities in a small group of patients (**Fig. 5**).[39]

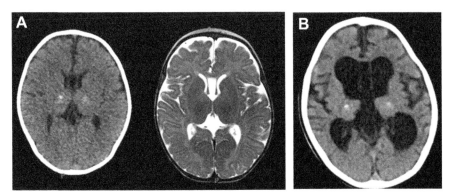

Fig. 5. (*A*) Axial non–contrast-enhanced computed tomography (CT) and matching axial T2-weighted MR images of a 5-year-old boy with confirmed Aicardi-Goutieres syndrome. Subtle hyperdense calcifications are noted within the bilateral thalami. The calcifications are barely visible as T2-signal alterations on the matching MRI. (*B*) Follow-up non–contrast-enhanced CT 2 years later shows progressive, global white matter volume loss with ex vacuo widening of the ventricular system and mild widening of the subarachnoid space.

SUMMARY

In conclusion, pediatric neuroinflammatory diseases encompass a wide range of disorders with varying clinical presentations, underlying pathophysiology, and treatments. Prompt evaluation for these conditions, with multidisciplinary involvement, should be initiated when neuroinflammation is suspected, as many are treatable with immunomodulating medications.

CLINICS CARE POINTS

- Clinical presentation of neuroinflammatory diseases can include encephalopathy/behavioral changes, seizures, focal neurologic deficits, or movement disorders.

- A multidisciplinary approach involving neurology, rheumatology, ophthalmology, psychiatry, and neuropsychology is critical to the diagnosis and management of children with neuroinflammatory conditions.

- Clinicians must exercise caution when interpreting results of antibody testing and should be aware of the possibility of overlapping neuroinflammatory syndromes.

DISCLOSURE

The authors have nothing to disclose.

REFERENCES

1. Chitnis T. Pediatric central nervous system demyelinating diseases. Continuum (Minneap Minn) 2019;25(3):793–814.
2. Pohl D, Alper G, Van Haren K, et al. Acute disseminated encephalomyelitis: updates on an inflammatory CNS syndrome. Neurology 2016;87(9 Suppl 2):S38–45.
3. Bar-Or A, Hintzen RQ, Dale RC, et al. Immunopathophysiology of pediatric CNS inflammatory demyelinating diseases. Neurology 2016;87(9 Suppl 2):S12–9.
4. Aubert-Broche B, Weier K, Longoni G, et al. Monophasic demyelination reduces brain growth in children. Neurology 2017;88(18):1744–50.

5. Papetti L, Figà Talamanca L, Spalice A, et al. Predictors of evolution into multiple sclerosis after a first acute demyelinating syndrome in children and adolescents. Front Neurol 2019;9:1156.

6. Iaffaldano P, Simone M, Lucisano G, et al. Prognostic indicators in pediatric clinically isolated syndrome. Ann Neurol 2017;81(5):729–39.

7. Metz LM. Clinically isolated syndrome and early relapsing multiple sclerosis. Continuum (Minneap Minn) 2019;25(3):670–88.

8. Dalmau J. NMDA receptor encephalitis and other antibody-mediated disorders of the synapse: the 2016 Cotzias Lecture. Neurology 2016;87(23):2471–82.

9. Erickson TA, Muscal E, Munoz FM, et al. Infectious and autoimmune causes of encephalitis in children. Pediatrics 2020;145(6):e20192543.

10. Srisupa-Olan T, Siritho S, Kittisares K, et al. Beneficial effect of plasma exchange in acute attack of neuromyelitis optica spectrum disorders. Mult Scler Relat Disord 2018;20:115–21.

11. Amato MP, Goretti B, Ghezzi A, et al. Neuropsychological features in childhood and juvenile multiple sclerosis: five-year follow-up. Neurology 2014;83(16):1432–8.

12. Krysko KM, Graves J, Rensel M, et al. Use of newer disease-modifying therapies in pediatric multiple sclerosis in the US. Neurology 2018;91(19):e1778–87.

13. Chitnis T, Ghezzi A, Bajer-Kornek B, et al. Pediatric multiple sclerosis: escalation and emerging treatments. Neurology 2016;87(9 Suppl 2):S103–9.

14. Fay AJ, Mowry EM, Strober J, et al. Relapse severity and recovery in early pediatric multiple sclerosis. Mult Scler 2012;18(7):1008–12.

15. Paolilo RB, Hacohen Y, Yazbeck E, et al. Treatment and outcome of aquaporin-4 antibody-positive NMOSD: a multinational pediatric study. Neurol Neuroimmunol Neuroinflamm 2020;7(5):e837.

16. Gombolay GY, Chitnis T. Pediatric neuromyelitis optica spectrum disorders. Curr Treat Options Neurol 2018;20(6):19.

17. Fernandez-Carbonell C, Vargas-Lowy D, Musallam A, et al. Clinical and MRI phenotype of children with MOG antibodies. Mult Scler 2016;22(2):174–84.

18. Hacohen Y, Banwell B. Treatment approaches for MOG-Ab-associated demyelination in children. Curr Treat Options Neurol 2019 Jan 22;21(1):2.

19. Pardo CA, Nabbout R, Galanopoulou AS. Mechanisms of epileptogenesis in pediatric epileptic syndromes: rasmussen encephalitis, infantile spasms, and febrile infection-related epilepsy syndrome (FIRES). Neurotherapeutics 2014;11(2):297–310.

20. Armangue T, Petit-Pedrol M, Dalmau J. Autoimmune encephalitis in children. J Child Neurol 2012;27(11):1460–9.

21. Gable MS, Sheriff H, Dalmau J, et al. The frequency of autoimmune N-methyl-D-aspartate receptor encephalitis surpasses that of individual viral etiologies in young individuals enrolled in the California Encephalitis Project. Clin Infect Dis 2012;54(7):899–904.

22. Dubey D, Pittock SJ, Kelly CR, et al. Autoimmune encephalitis epidemiology and a comparison to infectious encephalitis. Ann Neurol 2018;83(1):166–77.

23. Graus F, Titulaer MJ, Balu R, et al. A clinical approach to diagnosis of autoimmune encephalitis. Lancet Neurol 2016;15(4):391–404.

24. Armangue T, Spatola M, Vlagea A, et al. Frequency, symptoms, risk factors, and outcomes of autoimmune encephalitis after herpes simplex encephalitis: a prospective observational study and retrospective analysis. Lancet Neurol 2018;17(9):760–72.

25. Titulaer MJ, McCracken L, Gabilondo I, et al. Treatment and prognostic factors for long-term outcome in patients with anti-NMDA receptor encephalitis: an observational cohort study. Lancet Neurol 2013;12(2):157–65.

26. van Baalen A, Vezzani A, Häusler M, et al. Febrile infection-related epilepsy syndrome: clinical review and hypotheses of epileptogenesis. Neuropediatrics 2017; 48(1):5–18.

27. Gaspard N, Hirsch LJ, Sculier C, et al. New-onset refractory status epilepticus (NORSE) and febrile infection-related epilepsy syndrome (FIRES): state of the art and perspectives. Epilepsia 2018;59(4):745–52.

28. Kenney-Jung DL, Vezzani A, Kahoud RJ, et al. Febrile infection-related epilepsy syndrome treated with anakinra. Ann Neurol 2016;80(6):939–45.

29. Varadkar S, Bien CG, Kruse CA, et al. Rasmussen's encephalitis: clinical features, pathobiology, and treatment advances. Lancet Neurol 2014;13(2):195–205.

30. Pike M. Opsoclonus-myoclonus syndrome. Handb Clin Neurol 2013;112: 1209–11.

31. Pranzatelli MR, Tate ED. Dexamethasone, intravenous immunoglobulin, and rituximab combination immunotherapy for pediatric opsoclonus-myoclonus syndrome. Pediatr Neurol 2017;73:48–56.

32. Muscal E, Myones BL. The role of autoantibodies in pediatric neuropsychiatric systemic lupus erythematosus. Autoimmun Rev 2007;6(4):215–7.

33. Schwartz N, Stock AD, Putterman C. Neuropsychiatric lupus: new mechanistic insights and future treatment directions. Nat Rev Rheumatol 2019;15(3):137–52.

34. Gorman M, Muscal E. Immune- and inflammatory-mediated central nervous system syndromes in: Mark Kline. In: Rudolph's pediatrics, Vol 1, 23rd edition. USA: McGraw Hill; 2018.

35. Gowdie P, Twilt M, Benseler SM. Primary and secondary central nervous system vasculitis. J Child Neurol 2012;27(11):1448–59.

36. Twilt M, Benseler SM. CNS vasculitis in children. Mult Scler Relat Disord 2013; 2(3):162–71.

37. Beelen J, Benseler SM, Dropol A, et al. Strategies for treatment of childhood primary angiitis of the central nervous system. Neurol Neuroimmunol Neuroinflamm 2019;6(4):e567.

38. Adang LA, Gavazzi F, Jawad AF, et al. Development of a neurologic severity scale for Aicardi Goutières syndrome. Mol Genet Metab 2020;130(2):153–60.

39. Vanderver A, Adang L, Gavazzi F, et al. Janus kinase inhibition in the Aicardi-Goutières syndrome. N Engl J Med 2020;383(10):986–9.

Pediatric Neuro-Oncology

Fatema Malbari, MD

KEYWORDS

- Pediatric brain tumors • Gliomas • Medulloblastoma • ATRT • Ependymoma
- Craniopharyngioma • Cancer predisposition syndromes

KEY POINTS

- Central nervous system (CNS) tumors are the most common solid tumor in pediatrics and represent the largest cause of childhood cancer–related mortality.
- With the advances in molecular characterization of tumors considerable developments have occurred impacting diagnosis, management and refining prognostication of pediatric CNS tumors.
- Therapeutic approaches targeting the biology of these tumors are being investigated to improve overall survival and decrease treatment-related morbidity.

INTRODUCTION

Central nervous system (CNS) tumors are the most common solid tumor in pediatrics and represent the largest cause of childhood cancer–related mortality.[1] The incidence of CNS tumors in children and young adults, 0 to 19 years of age, is 6.06 per 100,000 population. Gliomas are the most common tumor histology reported in this age group and embryonal tumors have the highest incidence in children 0 to 4 years of age. Pituitary and craniopharyngeal duct tumors are the most common tumor location. The different pediatric CNS tumor types by histology and location are shown in **Fig. 1**. Risk factors for developing these tumors remain unknown aside from prior ionizing radiation exposure and genetic predisposition syndromes, such as neurofibromatosis (NF), tuberous sclerosis (TSC), Li Fraumeni syndrome (LFS), Gorlin syndrome, familial adenomatous polyposis (FAP) syndrome, and constitutional mismatch repair deficiency (CMMRD).

With the advances in molecular characterization of tumors, considerable advances have occurred in the field of pediatric neuro-oncology.[2] The understanding of the biology has impacted diagnosis and management, and refined prognostication of pediatric CNS tumors. Advances in management have led to better survival, but mortality remains high and significant morbidity persists. Patients often have deficits from the

Department of Pediatrics, Division of Pediatric Neurology and Developmental Neurosciences, Texas Children's Hospital, Baylor College of Medicine, 6701 Fannin Street, Suite 1250, Houston, TX 77030, USA
E-mail address: malbari@bcm.edu

Neurol Clin 39 (2021) 829–845
https://doi.org/10.1016/j.ncl.2021.04.005
neurologic.theclinics.com

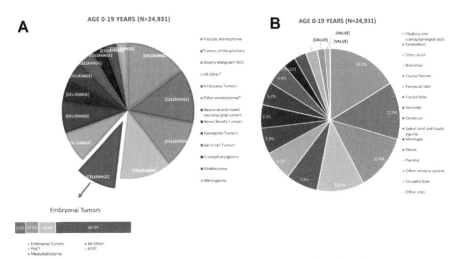

Fig. 1. Distribution in children and young adults (0–19 years of age) with primary CNS tumors based on (*A*) histology and (*B*) location from the Central Brain Tumor Registry in the United States. [a] All others include oligodendrogliomas, including anaplastic oligodendrogliomas, other neuroepithelial tumors, tumors of the pineal region, choroid plexus tumors, other tumors of cranial and spinal nerves, other tumors of the meninges, hemangioma, mesenchymal tumors, melanocytic lesions, hematopoietic neoplasms, and neoplasms unspecified. [b] Other astrocytomas includes diffuse astrocytoma, anaplastic astrocytoma and astrocytoma variants. [c] All other embryonal tumors include ICD-O3 histology codes 8963/3, 9364/3, 9480/0, 9480/3, 9490/0, 9490/3, 9500/3, 9501/3, 9502/3. (*Modified from* Ostrom, Q., Cioffi, G., Gittleman, H., Patil, N., Waite, K., Kruchko, C. and Barnholtz-Sloan, J., 2019. CBTRUS Statistical Report: Primary Brain and Other Central Nervous System Tumors Diagnosed in the United States in 2012–2016. Neuro-Oncology, 21(Supplement_5), pp.v1-v100.)

tumor or secondary to therapy. These include neurocognitive impairment, neuroendocrine dysfunction, and focal neurologic deficits, such as seizures; cranial nerve, motor, or sensory deficits; ataxia; and stroke. Molecular profiling of tumors has become incorporated in the most recent World Health Organization (WHO) 2016 classification and novel therapeutic approaches targeting the biology of these tumors are being investigated to improve overall survival (OS) and decrease treatment-related morbidity.[3] Further molecular understanding of pediatric CNS tumors will lead to continued refinement of tumor classification, management, and prognostication.

LOW-GRADE GLIOMA

Low-grade gliomas (LGG), the most common pediatric CNS tumor, represent 30% to 40% of all CNS tumors.[4,5] Histologically LGGs (WHO grade I and II) are composed of both astrocytic and mixed glial-neuronal tumors, with PA being the most common of all LGGs. Other histologies include pilomyxoid astrocytoma, pleomorphic xanthroastrocytoma (PXA), diffuse astrocytoma, ganglioma, dysembryoplastic neuroepithelial tumor (DNET), and subependymal giant cell astrocytoma (SEGA).[6] Clinical presentation is dependent on tumor location, which can arise anywhere in the CNS. Cortical tumors typically manifest with focal neurologic deficits, seizures, and headache. Cerebellar signs and increased intracranial pressure are most commonly seen with tumors in the posterior fossa. Diencephalic tumors can present with failure to thrive. Although LGGs are often localized, approximately 5% of patients at initial diagnosis and up to 12% of patients at time of progression will have disseminated disease.[7]

Management of LGG is dependent on tumor location and age of the patient. Gross total resection (GTR) can be curative and patients can be followed with serial imaging, with a low risk of recurrence, 5-year posterior fossa syndrome (PFS) of 94%.[8] Subtotal resection is also beneficial as tumors can become quiescent for extended periods. For patients in whom surgical resection cannot be achieved or if LGGs are progressive, chemotherapy, radiation, and targeted therapy are other treatment options with 10-year OS reported at approximately 90%.[9] Patients with residual or progressive disease often have a decrease in quality of life (QOL) due to the chronic nature of the disease and associated morbidity from the tumor and treatment. Radiation therapy (RT) can achieve comparable results, with 5-year PFS and OS of 87% and 96%, respectively.[9] However, due to potential adverse effects from RT, including neurocognitive effects, vasculopathies, secondary malignancies, endocrine and growth deficiencies, radiation is often reserved for children older than 10 in whom neurocognitive effects are not as significant, in children who have exhausted multiple treatment options, or in patients in whom RT may cause the least toxicity.[10] For these reasons, chemotherapy is usually the preferred treatment option when GTR is not feasible, although this may change with the recent advances in molecular characterization of pediatric CNS tumors and the availability of targeted therapy. Chemotherapy is not as effective as surgery or radiation but can achieve approximately 50% PFS at 5 years.[11,12] The most common chemotherapy regimens used are carboplatin and vincristine or single-agent vinblastine.

Pediatric LGG (pLGG) molecular alterations involve the RAS-MAPK pathway, with most involving the *BRAF* oncogene[13–19] (**Table 1**). In 70% to 80% of pediatric PAs, there is a tandem duplication on chromosome 7q34 resulting in a *BRAF-KIAA1549* fusion, which is almost universally found in midline and infratentorial PAs.[5] The other common alteration seen in 15% to 20% of pLGGs is a *BRAF* V600E mutation, which is frequently found in supratentorial hemispheric PAs, PXAs, gangliogliomas, and DNETs.[20] It suggests a poorer prognosis with an increased risk of tumor progression.[4,20] IDH mutations often observed in adults with LGG infrequently occur in adolescents with diffuse astrocytomas and the clinical significance in this population remains unclear. MAP/ERK kinase (MEK) inhibitors and BRAF inhibitors have shown promising results in patients with these alterations.[9,14] Results from phase I and II clinical trials using MEK and BRAF inhibitors in patients with recurrent or refractory pLGG has led to the development of upfront phase III clinical trials randomizing standard of care chemotherapy to these targeted therapies in patients with newly diagnosed or previously untreated pLGG with BRAF fusion alterations (NCT04166409) or mutations (NCT02684058).[21,22]

Patients with NF1 AND TSC have an increased risk of developing pLGGc (**Table 2**). PA of the optic pathway can occur in 15% to 20% of patients with NF1.[23–26] Treatment for symptomatic tumors are similar to non NF-1 PAs, with chemotherapy as the first option because surgery is generally not feasible and RT can cause an increased risk for secondary malignancies and vasculopathy; it is therefore reserved for patients with progressive tumors who have exhausted other therapeutic options. Targeted therapy with MEK inhibitors has shown promising results leading to a phase III clinical trial randomizing standard of care chemotherapy versus a MEK inhibitor (NCT03871257).[9] SEGAs can occur in 20% of patients with TSC. If a patient is symptomatic with acute focal neurologic deficits or obstructive hydrocephalus, surgical resection is indicated. Otherwise, targeted therapy with mammalian target of rapamycin inhibitors is recommended for unresectable tumors or multisystem involvement of TSC.[25,27,28]

Table 1
Molecular alterations of specific pediatric central nervous system tumors

Tumor	Molecular Alterations
Low-grade glioma	*BRAF* KIAA1549 fusion, *BRAF* V600E
	FGFR1
	NTRK
	MYB, MYBL1
	CDKN2A/B
	IDH
	NF1
	TSC1/2
High-grade glioma	H3.1 and H3.3 K27M, H3.3 G34R/V
Diffuse intrinsic pontine glioma	*IDH1, IDH2, MYCN, PDGFRA, EGFR, BRAF* V600E, *TP53, NF1, ATRX*
	PI3-kinase/Akt/mTOR
	H3.1 and H3.3 K27M, *ACVR1, PDGFRA, MYCN, ID2*
	PI3-kinase/Akt/mTOR
Medulloblastoma	Monosomy 6, *CTNNB1, TP53, DDX3X, APC* and *SMARCA4*
Wingless	*PTCH1, SUFU, SMO, GLI1, GLI2, TP53, PI3K, MYCN, TERT,* loss
Sonic hedgehog (SHH)	of chromosome 9q and 10q
Group 3	*MYC, MYCN, OTX2, SMARCA4, KBTBD4, CTDNEP1, KMT2D,*
Group 4	*GFI1, GFI1B*
	Isochromosome 17q gain of chromosomes 1q and 7, loss of
	chromosomes 8, 10q and 16q
	KDM6A, ZMYM3, KMT2C (MML3), MYCN, CDK6, OTX2
	isochromosome 17
	Gain of chromosome 7, 17
	Loss of chromosomes 8, 11 and 17 p
Atypical teratoid rhabdoid tumors (ATRT)	*SMARCB1, SMARCA4,SMARCB4*
ATRT-SHH	
ATRT-MYC	
ATRT-TYP	
Ependymoma	*C11ORF95-RELA, YAP1, CDKN2A/B* loss of either 9p or the
Supratentorial (excluding subependymoma)	entire chromosome 9
	CXorf67, Gain of chromosome 1q, histone 3 variants (H3.1
Posterior Fossa-A	and H3.3 K27M)
Posterior Fossa-B	Loss of chromosome 6 and 13q
Craniopharyngioma	*CTNNB1*
Adamantinomatous	*BRAF* V600E
Papillary	

HIGH-GRADE GLIOMA

High-grade gliomas (pHGG) in children represent approximately 15% to 20% of pediatric CNS tumors. These include anaplastic astrocytoma (WHO grade III), glioblastoma (WHO grade IV) and diffuse intrinsic pontine glioma (DIPG). Other less common histologies include anaplastic PXA, anaplastic ganglioglioma, and pilocytic astrocytoma with anaplasia. Despite advances in management, it still has a poor outcome, with OS at 5 years less than 20%.[29] Clinical presentation is dependent on tumor location. Patients can present with signs of increased intracranial pressure or focal neurologic deficits. Seizures are less common in pHGG.

Management of pHGG is maximal safe surgical resection followed by focal RT. The extent of resection is a predictor of overall outcome, with near to GTR associated with

Table 2

Hereditary cancer predisposition syndromes associated with central nervous system (CNS) tumors

Cancer Predisposition Syndrome	Germline Mutation	CNS Tumor Type
Neurofibromatosis 1	Chromosome 17q11, *NF1*	Pilocytic astrocytoma Low-grade glioma
Tuberous sclerosis	Chromosome 9q34, *TSC1* Chromosome 16p13, *TSC2*	Subependymal giant cell astrocytoma, Low-grade glioma
Gorlin syndrome	Chromosome 9q22, *PTCH1* chromosome 10q24, *SUFU*	Medulloblastoma, SHH subgroup
Constitutional mismatch repair deficiency	Biallelic mutations mismatch repair genes:	High-grade glioma
Lynch syndrome	Chromosome 7p22, *PMS2* Chromosome 3p22, *MLH1* Chromosomes 2p21–16, *MSH2* Chromosome 2p16, *MSH6* Monoallelic mutations in mismatch repair genes	
Familial adenomatous polyposis syndrome (Turcot syndrome 2)	Chromosome 5q21–22, *APC*	Medulloblastoma, WNT subgroup
Li Fraumeni Syndrome	Chromosome 17p13, *TP53*	High-grade glioma, choroid plexus carcinomas, medulloblastoma SHH subgroup
Neurofibromatosis 2	Chromosome 22q12, *NF2*	Ependymoma, meningioma, schwannoma

a greater than 5-year PFS.[30,31] Infants and very young children with HGG have better OS outcomes than older children.[32,33] Multiple chemotherapy regimens have been tried in pHGG without any significant improvement in OS.[14,34–36] Molecular profiling of pHGG has identified potential targetable therapeutic options that are currently being investigated.

Molecular characterization of pHGG has led to the discovery of unique characteristics that separate these tumors from adult HGG and has allowed for further subgrouping.[14,18] pHGGs have a novel oncogenic mutation in histone 3 variants including H3.1 K27M and H3.3 K27M as well as H3.3 G34R/V (see **Table 1**). The H3.1 and H3.3 K27M mutation are classically seen in diffuse midline HGGs.[14] Within the K27M mutated pHGG, the H3.3 K 27M mutation can be seen in all midline HGGs and in most DIPG tumors and is associated with a poorer outcome, whereas the H3.1 K27M mutation is unique to DIPG, frequently co-occurs with an *ACVR1* mutation, and portends a slightly better prognosis. H3.3 G34R/V mutations are seen in up to a third of hemispheric HGGs. As opposed to adult HGG, less than 5% of pHGGs have somatic mutations in *IDH1* or *IDH2*.[14,29,37–40] pHGG with wild-type Histone 3 and *IDH1/2* GBM can be subdivided further into 3 additional groups: (1) receptor tyrosine kinase, (2) mesenchymal, and (3) PXA-like, distinguished by *BRAF* V600E mutation and deletion of *CKDN2A*.[14,18,37,39] PXA-like pHGG, which represents 5% to 10% of pHGGs, have *BRAF* V600E mutations similar to LGGs and tend to have a better prognosis with slightly prolonged survival. They can be treated with targeted BRAF inhibitors.[14,29,39]

The discovery of these somatic mutations in pHGG has led to clinical trials using targeted agents to different molecular alterations. Histone deacetylate inhibitors, dopamine receptor 2 antagonist, and GD2 chimeric antigen therapy are being investigated in H3K27M mutated tumors (NCT02717455, NCT04196413, NCT03416530, NCT04099797).[41–43] Tyrosine kinase inhibitors targeting epidermal growth factor receptor, platelet-derived growth factor receptor, vascular endothelial growth factor receptor, and c-met are being explored in addition to PD-1 inhibitors for hypermutant gliomas.[20] Other treatment options include immune therapy using vaccines with glioma-associated antibodies and other different delivery approaches of novel agents to bypass the blood brain barrier (intra-arterial, convection enhanced delivery, intranasal, intracavitary).[29]

Diffuse Midline Glioma and Diffuse Intrinsic Pontine Glioma

Diffuse midline gliomas are a distinct entity of pHGG, with most of these tumors arising in the pons (DIPG). Other common locations include the thalamus and spinal cord. DIPG typically occurs in school-aged children and is universally fatal. Patients present with rapid onset of cranial nerve deficits, long tract signs, ataxia, and obstructive hydrocephalus in a third of patients. DIPGs are radiologically defined as an expansile diffusely infiltrative T1 hypointense and T2 hyperintense mass involving the pons.[44] Histologically, these tumors can be WHO grade II-IV but prognosis remains dismal, with median survival of 11 months.[45] Diagnosis is generally a combination of both clinical symptoms and radiographic appearance, although biopsies are being offered more routinely and are required for enrollment on some clinical trials. RT is standard of care and only provides transient relief of symptoms without any significant improvement in OS. Multiple therapeutic strategies have been investigated, including radiosensitizers and chemotherapy, but all have been ineffective.[46–48]

LFS, CMMRD, and Lynch syndrome are genetic cancer predisposition syndromes associated with the development of HGGs (see **Table 2**). Patients with LFS are predisposed to a variety of childhood malignancies including HGGs, choroid plexus carcinomas, and sonic hedgehog (SHH) medulloblastoma (MB).[29,49,50] Treatment is generally the standard therapy for sporadic cases. CMMRD and Lynch syndrome are associated with the development of glioblastoma. Patients with pHGG due to mismatch repair deficiencies are treated similar to patients with sporadic GBM but are often resistant to therapy. However, clinical responses have been seen to checkpoint inhibition.[14,29,49,51]

MEDULLOBLASTOMA

MB is the most common CNS embryonal tumor, representing approximately 64% of all pediatric embryonal tumors.[1,52] It generally arises from the cerebellum, can invade the fourth ventricle, and can present with CNS metastases in a third of patients at diagnosis. As part of tumor staging, patients will get an MRI of the spine and lumbar puncture for CSF cytology. Clinically, patients will present with symptoms concerning for increased intracranial pressure and cerebellar dysfunction.

Management of MB is initiated with maximal safe surgical resection followed by risk adapted craniospinal irradiation (CSI) and adjuvant chemotherapy in children older than 3 years. Risk stratification is based on age of the patient, extent of surgical resection, and the presence of metastatic disease. In patients with average-risk MB, defined as GTR with no evidence of metastatic disease, 5-year OS is approximately 80% in comparison with 60% for high-risk MB, defined as residual tumor measuring larger than 1.5 cm^2 and the presence of metastatic disease.[52] In general, patients with average-risk MB will receive 23.4 Gy CSI with a boost to the tumor bed of 54 Gy followed by chemotherapy consisting of a combination of cisplatin, carboplatin, vincristine, cyclophosphamide, and lomustine. Patients with high-risk MB will receive 36 Gy CSI with a boost to the tumor bed of 54 Gy followed by the same conventional chemotherapy. In infants with MB (younger than 3 years), radiation sparing therapy is the standard of care due to potential devastating effects; this often leads to inferior survival. Infants will receive myeloablative chemotherapy followed by autologous stem cell rescue (ASCR).

Treatment of MB is not without toxicity. Approximately 25% of patients develop PFS after surgical resection of MB.[53] PFS is a constellation of symptoms including emotional lability, paucity of speech (mutism), cerebellar syndrome, and cranial nerve dysfunction. The underlying mechanism for the development of this syndrome is not completely understood but is felt to be secondary to disruption of the dentate-rubro-thalamic pathway. Patients with posterior fossa syndrome will eventually have some recovery of speech and cerebellar dysfunction, but most without a full recovery. They also have significant neurocognitive impairment, worse than their counterparts with MB without posterior fossa syndrome.[53] CSI can cause neurocognitive impairment in patients with MB in addition to secondary malignancies, vasculopathy, and endocrine deficiencies. The conventional chemotherapy used for MB can cause neuropathy and ototoxicity. Because of these toxicities, MB survivors often have an increased risk of poor QOL. Molecular characterization of MB has allowed for identification of different prognostic groups and molecular risk stratification is now being incorporated into clinical management (**Table 3**). Previously, classification of medulloblastoma was dependent on histopathology; however, now DNA methylation profiling has identified 4 molecular subgroups of MB.[3] The 4 different subgroups are wingless (WNT), SHH, group 3, and group 4.[52,54–56]

The WNT subgroup represents 10% of all MBs and are typically seen in older children. These tumors are centrally located near the brainstem, are nonmetastatic, and most frequently have classic histology. Patients classified as the WNT subgroup have the best prognosis, with 5-year OS of 95%, and are stratified as low risk (see

Table 3
Clinical risk groups for medulloblastoma

Low-Risk 5-Year OS >90%	Intermediate-Risk 5-Year OS 75%–90%	High-Risk 5-Year OS <60%
WNT, M0, M+	SHH, *TP53* wild type	Group 3, *MYC* and non *MYC* amplified Group 3, M+
SHH, MBEN	SHH, not MBEN	SHH β/I
SHH γ/II	Group 4	SHH, *TP53* mutant
Group 4 with chromosome 11 loss or 17 gain		Group 4, M+

Abbreviations: M0, no evidence of metastases in MRI or CSF cytology; M1, microscopic tumor cells in CSF; M2, gross intracranial metastasis beyond primary site; M3, gross metastasis in subarachnoid space; M4, metastasis outside cerebrospinal axis; MBEN, medulloblastoma with extensive nodularity; OS, overall survival; SHH, sonic hedgehog.
Data from Northcott PA, Robinson GW, Kratz CP, et al. Medulloblastoma. Nature reviews. Disease primers. 2019;5(1):11.

Table 3).[57] Molecular alterations specific to WNT include monosomy 6 and a mutation in *CTNNB1* (**Fig. 2**; see **Table 1**).[56] *APC* mutations are often associated with FAP (see **Table 2**). De-escalation of therapy consisting of decreased doses of both CSI and chemotherapy are being investigated in this subgroup, given the overall excellent prognosis, in attempt to decrease toxicity and late effects.[52]

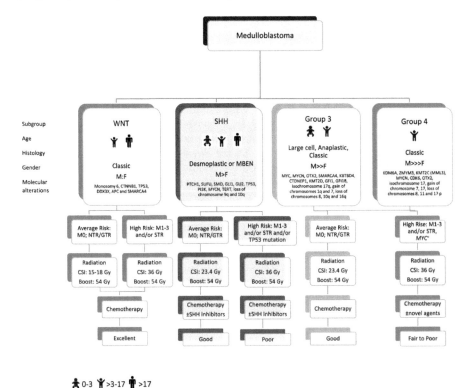

Fig. 2. MB subgroups and risk adapted management. (*Data from* Northcott PA, Robinson GW, Kratz CP, et al. Medulloblastoma. Nature reviews. Disease primers. 2019;5(1):11.)

The SHH subgroup accounts for approximately 30% of all MBs and has a bimodal age distribution, occurring more frequently in children younger than 3 or older than 16 years. These tumors usually arise from the cerebellar hemispheres and present with appendicular ataxia.[18] The most common histology seen is desmoplastic or MB with extensive nodularity.[18] SHH MB can be further categorized into 4 different subtypes: SHH β/I, SHH γ/II, SHHα, and SHHδ.[20,52,58] SHH β/I and SHH γ/II are the 2 predominant subtypes in infants. SHH β/I is associated with poorer outcomes, often with metastatic disease and molecularly have PTEN loss and SUFU mutations, whereas infants with SHH γ/II subtype have excellent outcomes and SMO mutations.[59] SHHα is the most common subtype in older children and when associated with germline p53 mutation, portend a significantly worse prognosis. SHHδ is most commonly seen in adults and adolescents and is associated with PTCH, SMO, and TERT promoter mutations (see **Fig. 2**, **Table 1**).[56,60] SHHα and SHHδ patients will receive surgery, CSI, and chemotherapy with the addition of an SHH inhibitor in the setting of a clinical trial (NCT01878617).

Group 3 MB represents approximately 25% of all MBs and are seen in young infants and children. Tumors are often midline near the fourth ventricle and metastatic in 40% of patients at initial diagnosis.[61] This subgroup is associated with the worst prognosis, with 5-year OS less than 60%.[52] Histology is frequently large cell, anaplastic, or classic. Three different subtypes of group 3 are being proposed based on genetic alterations and outcomes.[52,56,61] MYC amplification can be seen in 20% of patients, which is associated with poor outcomes (see **Table 3**). Isochromosome 17q is also seen frequently in this subgroup (see **Fig. 2**, **Table 1**). Treatment for high-risk patients includes surgery, CSI, and chemotherapy, with the addition of novel agents through a clinical trial (NCT01878617) and high-dose chemotherapy with ASCR for infants.[59,62,63]

Group 4 MB, the most common subgroup, represents 35% of all MB and is seen in late childhood, early adolescence. These tumors typically arise from the midline adjacent to the fourth ventricle and are metastatic in a third of patients. Histology is often classic and based on molecular features, and can be further subdivided into 3 subtypes. Prognosis is intermediate, with 5-year OS reported at 70%. The low-risk group has chromosome 11 loss or 17 gain and the high-risk group has metastatic disease at diagnosis (see **Table 3**).[57] Isochrome 17q is seen in 80% of patients in this subgroup (see **Fig. 2**, **Table 1**).[20] MYCN amplification can be seen in a small subset and is associated with poorer outcomes. Treatment includes surgery, CSI, and chemotherapy with the potential addition of novel agents for high-risk patients (NCT01878617).

Gorlin, FAP, and LFS are cancer predisposition syndromes associated with the development of MB. SHH MB typically develops in infants with Gorlin syndrome. Treatment is the same as infant SHH MB, specifically avoiding radiation, as there is a significantly higher risk for developing secondary basal cell carcinoma in the radiation field. FAP is characterized by the development of multiple adenomatous polyps and WNT MB in adolescence (see **Table 2**).[24,64,65] Patients are treated the same as sporadic cases of WNT MB.

ATYPICAL TERATOID RHABDOID TUMORS

Atypical teratoid rhabdoid tumors (ATRT) are highly aggressive tumors that affect children younger than 3 years, with a 5-year OS of 30% to 40%.[66] These tumors represent about 15% of all CNS embryonal tumors (see **Fig. 1**).[1,67] They can arise most commonly in the infratentorial region, followed by supratentorial and rarely in the spinal cord. Approximately 20% to 40% of patients will have metastatic disease at the time of diagnosis and require extent of disease evaluation with CSF analysis and MRI of the spine. Clinical presentation is dependent on tumor location, with infratentorial tumors presenting with increased intracranial pressure and cranial nerve deficits and supratentorial tumors with headaches and focal deficits.

Management of ATRT has been challenging due to the aggressive nature and young age of patients. Multimodal therapy with surgery, conventional chemotherapy, high-dose chemotherapy with ASCR, and focal radiation has shown dramatic improvement in OS compared with historical therapies that included dose-intensive multi-agent chemotherapy without radiation.[66] RT has been avoided due to age; however, some studies have shown that focal RT may not have as significant neurocognitive affects.[68] A recent Children's Oncology Group (COG) trial used this multimodal approach in addition to age-stratified RT, which resulted in a 4-year OS of 43%.

Mutations associated with ATRT include biallelic inactivation of *SMARCB1* on chromosome 22, which histologically can be identified as loss of INI1 nuclear staining. Less frequently you can see a *SMARCB4* mutation.[69] In addition to these somatic mutations, a third of patients will have germline mutations in *SMARCB1* and less commonly *SMARCA4*.[70] Further molecular analyses of ATRT has identified 3 main subgroups.[69] Targeted therapies are under investigation through clinical trials (NCT02114229).

EPENDYMOMA

Ependymoma is the third most common malignant CNS tumor and represents approximately 5% of all pediatric CNS tumors.[1] They can arise anywhere in the neuroaxis, but 90% of pediatric cases occur intracranially, with two-thirds in the posterior fossa and one-third supratentorially. There is a peak incidence in early childhood. Fewer than 10% of patients will present with metastatic disease at diagnosis and therefore require MRI spine and CSF analyses for further evaluation.[71,72] Clinical symptoms are dependent on tumor location with infratentorial tumors often presenting with signs of increased intracranial pressure, cranial nerve palsies, and ataxia and supratentorial tumors presenting with focal neurologic deficits, headaches, and seizures. Histologically, ependymomas can be WHO grade I (myxopapillary ependymoma, subependymoma), grade II (classic ependymoma), or grade III (anaplastic ependymoma).[73]

Treatment is similar for all tumor locations, with maximal safe surgical resection followed by focal RT in children older than 1. Chemotherapy is currently used for children younger than 1, as a bridge to focal RT. A Phase III COG study was recently completed to determine if chemotherapy provides any additional benefit after surgery; these data are currently being analyzed. The 10-year OS is approximately 60%, but patients diagnosed in infancy have the lowest survival.[74]

Nine molecular subgroups of ependymoma have been identified, 3 in each anatomic location: supratentorial, posterior fossa, and spinal cord (**Fig. 3**). Sub-ependymomas, which primarily occur in adults, represent one molecular subgroup in each anatomic region. The other 2 molecular subgroups for spinal cord ependymomas are distinguished by pathology: myxopapillary, and WHO grade II/III ependymomas. Supratentorial ependymomas (ST-EPN) can be subdivided by the presence of fusion oncoproteins: *C11ORF95-RELA* and *YAP1* (ST-EPN-RELA and ST-EPN-YAP1, respectively) (see **Table 1**). The ST-RELA subgroup represents 85% of supratentorial ependymomas and occurs in all ages, whereas the ST-YAP1 subgroup is found mostly in pediatric patients.[73,74] The ST-RELA subgroup is believed to have a poorer prognosis but prospective studies did not show any differences in event-free survival between the different subgroups.[72-76] The ST-YAP1 subgroup is said to have an

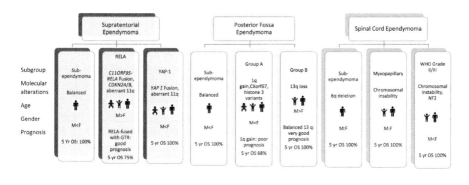

♦ 0-10 ♀ 10-18 ♦ >18

Fig. 3. Ependymoma molecular subgroups. (*Data from* Pajtler KW, Witt H, Sill M, et al. Molecular Classification of Ependymal Tumors across All CNS Compartments, Histopathological Grades, and Age Groups. Cancer cell. 2015;27(5):728-743.)

excellent prognosis while homozygous deletion of *CDKN2A/B* is associated with inferior outcomes in ST-RELA tumors.[20,74,76] Posterior fossa ependymomas (PF-EPN) have 2 additional subgroups identified as PF-EPN Group A (PF-EPN-A) and PF-EPN Group B (PF-EPN-B). PF-EPN-A tumors primarily occur in infants and young children, whereas PF-EPN-B ependymomas are predominant in adolescents and young adults.[73,74] PF-EPN-A subgroup is associated with a poorer prognosis and in a small proportion of tumor mutations in *CXorf67* and histone 3 variants have been described.[77,78] Gain of chromosome 1q in the PF-EPN-A subgroup and loss of chromosome 13q in the PF-EPN-B subgroup are also associated with poorer outcomes in PF-EPN.[74,76] Management is standard for all subgroups; however, observation-only clinical trials will be implemented for PF-EPN-B without loss of chromosome 13q and ST-EPN-RELA after GTR.[20,73]

Approximately 50% of patients with NF2 can develop ependymomas in addition to meningiomas, gliomas, schwannomas, and neurofibromas.[79] Treatment of NF2 CNS-associated tumors are similar to sporadic counterparts; however, molecularly targeted therapies are currently being investigated (NCT04374305, NCT04283669, NCT03095248).

CRANIOPHARYNGIOMA

Craniopharyngiomas occur in the sellar/parasellar region and represent 2% to 6% of all pediatric brain tumors.[80] There are 2 histologic subtypes, adamantinomatous (ACP) and papillary (PCP). In childhood and adolescence, the predominant histologic subtype is ACP, with peak age of incidence at 5 to 15 years (bimodal peak with second peak at 45–60 years). PCP is most frequently seen in adults. Children with ACP often present with visual disturbances, headaches, and endocrine deficiencies. Current treatment options for craniopharyngioma include GTR or partial resection followed by RT. Both treatment options achieve comparable results and decrease the risk of tumor recurrence. Although histologically these tumors are considered benign, they are associated with significant morbidity and poor QOL. Overall, mortality is also 3 to 5 times greater than the general population in patients with CP.[80] As such, more effective, novel therapeutic strategies are being investigated.

ACP tumors frequently carry mutations in *CTNNB1*, whereas PCP subtypes carry *BRAF* V600E mutations. In addition, activation of the MAPK, immune, and inflammatory pathways has been demonstrated, such as elevation of interleukin-6 and increased expression of PD-1, PD-LI, and CTLA-4.[81–85] Clinical trials using targeted therapy to address some of these pathways are currently ongoing, whereas others are being designed (NCT03224767, NCT03970226).

CLINICS CARE POINTS

- Molecular profiling of CNS tumors are changing the current tumor classification, management, and prognostication of these patients.
- The goal of management of pediatric brain tumors is to continue to improve survival, decrease morbidity, and improve QOL.
- In patients who have received RT, recommend monitoring for potential neurologic side effects, including neurocognitive outcomes, radiation vasculopathy, and secondary CNS malignancies.
- Targeted therapy for pediatric brain tumors is currently being investigated for different tumor types and may be the future direction of care for these patients.

DISCLOSURE

None.

REFERENCES

1. Ostrom QT, Cioffi G, Gittleman H, et al. CBTRUS statistical report: primary brain and other central nervous system tumors diagnosed in the United States in 2012-2016. Neuro Oncol 2019;21(Suppl 5):v1–100.
2. Kumar R, Liu APY, Orr BA, et al. Advances in the classification of pediatric brain tumors through DNA methylation profiling: from research tool to frontline diagnostic. Cancer 2018;124(21):4168–80.
3. Louis DN, Perry A, Reifenberger G, et al. The 2016 World Health Organization classification of tumors of the central nervous system: a summary. Acta Neuropathol 2016;131(6):803–20.
4. Jones DTW, Kieran MW, Bouffet E, et al. Pediatric low-grade gliomas: next biologically driven steps. Neuro Oncol 2018;20(2):160–73.
5. Packer RJ, Pfister S, Bouffet E, et al. Pediatric low-grade gliomas: implications of the biologic era. Neuro Oncol 2017;19(6):750–61.
6. Bergthold G, Bandopadhayay P, Bi WL, et al. Pediatric low-grade gliomas: how modern biology reshapes the clinical field. Biochim Biophys Acta 2014; 1845(2):294–307.
7. Chamdine O, Broniscer A, Wu S, et al. Metastatic low-grade gliomas in children: 20 years' experience at St. Jude Children's Research Hospital. Pediatr Blood Cancer 2016;63(1):62–70.
8. Stokland T, Liu JF, Ironside JW, et al. A multivariate analysis of factors determining tumor progression in childhood low-grade glioma: a population-based cohort study (CCLG CNS9702). Neuro Oncol 2010;12(12):1257–68.
9. de Blank P, Bandopadhayay P, Haas-Kogan D, et al. Management of pediatric low-grade glioma. Curr Opin Pediatr 2019;31(1):21–7.
10. Merchant TE, Conklin HM, Wu S, et al. Late effects of conformal radiation therapy for pediatric patients with low-grade glioma: prospective evaluation of cognitive, endocrine, and hearing deficits. J Clin Oncol 2009;27(22):3691–7.

11. Ater JL, Zhou T, Holmes E, et al. Randomized study of two chemotherapy regimens for treatment of low-grade glioma in young children: a report from the Children's Oncology Group. J Clin Oncol 2012;30(21):2641–7.

12. Lassaletta A, Scheinemann K, Zelcer SM, et al. Phase II weekly vinblastine for chemotherapy-naive children with progressive low-grade glioma: a Canadian Pediatric Brain Tumor Consortium Study. J Clin Oncol 2016;34(29):3537–43.

13. Hoffman LM, Salloum R, Fouladi M. Molecular biology of pediatric brain tumors and impact on novel therapies. Curr Neurol Neurosci Rep 2015;15(4):10.

14. Sturm D, Pfister SM, Jones DTW. Pediatric gliomas: current concepts on diagnosis, biology, and clinical management. J Clin Oncol 2017;35(21):2370–7.

15. Northcott PA, Pfister SM, Jones DT. Next-generation (epi)genetic drivers of childhood brain tumours and the outlook for targeted therapies. Lancet Oncol 2015; 16(6):e293–302.

16. Ichimura K, Nishikawa R, Matsutani M. Molecular markers in pediatric neuro-oncology. Neuro Oncol 2012;14(Suppl 4):iv90–9.

17. Chen YH, Gutmann DH. The molecular and cell biology of pediatric low-grade gliomas. Oncogene 2014;33(16):2019–26.

18. Gajjar A, Bowers DC, Karajannis MA, et al. Pediatric brain tumors: innovative genomic information is transforming the diagnostic and clinical landscape. J Clin Oncol 2015;33(27):2986–98.

19. Pollack IF, Jakacki RI. Childhood brain tumors: epidemiology, current management and future directions. Nat Rev Neurol 2011;7(9):495–506.

20. Cacciotti C, Fleming A, Ramaswamy V. Advances in the molecular classification of pediatric brain tumors: a guide to the galaxy. J Pathol 2020;251(3):249–61.

21. Hargrave DR, Bouffet E, Tabori U, et al. Efficacy and safety of dabrafenib in pediatric patients with BRAF V600 mutation-positive relapsed or refractory low-grade glioma: results from a phase I/IIa study. Clin Cancer Res 2019;25(24): 7303–11.

22. Nicolaides T, Nazemi KJ, Crawford J, et al. Phase I study of vemurafenib in children with recurrent or progressive BRAF(V600E) mutant brain tumors: Pacific Pediatric Neuro-Oncology Consortium study (PNOC-002). Oncotarget 2020;11(21): 1942–52.

23. Daras M, Kaley TJ. Benign brain tumors and tumors associated with phakomatoses. Continuum (Minneap Minn) 2015;21(2 Neuro-oncology):397–414.

24. Ranger AM, Patel YK, Chaudhary N, et al. Familial syndromes associated with intracranial tumours: a review. Childs Nerv Syst 2014;30(1):47–64.

25. Ullrich NJ. Neurocutaneous syndromes and brain tumors. J Child Neurol 2016; 31(12):1399–411.

26. Hottinger AF, Khakoo Y. Neurooncology of familial cancer syndromes. J Child Neurol 2009;24(12):1526–35.

27. Franz DN, Belousova E, Sparagana S, et al. Efficacy and safety of everolimus for subependymal giant cell astrocytomas associated with tuberous sclerosis complex (EXIST-1): a multicentre, randomised, placebo-controlled phase 3 trial. Lancet 2013;381(9861):125–32.

28. Franz DN, Belousova E, Sparagana S, et al. Long-term use of everolimus in patients with tuberous sclerosis complex: final results from the EXIST-1 study. PLoS One 2016;11(6):e0158476.

29. Braunstein S, Raleigh D, Bindra R, et al. Pediatric high-grade glioma: current molecular landscape and therapeutic approaches. J Neurooncol 2017;134(3): 541–9.

30. Pollack IF. The role of surgery in pediatric gliomas. J Neurooncol 1999;42(3): 271–88.
31. Wisoff JH, Boyett JM, Berger MS, et al. Current neurosurgical management and the impact of the extent of resection in the treatment of malignant gliomas of childhood: a report of the Children's Cancer Group trial no. CCG-945. J Neurosurg 1998;89(1):52–9.
32. Espinoza JC, Haley K, Patel N, et al. Outcome of young children with high-grade glioma treated with irradiation-avoiding intensive chemotherapy regimens: final report of the Head Start II and III trials. Pediatr Blood Cancer 2016;63(10): 1806–13.
33. Sanders RP, Kocak M, Burger PC, et al. High-grade astrocytoma in very young children. Pediatr Blood Cancer 2007;49(7):888–93.
34. Turner CD, Chi S, Marcus KJ, et al. Phase II study of thalidomide and radiation in children with newly diagnosed brain stem gliomas and glioblastoma multiforme. J Neurooncol 2007;82(1):95–101.
35. Wolff JE, Wagner S, Reinert C, et al. Maintenance treatment with interferon-gamma and low-dose cyclophosphamide for pediatric high-grade glioma. J Neurooncol 2006;79(3):315–21.
36. Grill J, Massimino M, Bouffet E, et al. Phase II, open-label, randomized, multi-center trial (HERBY) of bevacizumab in pediatric patients with newly diagnosed high-grade glioma. J Clin Oncol 2018;36(10):951–8.
37. Korshunov A, Schrimpf D, Ryzhova M, et al. H3-/IDH-wild type pediatric glioblas-toma is comprised of molecularly and prognostically distinct subtypes with asso-ciated oncogenic drivers. Acta Neuropathol 2017;134(3):507–16.
38. Chamdine O, Gajjar A. Molecular characteristics of pediatric high-grade gliomas. CNS Oncol 2014;3(6):433–43.
39. Jones C, Karajannis MA, Jones DTW, et al. Pediatric high-grade glioma: biolog-ically and clinically in need of new thinking. Neuro Oncol 2017;19(2):153–61.
40. Panditharatna E, Yaeger K, Kilburn LB, et al. Clinicopathology of diffuse intrinsic pontine glioma and its redefined genomic and epigenomic landscape. Cancer Genet 2015;208(7–8):367–73.
41. Lin GL, Wilson KM, Ceribelli M, et al. Therapeutic strategies for diffuse midline gli-oma from high-throughput combination drug screening. Sci Transl Med 2019; 11(519):eaaw0064.
42. Chi AS, Tarapore RS, Hall MD, et al. Pediatric and adult H3 K27M-mutant diffuse midline glioma treated with the selective DRD2 antagonist ONC201. J Neurooncol 2019;145(1):97–105.
43. Mount CW, Majzner RG, Sundaresh S, et al. Potent antitumor efficacy of anti-GD2 CAR T cells in H3-K27M(+) diffuse midline gliomas. Nat Med 2018;24(5):572–9.
44. Grimm SA, Chamberlain MC. Brainstem glioma: a review. Curr Neurol Neurosci Rep 2013;13(5):346.
45. Hoffman LM, Veldhuijzen van Zanten SEM, Colditz N, et al. Clinical, radiologic, pathologic, and molecular characteristics of long-term survivors of Diffuse Intrinsic Pontine Glioma (DIPG): a collaborative report from the International and European Society for Pediatric Oncology DIPG Registries. J Clin Oncol 2018;36(19):1963–72.
46. Korones DN, Fisher PG, Kretschmar C, et al. Treatment of children with diffuse intrinsic brain stem glioma with radiotherapy, vincristine and oral VP-16: a Chil-dren's Oncology Group phase II study. Pediatr Blood Cancer 2008;50(2):227–30.

47. Massimino M, Spreafico F, Biassoni V, et al. Diffuse pontine gliomas in children: changing strategies, changing results? A mono-institutional 20-year experience. J Neurooncol 2008;87(3):355–61.
48. Cohen KJ, Heideman RL, Zhou T, et al. Temozolomide in the treatment of children with newly diagnosed diffuse intrinsic pontine gliomas: a report from the Children's Oncology Group. Neuro Oncol 2011;13(4):410–6.
49. Michaeli O, Tabori U. Pediatric high grade gliomas in the context of cancer predisposition syndromes. J Korean Neurosurg Soc 2018;61(3):319–32.
50. Kratz CP, Achatz MI, Brugieres L, et al. Cancer screening recommendations for individuals with Li-Fraumeni syndrome. Clin Cancer Res 2017;23(11):e38–45.
51. Johnson A, Severson E, Gay L, et al. Comprehensive genomic profiling of 282 pediatric low- and high-grade gliomas reveals genomic drivers, tumor mutational burden, and hypermutation signatures. Oncologist 2017;22(12):1478–90.
52. Northcott PA, Robinson GW, Kratz CP, et al. Medulloblastoma. Nat Rev Dis Primers 2019;5(1):11.
53. Lanier JC, Abrams AN. Posterior fossa syndrome: review of the behavioral and emotional aspects in pediatric cancer patients. Cancer 2017;123(4):551–9.
54. Gottardo NG, Hansford JR, McGlade JP, et al. Medulloblastoma down under 2013: a report from the third annual meeting of the International Medulloblastoma Working Group. Acta Neuropathol 2014;127(2):189–201.
55. Northcott PA, Shih DJ, Remke M, et al. Rapid, reliable, and reproducible molecular sub-grouping of clinical medulloblastoma samples. Acta Neuropathol 2012;123(4):615–26.
56. Cavalli FMG, Remke M, Rampasek L, et al. Intertumoral heterogeneity within medulloblastoma subgroups. Cancer Cell 2017;31(6):737–54.e6.
57. Ramaswamy V, Remke M, Bouffet E, et al. Risk stratification of childhood medulloblastoma in the molecular era: the current consensus. Acta Neuropathol 2016;131(6):821–31.
58. Suva ML, Louis DN. Next-generation molecular genetics of brain tumours. Curr Opin Neurol 2013;26(6):681–7.
59. Robinson GW, Rudneva VA, Buchhalter I, et al. Risk-adapted therapy for young children with medulloblastoma (SJYC07): therapeutic and molecular outcomes from a multicentre, phase 2 trial. Lancet Oncol 2018;19(6):768–84.
60. Taylor MD, Northcott PA, Korshunov A, et al. Molecular subgroups of medulloblastoma: the current consensus. Acta Neuropathol 2012;123(4):465–72.
61. Liu KW, Pajtler KW, Worst BC, et al. Molecular mechanisms and therapeutic targets in pediatric brain tumors. Sci Signal 2017;10(470):eaaf7593.
62. Dhall G, Grodman H, Ji L, et al. Outcome of children less than three years old at diagnosis with non-metastatic medulloblastoma treated with chemotherapy on the "Head Start" I and II protocols. Pediatr Blood Cancer 2008;50(6):1169–75.
63. HeadStart4: Newly diagnosed children (<10 y/o) with medulloblastoma and other CNS embryonal tumors. 2019. Available at: https://clinicaltrials.gov/ct2/show/NCT02875314. Accessed January 10, 2021.
64. Johansson G, Andersson U, Melin B. Recent developments in brain tumor predisposing syndromes. Acta Oncol 2016;55(4):401–11.
65. Septer S, Lawson CE, Anant S, et al. Familial adenomatous polyposis in pediatrics: natural history, emerging surveillance and management protocols, chemopreventive strategies, and areas of ongoing debate. Fam Cancer 2016;15(3):477–85.
66. Reddy AT, Strother DR, Judkins AR, et al. Efficacy of high-dose chemotherapy and three-dimensional conformal radiation for atypical teratoid/rhabdoid tumor:

a report from the children's oncology group trial ACNS0333. J Clin Oncol 2020; 38(11):1175–85.

67. Nesvick CL, Lafay-Cousin L, Raghunathan A, et al. Atypical teratoid rhabdoid tumor: molecular insights and translation to novel therapeutics. J Neurooncol 2020; 150(1):47–56.

68. Merchant TE, Mulhern RK, Krasin MJ, et al. Preliminary results from a phase II trial of conformal radiation therapy and evaluation of radiation-related CNS effects for pediatric patients with localized ependymoma. J Clin Oncol 2004;22(15): 3156–62.

69. Ho B, Johann PD, Grabovska Y, et al. Molecular subgrouping of atypical teratoid/ rhabdoid tumors-a reinvestigation and current consensus. Neuro Oncol 2020; 22(5):613–24.

70. Eaton KW, Tooke LS, Wainwright LM, et al. Spectrum of SMARCB1/INI1 mutations in familial and sporadic rhabdoid tumors. Pediatr Blood Cancer 2011;56(1):7–15.

71. Fangusaro J, Van Den Berghe C, Tomita T, et al. Evaluating the incidence and utility of microscopic metastatic dissemination as diagnosed by lumbar cerebrospinal fluid (CSF) samples in children with newly diagnosed intracranial ependymoma. J Neurooncol 2011;103(3):693–8.

72. Upadhyaya SA, Robinson GW, Onar-Thomas A, et al. Molecular grouping and outcomes of young children with newly diagnosed ependymoma treated on the multi-institutional SJYC07 trial. Neuro Oncol 2019;21(10):1319–30.

73. Pajtler KW, Mack SC, Ramaswamy V, et al. The current consensus on the clinical management of intracranial ependymoma and its distinct molecular variants. Acta Neuropathol 2017;133(1):5–12.

74. Pajtler KW, Witt H, Sill M, et al. Molecular classification of ependymal tumors across all CNS compartments, histopathological grades, and age groups. Cancer Cell 2015;27(5):728–43.

75. Ramaswamy V, Hielscher T, Mack SC, et al. Therapeutic impact of cytoreductive surgery and irradiation of posterior fossa ependymoma in the molecular era: a retrospective multicohort analysis. J Clin Oncol 2016;34(21):2468–77.

76. Merchant TE, Bendel AE, Sabin ND, et al. Conformal radiation therapy for pediatric ependymoma, chemotherapy for incompletely resected ependymoma, and observation for completely resected, supratentorial ependymoma. J Clin Oncol 2019;37(12):974–83.

77. Mack SC, Witt H, Piro RM, et al. Epigenomic alterations define lethal CIMP-positive ependymomas of infancy. Nature 2014;506(7489):445–50.

78. Pajtler KW, Wen J, Sill M, et al. Molecular heterogeneity and CXorf67 alterations in posterior fossa group A (PFA) ependymomas. Acta Neuropathol 2018;136(2): 211–26.

79. Evans DGR, Salvador H, Chang VY, et al. Cancer and central nervous system tumor surveillance in pediatric neurofibromatosis 2 and related disorders. Clin Cancer Res 2017;23(12):e54–61.

80. Muller HL, Merchant TE, Warmuth-Metz M, et al. Craniopharyngioma. Nat Rev Dis Primers 2019;5(1):75.

81. Apps JR, Carreno G, Gonzalez-Meljem JM, et al. Tumour compartment transcriptomics demonstrates the activation of inflammatory and odontogenic programmes in human adamantinomatous craniopharyngioma and identifies the MAPK/ERK pathway as a novel therapeutic target. Acta Neuropathol 2018; 135(5):757–77.

82. Donson AM, Apps J, Griesinger AM, et al. Molecular analyses reveal inflammatory mediators in the solid component and cyst fluid of human adamantinomatous craniopharyngioma. J Neuropathol Exp Neurol 2017;76(9):779–88.
83. Grob S, Mirsky DM, Donson AM, et al. Targeting IL-6 is a potential treatment for primary cystic craniopharyngioma. Front Oncol 2019;9:791.
84. Whelan R, Prince E, Gilani A, et al. The inflammatory milieu of adamantinomatous craniopharyngioma and its implications for treatment. J Clin Med 2020;9(2):519.
85. Coy S, Rashid R, Lin JR, et al. Multiplexed immunofluorescence reveals potential PD-1/PD-L1 pathway vulnerabilities in craniopharyngioma. Neuro Oncol 2018; 20(8):1101–12.

Neurocritical Care and Brain Monitoring

James J. Riviello Jr, MD[a],*, Jennifer Erklauer, MD[a,b]

KEYWORDS

- Pediatric neurocritical care • Brain monitoring: noninvasive and invasive
- Multimodality monitoring • Continuous EEG monitoring
- The ictal-interictal continuum

KEY POINTS

- "To Detect and Protect" refers to the prevention of secondary brain injury.
- Neuromonitoring relies on many modalities, therefore the term "multimodality monitoring".
- Continuous electroencephalogram (CEEG) monitoring is used in many Neurocritical Care Units.
- Quantified EEG helps to interpret the massive data generated by CEEG monitoring.
- The ictal-interictal continuum consists of rhythmic and periodic patterns that lie in the spectrum between the ictal and the interictal states.

INTRODUCTION

The goal of neurocritical care (NCC) is to improve the outcome of patients with life-threatening neurologic illness. NCC includes the management of primary and secondary central nervous system (CNS) injury. The CNS response to the primary injury, through ischemia, inflammation, edema, or iatrogenic, may cause secondary injury, which may be detected by CNS monitoring. The word "monitor" means to observe and check the progress or quality over time. The derivation of monitor comes from the Latin word, monere, to warn. The purpose of monitoring is to identify neurologic compromise or deterioration and intervene before the insult becomes irreversible. The term "To detect and protect," referring to the continuous electroencephalogram (CEEG) monitoring, can be applied to the prevention of secondary brain injury.[1]

Neuromonitoring uses many modalities. Neuromonitoring starts with a baseline neurologic examination, performed on admission, with then serial examinations used to detect progression or improvement. These include an assessment of baseline

[a] Section of Pediatric Neurology and Developmental Neuroscience, Department of Pediatrics, Baylor College of Medicine, Texas Children's Hospital, 6701 Fannin Street, Suite 1250, Houston, TX 77030, USA; [b] Section of Pediatric Critical Care Medicine, Baylor College of Medicine, Texas Children's Hospital, 6701 Fannin Street, Suite 1250, Houston, TX 77030, USA
* Corresponding author.
E-mail address: riviello@bcm.edu

Neurol Clin 39 (2021) 847–866
https://doi.org/10.1016/j.ncl.2021.04.006
neurologic.theclinics.com

mental status with level of alertness; brain stem function, especially the pupillary and oculomotor findings; and motor responses. If progression occurs, treatment needs to be reevaluated and possibly modified.

The Glasgow Coma Scale is one example of a monitoring tool. Others include EEG, neuroimaging, evoked potentials, transcranial doppler for cerebral blood flow (CBF), and various physiologic parameters. These tests vary in spatial and temporal resolution, ease of performance, and bedside interpretation and are either invasive or noninvasive and determine their use in a given patient; for example, portable bedside computed axial tomography (CAT) scanning makes it safer to obtain a cranial CAT scan on a critically ill patient, especially those on extracorporeal membrane oxygenation (ECMO). The neurologic examination itself, and therefore the clinical detection of deterioration, is frequently limited in the NCC unit by coma, sedation, and pharmacologic neuromuscular blockade. Therefore, other methods such as real-time neurophysiologic monitoring is necessary in these patients to detect brain injury early and act in time to prevent irreversible injury.

Pediatric Neurocritical Care

Pediatric NCC is a relatively new field. We have created our NCC program as a collaborative effort among pediatric critical care medicine (CCM), child neurology, and pediatric neurosurgery. Each field has identified a director for its NCC program. CCM and child neurology each have a dedicated group of subspecialists with NCC as their primary interest. The CCM service functions as the primary team with the neuroscience services providing consultations. In the dedicated NCC unit, the CCM and NCC teams make combined mutual rounds, along with the families. Neurophysiology is actively involved in neuromonitoring, with CEEG, working directly with the NCC and pediatric intensive care unit (PICU) teams.

The first program started in 1996 at Boston Children's Hospital with a dedicated team of child neurologists providing consultative services to the multidisciplinary PICU, the surgical PICU, the cardiac ICU, and the neonatal ICU.[2] The second started in 2003 at Children's National Medical Center, with a multidisciplinary team of neurologists, CCM specialists, and neurosurgeons who consulted on about 25% of all ICU admissions.[3]

The delivery of pediatric NCC has changed over time, analogous to that occurring in adult NCC. Pediatric NCC has evolved from the general child neurologist performing a consult to the development of dedicated pediatric NCC teams. In 2008, a survey of pediatric neurology programs revealed that only 5 of 48 pediatric neurology programs in academic children's hospitals had dedicated NCC services.[4] In 2018, a survey of PICU medical directors and program directors of pediatric neurosurgery and child neurology training programs revealed that 45/128 had a pediatric NCC service.[5] Tasker described 3 models for pediatric NCC: a combined venture with neurology and neurosurgery providing care to the PICU patients; neuroscience specialists (neurologists and neurosurgeons) interacting directly with the CCM specialists; or a combination of these 2, with the caveat that all PICU admissions require consideration of brain-oriented critical care.[6]

Pediatric Neurocritical Care Is Not Limited to the Dedicated Intensive Care Unit

The practice of NCC extends beyond the actual physical location of the NCC unit: the principles of NCC must be practiced wherever neuroprotective treatment is needed to treat a specific disorder that causes primary or secondary CNS injury. Therefore, NCC is a continuum from the prehospital setting to the ICU.[7] Treatment guidelines must consider all steps in the treatment sequence,[7] as providers in various fields (emergency physicians, pediatricians, child neurology consultants, CCM and NCC specialists) and locations (community, academic hospitals) may care for a given patient or for specific disorders. This concept is addressed by the Emergency Neurological Life Support (ENLS) course, a joint venture between emergency medicine and NCC specialists, offered by the Neurocritical Care Society. The goal of the ENLS course is to improve the neurologic care during the first critical hour of a neurologic emergency[8] and is now in its fifth version.

The delivery of NCC has evolved at Texas Children's Hospital (TCH). In 2009, we created a dedicated NCC service, consisting of a separate team of child neurologists and residents providing consultations only in the various ICUs: the multidisciplinary PICU, cardiovascular ICU, and the neonatal ICU (NICU). Only one child neurologist had NCC experience. Before this, the general neurology consult team provided all neurologic consultations to all services throughout our institution. In 2018, a dedicated 12-bed NCC unit for children with primary neurologic diagnoses was opened in a new ICU tower. The NCC service provides consultations to the various ICUs that now include the NCC ICU, a multidisciplinary general PICU, a pulmonary ICU, hematology/oncology ICU, surgical ICU including transplantation and hepatic, and the cardiovascular ICU, which now consists of dedicated cardiac failure and postoperative cardiac surgery ICUs.

Our NCC team consists of 6 child neurologists with additional subspecialty expertise: a CCM/NCC specialist; 2 neurophysiologist/NCC specialists, one with additional stroke training; and 2 with a neurodevelopmental disability background, one specializing in traumatic brain injury (TBI) and the other in neurogenetics. All TCH specialties provide care in the ICU, but we especially rely on our neuroimmunology and rheumatology partners. TCH has 2 community hospitals around Houston, with the neurologic care provided locally by the neurology consultants, with back-up from our dedicated NCC team. We have developed a telehealth outreach for NCC consultations in these hospitals and protocols to transfer the children who need a higher level of neurologic care to the NCC unit at the main campus. The goal is to provide excellent care to children with acute neurologic disorders in all locations. This requires standardization of care and integration of care across the TCH system.

Continuous EEG monitoring (CEEG) is an integral part of our NCC service and neuromonitoring. Eight beds are equipped with hard-wired CEEG with digital trending capabilities, and there are 16 portable EEG machines and 3 portable multimodality monitors for those not in the wired beds. In 2009, we started monitoring the ICU CEEGs in the epilepsy monitoring unit. Our EEG service had 10 reading sessions per week (AM and PM every day) with the interpreter for each occasion responsible for the ICU EEGs. As EEG interpretation is subjective, having many providers resulted in inconsistent interpretations. With opening of the new ICU tower in 2018, we created a dedicated CEEG service, with the same neurophysiologist interpreting the study through the week, resulting in more consistent EEG interpretation. We also created a dedicated critical care EEG monitoring unit within the NCC unit with dedicated specially trained neurodiagnostic technologists monitoring the EEGs 24/7. Notification criteria are established for each patient, and if these criteria are met, the neurophysiologist notifies the ICU team. CEEG monitoring can detect seizures and other changes that indicate deterioration, such as new-onset slowing.

What Disorders Are Encountered in Pediatric Neurocritical Care?

Pediatric NCC is practiced in different settings: community hospitals, regional referral centers, and large and small pediatric hospitals and academic centers, some with dedicated NCC teams. A Spanish regional referral center reported that 711/2198 (32%) of their PICU admissions were for primary neurologic disorders. Thirty percent of these were head trauma, 18% were neurosurgical, and 15% were for seizures.[9] The NCC service at Children's National Medical Center reported on their experience with NCC. Two hundred thirty-nine of one thousand four hundred twenty-three or 26% of PICU admissions had a primary neurologic disorder. Status epilepticus (SE) accounted for 70 of these (18.9%), TBI accounted for 53 (14.2%), and brain tumor accounted for 48 (12.8%) (**Table 1**). Coma from an unknown cause only occurred in 14 (3.8%) (**Table 2**). The remaining 134 cases required consultation for the neurologic manifestations of systemic medical disorders (see **Table 2**).[3] From Boston Children's Hospital, of 3719 children admitted to the PICU, 689 (19%) were seen by the NCC team. Complete data were available for 615 children, in whom 900 diagnostic codes were used. Four hundred thirty-six of nine hundred (48%) of the NCC consultations were for seizures and SE, 126/900 (14%) were for cerebrovascular disorders, 75/900 (8%) were for coma or brain death, 44/900 (5%) were for CNS infection, and 42/900 (5%) were for demyelinating diseases.[10]

The disorders seen in pediatric NCC differ from those seen in adult NCC. In one adult NCC unit with 1155 consecutive admissions, cerebrovascular disease was the predominant reason for admission, with intracerebral hemorrhage in 20%, subarachnoid hemorrhage in 16%, and malignant ischemic stroke in 15%, TBI in 19%, meningitis/encephalitis in 7%, and SE in only 6%.[11] Williams (2018) analyzed the Kids Inpatient database, a pediatric inpatient care database for the United States, for NCC disorders.[12] The major categories were TBI, infection/inflammation, SE, stroke, hypoxic-ischemic injury, and spinal cord injury. At least one critical care intervention was recorded in 23% (67,058) children with a primary neurologic diagnosis (**Table 3**). More than half of the PNCC admissions had at least one chronic condition and 23% were treated at a children's hospital. Twelve percent of the admissions died and 21% had poor functional outcomes.[12] Williams then studied hospital mortality and functional outcomes over 2 years from their own institution. Three hundred twenty-five patients had a primary PNCC diagnosis, accounting for 16% of all ICU admissions: 154 with TBI, 71 with SE, 40 with infectious or inflammatory disorders, 37 with cardiac arrest, and 23 with stroke. The largest group in which the outcome was death was cardiac arrest (**Table 4**).[13]

Table 1 Primary neurologic diagnoses seen by the neurocritical care service	
Status Epilepticus	70 (18.9%)
Traumatic Brain Injury	53 (14.2%)
Tumor	48 (12.8%)
Neurosurgical Procedure	24 (6.4%)
Hydrocephalus	17 (4.6%)
Subarachnoid/Intracranial Hemorrhage	13 (3.5%)
Stroke	7 (1.9%)
Meningitis	5 (1.3%)
Other	2 (0.5%)
Total	239 (64.1%)

Data from Bell MJ, Carpenter J, Au AK, Keating RF, Myseros JS, Yaun A, Weinstein S. Development of a pediatric neurocritical care service. Neurocrit Care 2009:10:4-10.

Table 2 Primary medical diagnoses seen by the neurocritical care service	
Respiratory Failure	41 (11%)
Cardiovascular	27 (7.2%)
Shock	22 (5.9%)
Cardiac Arrest	14 (3.8%)
Coma (Unknown Cause)	14 (3.8%)
Ingestion	5 (1.3%)
Diabetic Ketoacidosis	5 (1.3%)
Other	6 (1.6%)
Total	134 (35.9%)

Data from Bell MJ, Carpenter J, Au AK, Keating RF, Myseros JS, Yaun A, Weinstein S. Development of a pediatric neurocritical care service. Neurocrit Care 2009:10:4-10.

In general, children with underlying neurologic disorders account for a high proportion of the PICU admissions. Over the course of 1 year in the PICU at Boston Children's Hospital, 427/1820 (23%) of children admitted to the PICU had an underlying neurodevelopmental disorder; the 2 most common reasons for admission were either a surgical procedure or an acute respiratory illness.[14] Although not admitted for an acute neurologic illness, the expertise of the child neurologist is needed for optimal care. In addition, neurologic disorders account for a large percentage of PICU mortality. Over a 21-month period at Children's Hospital, Pittsburgh, brain injury occurred in 51 of the 78 (65%) deaths out of 4694 admissions.[15]

What Expertise Is Required for Neurocritical Care?

Adult NCC units are now staffed by NCC-trained adult neurologists who manage all aspects of care. Their training involves NCC and general critical care. This is not the case in pediatric NCC. From the Boston PICU experience in patients with an acute neurologic disorder, 57% required ventilation and 45% had coexisting medical or surgical diagnoses.[10] Therefore, the additional expertise needed to care for these children is beyond the training or experience of the child neurologist and requires pediatric CCM. For the child neurologist to assume a role analogous to the adult NCC specialist, additional training is needed in pediatric CCM or even adult NCC. It is unlikely that enough child neurologists would be willing to train an additional 3 years in pediatric CCM to develop an analogous NCC unit. The director of our NCC unit has

Table 3 Disorders with critical care interventions from the kid inpatient database	
Disorder	%
TBI	14.8
Infection/Inflammation	4.3
Status Epilepticus	3.6
Stroke	2.4
Hypoxic-Ischemic	1.3
Spinal Cord Injury	0.6

Data from Williams CN, Piantino J, McEvoy C, Fino N, Eriksson. The burden of pediatric neurocritical care in the United States. Pediatr Neurol 2018;89:31-38.

Table 4	
Primary neurologic diagnoses in the pediatric intensive care unit	
Traumatic Brain Injury	154 (47.4%)
Status Epilepticus	71 (21.8%)
Infectious/Inflammatory	40 (12.3%)
Cardiac Arrest	37 (11.4%)
Stroke	23 (7.1%)
Total	325

Data from Williams CN, Eriksson CO,Kirby A, Piantino JA, Hall TA, Luther M, McEvoy CT. Hospital mortality and functional outcomes in pediatric neurocritical care. Pediatrics 2019;9:958-966.

this dual training. Even for a child neurologist that trains in NCC, the NCC training does not provide the technical expertise needed for children.

The Section of Child Neurology of the American Academy of Neurology and the Professors of Child Neurology delineated the training needed for the Child Neurologist in the twenty-first century, including NCC.[7] **Box 1** lists the specific NCC disorders in which the child neurologist must become proficient.[7] A different skill set is required for the child neurologist to function as a consultant to the PICU, compared with the outpatient practice of pediatric neurology. **Box 2** lists the specific competencies in pediatric NCC needed during the child neurology residency.[7]

Advanced training in pediatric NCC must be available for those who practice NCC as their primary subspecialty; this is especially important for the NCC teams that provide care in larger children's hospitals.[2,6,16]

A required competency for pediatric NCC is to be aware of the current guidelines and practice parameters. The production of evidence-based practice guidelines ensures that patient care is standardized across institutions that provide pediatric NCC: from the emergency department of a local community hospital to the children's hospital.

Multimodality Monitoring

Brain monitoring is important in NCC. The use of MMM has been developed using a combination of multiple monitoring techniques including hemodynamic parameters and specific noninvasive and invasive neuromonitoring techniques.[17,18] MMM helps to individualize patient management, assess response to treatment, and modify subsequent treatment to maintain certain parameters to prevent injury.[19] A recent consensus on MMM in NCC identified the physiologic processes important to NCC (**Box 3**).[17] MMM is currently used in pediatric NCC.[20]

MMM uses both invasive and noninvasive monitoring techniques. Noninvasive monitoring techniques include CEEG, near-infrared spectroscopy (NIRS), and transcranial doppler (TCD) ultrasonography. Invasive monitoring techniques include intracranial pressure (ICP), cerebral perfusion pressure (CPP), CBF, brain tissue oxygenation (PbtO$_2$), microdialysis, and depth electrodes (DE). The following reviews were used for background information on various physiologic parameters and MMM.[18,21,22]

Noninvasive Monitoring Techniques

Systemic hemodynamics include heart rate, blood pressure, mean arterial pressure, pulse oximetry, and end-tidal carbon dioxide. These measurements are important for monitoring cardiorespiratory function and intracranial hemodynamics.[23,24] hyperthermia and worsening outcomes in NCC.[25]

Box 1
Proficiency needed for specific disorders: neonate and child

Neonatal Neurology:
  Neonatal seizures
  Intraventricular hemorrhage, periventricular leukoencephalopathy, intracranial hemorrhage, subarachnoid hemorrhage
  Neonatal stroke
  Hypoxic-ischemic encephalopathy and its treatment
  Neonatal weakness, exclude treatable spinal cord trauma

Older Child:
  Alteration of awareness, altered mental status
  Coma, especially with increased intracranial pressure and herniation
  Increased intracranial pressure
  Hydrocephalus
  Intracranial hemorrhage (hematoma), subarachnoid hemorrhage, subdural and epidural hemorrhage.
  Stroke
  Seizures and status epilepticus
  Infections (meningitis, encephalitis), inflammatory disorders, postinfectious and autoimmune disorders acute disseminated encephalomyelitis (ADEM), CNS vasculitis
  Traumatic Brain Injury (TBI)
  Spinal Cord Injury
  Acute weakness
  Malignant hyperthermia syndrome, malignant neuroleptic syndrome, serotonin syndrome (Call-Fleming syndrome)

Data from Lee JC, Riviello JJ Jr. Education of the child neurologist: Pediatric Neurocritical Care. Semin Pediatr Neurol 2011;18:128-130.

NIRS uses infrared light to estimate $PbtO_2$ using the relative absorption of oxygenated and unoxygenated hemoglobin. The ratio of oxygenated Hb to total Hb, the tissue oxygenation index, is related to regional CBF. NIRS has a long history of use in the neonatal and cardiac ICUs and during cardiac surgery. NIRS is an indirect measurement of CBF.

Box 2
Essential competencies in neurocritical care for the child neurologist

Recognize the special disorders that constitute a neurologic emergency and place the brain at risk (high risk of secondary injury). Includes NICU and PICU.

Perform a neurologic examination in the critically ill child.

Understand proper use of ancillary tools used or brain monitoring techniques.

Be aware of neurology and critical care guidelines and practice parameters, including those regarding adults.

Understand evidence-based medicine, as it applies to child neurology and CCM, quality improvement, and patient safety.

Be proficient in ethical issues of the ICU, especially evidence-based neuroprognostication.

Synthesize the information obtained from to predict the neurologic outcome (make a prognosis).

Data from Lee JC, Riviello JJ Jr. Education of the child neurologist: Pediatric Neurocritical Care. Semin Pediatr Neurol 2011;18:128-130.

Box 3
Physiologic processes important in neurocritical care

The clinical examination

Systemic hemodynamics

Intracranial pressure

Cerebral perfusion pressure

Cerebrovascular autoregulation

Systemic and brain oxygenation

Cerebral blood flow and ischemia

Electrophysiology

Cerebral metabolism

Glucose and nutrition

Hemostasis and hemoglobin

Temperature and inflammation

Biomarkers of cellular damage and degeneration

Data from Le Roux P, Menon DK, Citerio G, et al. Consensus summary statement of the International Multidisciplinary Consensus Conference on Multimodality Monitoring in Neurocritical Care. Intensive Care Med 2014;40:1189-1209. https://doi.org/10.1007/s00134-014-3369-6.

TCD ultrasonography indirectly measures the mean blood flow velocity of red blood cells in major cerebral vessels.[26–28] TCD has been used in children with TBI, intracranial hypertension, vasospasm, stroke, cerebrovascular disorders, CNS infections,[29] ECMO,[30] and brain death.

Pupilometer is a hand-held device that provides objective measurement of pupil size and reactivity before and after a light stimulus. Abnormalities of pupil reactivity are often associated with neurologic deterioration and poor outcome[31] in patients with increased ICP, especially in cerebral herniation, third nerve compression, and brainstem perfusion.[32] Traditional means of monitoring pupil size and reactivity by gross inspection are highly subjective,[33] making it difficult for ongoing monitoring. Aside from providing objective measurements of pupil size, the pupilometer can calculate pupil reactivity, latency time, and constriction and latency velocities.[34] In specific patients, the monitoring of changes in these variables may be helpful in distinguishing pathologic increase in ICP.

The use of *CEEG monitoring* for neuromonitoring in the PICU markedly expanded when digital technology became available for EEG. With analog paper EEG recording, it was a typical practice to do intermittent "routine" EEGs to identify seizures or assess background; this introduced sampling error, as seizures could be missed. CEEG monitoring is better to identify seizures, subclinical seizures, or acute changes, as CEEG is used in certain high-risk situations, such as stroke, subarachnoid hemorrhage (SAH), intracranial hemorrhage, or CNS infections (meningitis, encephalitis).

The addition of quantified EEG (QEEG), or digital trending analysis (DTA), to CEEG monitoring has greatly enhanced the ability to identify seizure activity or changes indicating ischemia, such as the alpha-delta ratio to detect vasospasm in SAH. QEEG allows performance of spectral analysis, which can display the EEG signal by its frequency or amplitude components. It can be displayed in various time windows, showing the entire EEG segment over a specific time period, allowing the reader to identify recurrent seizures over time. It also permits the nonneurophysiologist at the bedside to identify significant changes. Digital trending is derived from the CEEG and is time-locked to CEEG. The raw EEG must be available to review at the same time as the digital trend, in order to identify and exclude artifact. MMM is performed concomitantly with CEEG and the digital trending. Certain software packages can visualize EEG, the digital trends, and other physiologic parameters at the same time.

Invasive Monitoring Techniques

The major invasive MMM techniques include ICP, $PbtO_2$, cerebral microdialysis, and invasive EEG monitoring. These yield measurement such as the ICP, CPP, $PbtO_2$, pressure reactivity, and chemical concentrations of the dialysate.

ICP is typically measured from the brain parenchyma or intraventricular space through an intraparenchymal probe or external ventricular drain, respectively. The ICP is the pressure generated by the major contents of the intracranial space: brain tissue, ventricular fluid, arterial and venous blood volume. Intracranial pathology, such as a space-occupying lesion, increases the volume of the intracranial contents and can result in increased ICP. The skull is a fixed space, so when the volume of one component increases, there must be a compensatory decrease in the other components, or else, the ICP will increase.

In adults, the threshold for treating an elevated ICP is set as between 20 and 25 mm Hg.[35] In children, the Brain Trauma Foundation Guidelines "supports the use of less than 20 mm Hg as the initial ICP target," and "supports the need for intervention when ICP is raised greater than 20 mm Hg for 5 minutes." Increases for less than 5 minutes may not be significant but increases for greater than 5 minutes may be significant and treatment should be considered.[35]

CBF is determined, in part, by the ICP along with the mean arterial pressure (MAP). The venous pressure also contributes to the ICP. Brain perfusion reaches zero when the ICP exceeds the MAP.

CPP is the perfusion pressure across the brain, related to MAP and ICP. $CPP = MAP - ICP$. The optimal CPP is between 50 and 70 mm Hg in adults. A CPP of 45 to 60 mm Hg may be targeted in children, with lower values in younger children.[36] In the TBI guidelines, CPP should be greater than 40 mm Hg in children younger than 5 years[37] and greater than 50 mm Hg in children aged 6 to 17 years.[38]

Cerebral autoregulation (CA) refers to the maintenance of CBF across a range of the MAP; this is mediated by sympathetic innervation and local tissue factors, such as ischemia. A common method of determining CA is the pressure-reactivity index (PRx). The PRx is a model-based index derived from the relationship of ICP with MAP and assumes that changes in intracranial blood flow are being driven fundamentally by changes in cerebrovascular motor responses.[39] CA is reported with values between −1 and +1. A positive result represents a passive nonreactive cerebral vascular bed; a negative result represents a normally reactive vascular bed. An "optimal cerebral perfusion pressure" can be formulated, representing the lower threshold at which CPP may be maintained for the an optimal autoregulatory state.[40]

$PbtO_2$: it is the partial pressure of O_2 in brain tissue, measured by either a polarographic method or the oxygen diffusion across a semipermeable membrane. $PbtO_2$ has been used the most in trauma. In adults, the monitoring device is typically placed along with ICP and cerebral microdialysis catheters. A recent trial (BOOST-II), in adult TBI, showed a significant reduction in cerebral hypoxia with therapy guided by $PbtO_2$ and ICP monitoring as compared with ICP-based therapy alone; there was a trend toward improved functional outcome.[41] At least for TBI in children, the $PbtO_2$ should be targeted as the "goal."[36] Normal values range from 25 to 35 but may be regional: white matter 20 and 35 to 40 in gray matter. The 2019 guidelines state that the minimum value should be 10 mm Hg in children.[37]

Microdialysis: cerebral microdialysis is a real-time measurement of cerebral interstitial space extracellular fluid analyte concentrations, using a dialysis catheter with a semipermeable membrane typically placed in the white matter. The usual analytes measured are glucose, pyruvate, lactate, glycerol, and glutamate. The term "metabolic crisis" has been applied to elevations in the lactate/pyruvate ratio (LPR). Existing studies in pediatric TBI show an association among anaerobic metabolites and a poor outcome.[42–44]

Depth electrodes: intracortical EEG has been used in acute brain injury, including trauma and SAH. Electrographic seizures may be detected on DE that do not show up on scalp recording.[45] The DE should be placed into the tissue at maximal risk. In an adult study, DE were placed in 14 patients with TBI along with conventional CEEG monitoring.[45] Clinically important findings were detected in 12/14, including electrographic seizures in 10 and acute changes related to secondary neurologic injury in 2 patients, one with ischemia, and 1 with hemorrhage. In the 10 with electrographic seizures detected on DE, no surface EEG correlate was seen in 6, and rhythmic delta activity in 2. In 2 patients with secondary injury, EEG attenuation was seen 2 to 6 hours before changes in other parameters and 8 hours before clinical deterioration. In a follow-up multicenter study, Vespa and colleagues reported seizures in 62% of patients with severe TBI; seizures were seen only on the intracortical or invasive electrodes in 43%. Metabolic crisis detected by microdialysis was more severe when epileptiform was present.[46]

Appavu used intracranial EEG in 11 children with severe TBI, using a 6 contact DE in conjunction with surface CEEG. Four patients had epileptiform activity on DE, 2 had epileptiform abnormalities noted only on DE, and 1 patient had seizures originating on DE before those seen on surface EEG. Epileptiform abnormalities were associated with stroke or malignant cerebral edema.[47]

Cortical spreading depressions represent transient and terminal cortical depolarizations.[48] These EEG waveforms can be seen on conventional surface EEG or invasive EEG monitoring, including subdural grids, strips, or DE.

Neuroimaging is included, as it is a data point in time to assesses brain anatomy and function and has been correlated with other MMM techniques. Neuroimaging has poor temporal resolution.[49]

Continuous Electroencephalogram Monitoring

EEG consists of various frequencies of which the waveforms depend on CBF.[50] Normal CBF is approximately 50 mL/100 g/min. With ischemia, as CBF decreases, EEG changes occur: as CBF decreases to 25 to 35 mL/100 g/min, there is a loss of the faster frequencies; at 18 to 25 mL/100 g/min, there is increased slowing (4–7 Hz), which may be rhythmic; at 12 to 18 mL/100 g/min, there is an increase in slower frequencies (1–4 Hz); and at less than 10 to 12 mL/100 g/min, there is EEG suppression and loss of electrocerebral activity. Therefore, sequential changes in EEG are an indirect indicator of decreased CBF. Not all EEG changes are related to decreased CBF, and EEG changes are independent of cause, as EEG slowing can also be caused by brain injury.

EEG changes may be markers of neurologic deterioration. New-onset seizures signify a change, such as a stroke, especially in the newborn. New-onset spikes or sharp waves, or periodic features, could indicate deterioration. A sudden change in background, especially if lateralized or focal, could indicate a new focal lesion. A loss of faster frequencies can indicate ischemia.[50] Generalized discontinuity could indicate increased ICP or herniation; this is especially so in the patient with increased ICP, in whom there are changes in EEG, such as with the EEG suppression seen during a plateau wave,[51,52] or increasing ICP.[53] These findings may occur before a clinical change.[53,54] The worsening of the EEG background, such as the development of delayed EEG suppression after cardiac arrest, carries a poor prognosis.[55]

The EEG changes in our CEEG monitoring program at TCH considered "actionable" are included in **Box 4**.[22] When "actionable" changes are detected by our monitoring team, the clinical teams are notified: the PICU team if immediate intervention is needed, because they are at the bedside, or the NCC team if immediate intervention not required.

Status Epilepticus

CEEG is not needed to identify overt convulsive SE. However, there is a continuum in the clinical and electrographic findings in SE. As a clinical seizure continues, or after treatment, the convulsive movements may stop, but the electrical activity continues; this is the state of nonconvulsive SE (NCSE) and results from electromechanical dissociation.[56] Generalized convulsive SE is always associated with overt electrographic seizure activity. Nonconvulsive SE may be associated with EEG patterns that are overtly ictal patterns or patterns in which it is not absolutely clear. Careful clinical examination of patients with NCSE may reveal subtle clinical manifestations.[57]

Electrographic seizures are more common in the sick brain, especially in the newborn, and nonconvulsive seizures, especially if frequent, may cause altered awareness. The burden of electrographic seizure activity has been correlated with outcomes: the greater the seizure "burden," the more likely there will be a poor outcome.[58]

The Ictal-Interictal Continuum

EEG waveforms (patterns) may be ictal, indicating an overt electrographic seizure, or interictal, indicating the nonictal state. CEEG monitoring has identified EEG waveforms with a less certain significance than overt electrographic SE. These waveforms are referred to as the ictal-interictal continuum (IIC) (**Box 5**). Waveforms in the IIC are

---

Box 4
Actionable electroencephalogram changes indicating intervention

Seizures: new-onset seizures; increasing nonconvulsive seizures; a new seizure type, such as a different location.

Spikes: no spikes to new-onset spies; increasing spikes, spreading spikes, or new location.

Background: continuous to discontinuous; discontinuity suggests disease progression or sedation.

Slowing: new-onset slowing, increasing slowing, new location of slowing.

Frequency changes: loss of fast frequencies, loss of alpha activity, development of slowing, rhythmic slowing; development of attenuation or discontinuity; QEEG: the alpha-delta ratio (stroke, subarachnoid hemorrhage, vasospasm).

Attenuation: regional attenuation without delta (RAWOD); focal or generalized.

Any sudden change: sudden slowing, attenuation.

Data from Riviello JJ, Appavu B. Multimodal monitoring and the ictal-interictal continuum. Sansavere AJ, Harrar DB, editors, Atlas of Pediatric and Neonatal ICU EEG. Springer, New York, 2021, pages 411-434.

Box 5
Electroencephalogram patterns in the ictal-interictal continuum

Ictal EEG Patterns: Status Epilepticus, Convulsive or Nonconvulsive:
  Focal (epilepsia partialis continua)

Patterns in the Ictal-Interictal Continuum:
  Periodic discharges (PDs):
    Generalized (GPDs); lateralized (focal) LPDs
    LPDs plus
    Bilateral independent periodic discharges (BIPDs)
  Rhythmic delta activity (RDA):
    Generalized RDA; lateralized RDA
    Intermittent rhythmic delta activity (IRDA)
  Stimulus-induced rhythmic, periodic or ictal discharges (SIRPIDs)
  Brief, potentially ictal, rhythmic discharges (BIRDS)
  Extreme delta brush pattern (beta-delta complex)
  Triphasic waves (TW): now called "GPDs with triphasic morphology"
  Suppression-burst background

Interictal EEG Patterns:
  Slowing or suppression

---

characteristically rhythmic or periodic.[59–62] These waveforms may occur between the clearly ictal and interictal states.

The IIC is a dynamic pathophysiological state of unstable neurologic processes that suggests an increased risk toward evolution to the ictal state and a greater potential for neuronal injury. The therapeutic question for these IIC waveforms is, do they indicate the potential for secondary neuronal injury, which would then require aggressive therapy or are these IIC waveforms an epiphenomenon, arising because of the insult and not causing ongoing neuronal injury, which would then not require aggressive therapy, or could they be both? Aggressive therapy must be considered when clinical deterioration is associated with one of these IIC patterns.

Waveforms within the IIC are typically rhythmic and periodic. Rhythmic waveforms are described as repetitive waveforms with a relatively uniform morphology and duration, without an interval between consecutive waveforms. Periodic waveforms are defined as repetitive waveforms with a relatively uniform morphology and duration with a quantifiable interdischarge interval between consecutive waveforms and recurrence of the waveforms at nearly regular intervals. Rhythmic and periodic waveforms must continue for at least 6 cycles.[63,64]

Periodic discharges (PDs) are stereotyped, repetitive discharges occurring at regular intervals.[65] PDs are classified as generalized periodic discharges (GPDs) when they are generalized, synchronous, and have relatively equal amplitudes across homologous brain regions.[63,64] When maximally involving one hemisphere, PDs are classified as lateralized periodic discharges (LPDs). These were previously called generalized periodic epileptiform discharges or periodic lateralized epileptiform discharges. The descriptor "epileptiform" was removed because these patterns are not always associated with seizures. PDs subtypes have been described: LPDs plus is a modified term describing LPDs with superimposed rhythmic fast activity and/or sharp waves; bilateral independent periodic discharges represent asynchronous periodic discharges occurring over both hemispheres.[63,64] Stimulus-induced rhythmic, periodic, or ictal discharges (SIRPIDs) occur in patients with altered awareness on physical stimulation, notably percussion.[66]

Standard terminology for the interpretation of repetitive of periodic EEG patterns in the ICU has been introduced.[63,64] The EEG patterns included in the IIC are GPDs, LPDs, and LPDs plus (plus refers to admixed spike and sharp waves), GRDA OR LRDA, SIRPIDS, BIRDs, triphasic waves, and burst-suppression background. One important criterion for identifying an ictal pattern is the frequency of the rhythmic or periodic waveform. The higher the frequency, the more likely that the pattern represents an ictal pattern: 3 Hz for the Young criteria[67] and 2.5 Hz for the Salzburg criteria.[68]

Rhythmic Delta Activity

Rhythmic delta activity (RDA) represents repetitive activity in the delta frequency with a relatively uniform morphology, referred to as "monomorphic delta," and a frequency of 4 Hz or less, without an interval between consecutive waveforms.[64] RDA can seem either generalized (GRDA) or lateralized (LRDA). As PDs, RDA may use modifiers including fast activity (RDA + F), sharply contoured waveforms (RDA + S), or both (RDA, +FS). Intermittent rhythmic delta activity occurs when these rhythmic patterns occur with an intervening interval.

The cause, association with seizures, and prognostic utility of PEDs have been studied. GPDs occur in diverse settings, whereas LPDs are commonly associated with acute structural lesions.[69,70] A correlation has been observed between GPDs and seizures.[65] In children with refractory SE, GPDs occurring after the control of SE are still considered in an active epileptic state and have a lower mortality compared with adults.[71] LPDs also correlate with clinical seizures,[69,70] and LPDs plus are more likely associated with clinical or electrographic seizures than LPDs alone.[72] A recent multicenter cohort study found that LPDs were associated with seizures at all frequencies with and without a plus modifier.[73]

There is evidence to suggest that LRDA confers similar pathogenicity to LPDs. A retrospective analysis found that LPDs occurred in 44% of patients who exhibited LRDA and that both features carry a similar risk of seizure occurrence.[74] The seizures seen were most likely nonconvulsive seizures. LRDA was commonly associated with a cause of intracranial hemorrhage and SAH. It is not yet determined if the "plus" modifier for LPDs confers increased pathogenicity.

The addition of QEEG and DTA to the CEEG has greatly added to our monitoring capabilities.[75] DTA has helped to identify seizures, subtle seizures, and exclude artifact, which may obscure seizure activity. It can also display a specified EEG segment over time. **Fig. 1** shows a portion of a single seizure, whereas the DTA shows 11 seizures over a 2-hour segment. **Fig. 2**A shows a predominantly right-sided seizure obscured by movement artifact, whereas as the DTA **Fig. 2**B shows 9 seizures over 4 hours.

A subtype of SE, cyclic seizures, occurring in both adults and children, is detected easily by DTA, whereas it may be difficult to appreciate on convention CEEG. CS is a discrete EEG pattern seen during SE, constituting NCSE and usually associated with an acute symptomatic cause. These occur in a cyclic fashion, typically in regular intervals, in a periodic manner.[76] We have seen CS in 28 of 279 (10%) of pediatric SE.[77] Although not typically included in the IIC, this pattern should be considered SE.

Multimodality Monitoring to Determine Factors Requiring Treatment

Does MMM help determine which EEG patterns require treatment? This has been evaluated with CEEG in combination with functional neuroimaging, PET, single-photon emission computerized tomography (SPECT), and magnetic resonance (MR) perfusion. PET measures the cerebral metabolism of glucose and SPECT, and MR perfusion measures CBF. Cerebral metabolism and CBF should increase during a

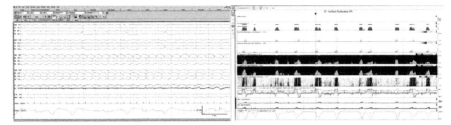

Fig. 1. The EEG segment on the left displays the right hemisphere seizure activity over an 18-second segment. The digital trending analysis shows 11 recurrent seizures over a 2-hour period.

seizure because cerebral metabolic demands increase. PET scans obtained in 18 patients with IIC patterns, such as PDs, demonstrated that hypermetabolism was common and predicted SE.[78] SPECT has shown increased CBF in regions in which PDs were actively occurring, suggesting that PDs may represent an ictal pattern.[79,80] A high correlation with the location of elevated regional CBF (rCBF) to PDs was found in SPECT scan following convulsive seizures; regions with decreased rCBF had little correlation with PEDs.[81]

Witsch and colleagues[82] used MMM, including CEEG and depth EEG, to study the relationship between PD frequency and the CBF and $PbtO_2$ in order to determine if

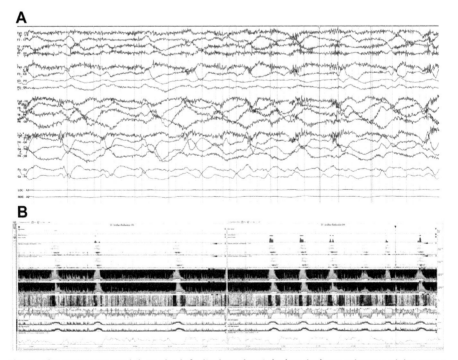

Fig. 2. The EEG segment (A) on the left displays the right hemisphere seizure activity over a 12-second segment, with admixed muscle artifact. The digital trending analysis (B) shows 9 recurrent seizures over a 4-hour period.

there is a threshold frequency for tissue hypoxia in aneurysmal SAH. The median PbtO2 was 23 mm Hg without PDs, compared with 16 mm HG at 2.0 Hz and 14 mm Hg at 2.5 Hz. The rCBF also increased with increasing frequency of PDs. This study suggests that rCBF increases with PEDs in order to compensate for an increased metabolic demand. Subramaniam and colleagues correlated LPD frequency with glucose metabolism using CEEG and PET scanning. LPDs were stratified into those less than 1 Hz, 1 Hz, and greater than 1 Hz. Metabolism increased by 100% for LPD frequencies at 1 Hz and by 309% for LPD frequencies greater than 1 Hz.[83] In SAH, the time spent in a "supraoptimal" CPP range was higher in patients with seizures or in the IIC, and the supraoptimal CPP occurred an hour before the seizures or the IIC patterns and increased during these.[84]

Microdialysis has also been used to study the relationship between PDs and cerebral metabolism. A prospective study on patients with severe TBI-assessed time-locked neurochemical responses in relation to PEDs found that elevated LPRs were more likely to occur in seizures and PEDs as compared with interictal epochs.[46]

In summary, the pathogenicity conferred onto PEDs greater than 2.0 Hz is significant, considering previous criteria for nonconvulsive seizures that require repetitive epileptiform discharges to be equal or greater than 3.0 Hz in the absence of evolution in frequency, morphology, or location.[60] These studies all suggest that in acute brain injury, increases in CBF or metabolism may be associated with a more pathologic relationship with PDs.

CLINICS CARE POINTS

- Pediatric NCC is a collaborative effort among specialists in pediatric CCM, child neurologists, and pediatric neurosurgery.

- The clinical care of the patient relies on the monitoring of various physiologic parameters to detect neurologic dysfunction, with the goal of intervention before the dysfunction becomes irreversible.

- Multimodality monitoring refers to the simultaneous utilization of multiple monitoring techniques; these may be noninvasive or invasive.

- Seizures are a common manifestation of neurologic injury in the ICU. Seizures may have clinical manifestations or commonly may be subclinical (electrographic only) in the injured brain.

- CEEG monitoring in the ICU is used to detect subclinical seizures or ongoing ischemia related to the underlying brain insult.

REFERENCES

1. Vespa P. Continuous EEG monitoring for detection of seizures in traumatic brain injury, infarction, and intracerebral hemorrhage: "to detect and protect". J Clin Neurophysiol 2005;22(2):99–106.
2. LaRovere KL, Riviello JJ. Emerging subspecialties in neurology: building a career and a field, pediatric neurocritical care. Neurology 2008;70:e89–91.
3. Bell MJ, Carpenter J, Au AK, et al. Development of a pediatric neurocritical care service. Neurocrit Care 2009;10:4–10.
4. Riviello JJ Jr, Page T, Chang CWJ. The practice of pediatric neurocritical care by the child neurologist. Neurocrit Care 2008;9:S142.

5. LaRovere KL, Murohy SA, Horak R, et al. Pediatric neurocritical care: evolution of a new clinical service in PICUs across the United States. Pediatr Crit Care Med 2018;19:103901045.

6. Tasker RC. Pediatric neurocritical care: is it time to come of age? Curr Opin Pediatr 2009;39:1–5.

7. Lee JC, Riviello JJ Jr. Education of the child neurologist: pediatric neurocritical care. Semin Pediatr Neurol 2011;18:128–30.

8. Smith WS, Weingart S. Emergency Neurological Life Support (ENLS): what to do in the first hour of a neurological emergency. Neurocrit Care 2012;17:S1–3.

9. Lopez Pison J, Galvin Manso M, Rubio Morales L, et al. Descriptive analysis of neurological disorders in the pediatric neurocritical care unit of a regional referral hospital. An Esp Pediatr 2000;53:119–24 [in Spanish].

10. LaRovere KL, Graham RJ, Tasker RC. Pediatric neurocritical care: a neurology consultation model and implication for education and training. Pediatr Neurol 2013;48:206–11.

11. Broessner G, Helbok R, Lackner P, et al. Survival and long-term functional outcome in 1,155 consecutive neurocritical care patients. Crit Care Med 2007; 35:2015–30.

12. Williams CN, Piantino J, McEvoy C, et al. The burden of pediatric neurocritical care in the United States. Pediatr Neurol 2018;89:31–8.

13. Williams CN, Eriksson CO, Kirby A, et al. Hospital mortality and functional outcomes in pediatric neurocritical care. Pediatrics 2019;9:958–66.

14. Graham RJ, Dumas HM, O'Brien JE, et al. Congenital neurodevelopmental diagnoses and an intensive care unit: defining a population. Pediatr Crit Care Med 2004;5:321–8.

15. Au AK, Carcillo JA, Clark RSB, et al. Brain injuries and neurological system failure are the most common proximate causes of death in children admitted to a pediatric intensive care unit. Pediatr Crit Care Med 2011;12:566–71.

16. Scher MS. Proposed cross-disciplinary training in pediatric neurointensive care. Pediatr Neurol 2008;39:1–5.

17. Le Roux P, Menon DK, Citerio G, et al. Consensus summary statement of the international multidisciplinary consensus conference on multimodality monitoring in neurocritical care. Intensive Care Med 2014;40:1189–209.

18. Macial CB, Claassen J, Gilmore EJ. Multimodality monitoring. In: LaRoche SM, Haider HA, editors. Handbook of ICU EEG monitoring. 2nd edition. New York: Demos Medical; 2018. p. 366–80.

19. Korbakis G, Vespa PM. Multimodal neurologic monitoring. In: Wijdicks EFM, Kramer AH, editors. Critical care neurology, part 1. Amsterdam: Elsevier; 2017. p. 91–105.

20. Grinspan ZM, Pon S, Greenfield JP, et al. Multimodality monitoring in the pediatric intensive care unit: new modalities and informatics challenges. Semin Pediatr Neurol 2014;21:291–8.

21. Miller CM, Torbey MT. Neurocritical care monitoring. New York: Demos Medical; 2015.

22. Riviello JJ, Appavu B. Multimodal monitoring and the ictal-interictal continuum. In: Sansavere AJ, Harrar DB, editors. Atlas of pediatric and neonatal ICU EEG. New York: Springer; 2021. p. 411–34.

23. Smith ER, Madsen JR. Cerebral pathophysiology and critical care neurology: basic hemodynamic principles, cerebral perfusion, and intracranial pressure. Semin Pediatr Neurol 2004;11:89–104.

24. Smith ER, Madsen JR. Neurosurgical aspects of critical care neurology. Semin Pediatr Neurol 2004;11:169–78.

25. Provencio JJ, Badjatia N. Monitoring inflammation (including fever) in acute brain injury. Neurocrit Care 2014;21:S177–86.

26. LaRovere KL, O'Brien NF. Transcranial doppler sonography in pediatric neurocritical care. J Ultrasound Med 2015;34:2121–32.

27. LaRovere KL, O'Brien NF, Tasker RC. Current opinion and use of transcranial doppler ultrasonography in traumatic brain injury in the pediatric intensive care unit. J Neurotrauma 2016;33(23):1–10.

28. Fanelli A, Vonberg FW, LaRoverre KL, et al. Fully automated, real-time, calibration-free, continuous noninvasive estimation of intracranial pressure in children. J Neurosurg Pediatr 2019. https://doi.org/10.3171/2019.5.PEDS19178.

29. Ducharme-Crevier L, Mills MG, Mehta PM, et al. Use of transcranial doppler for management of central nervous system infections in critically ill children. Pediatr Neurol 2016;65:52–8.

30. Rilinger JF, Smith CM, deGegnier RAO, et al. Transcranial doppler identification of neurologic injury during pediatric extracorporeal membrane oxygenation therapy. J Stroke Cerebrovasc Dis 2017;26(10):2336–45.

31. Litvan I, Saposnik G, Maurino J, et al. Pupillary diameter assessment: need for a graded scale. Neurology 2000;54(2):530–1.

32. Ritter AM, Muizelaar JP, Barnes T, et al. Brain stem blood flow, pupillary response, and outcome in patients with severe head injury. Neurosurgery 1999;44(5):941–8.

33. Boev AN, Fountas KN, Karampelas I, et al. Quantitative pupillometry: normative data in healthy pediatric volunteers. J Neurosurg 2005;103(6 Suppl):496–500.

34. Martinez-Ricarte F, Castro A, Poca MA, et al. Infrared pupillometry. Basic principles and their application in the non-invasive monitoring of neurocritical care patients. Neurologia 2013;28(1):41–51.

35. Tasker RC. Intracranial pressure and cerebrovascular autoregulation in pediatric critical illness. Semin Pediatr Neurol 2014;21:255–62.

36. Garvin R, Mangat HS. Emergency neurological life support: severe traumatic brain injury. Neurocrit Care 2017 Sep;27(Suppl 1):159–69.

37. Kochanek PM, Tasker RC, Bell MJ, et al. Management of pediatric severe traumatic brain injury: 2019 consensus and guidelines-based algorithm for first and second tier therapies. Pediatr Crit Care Med 2019;20(3):269–79.

38. Allen BB Chiu YL, Gerber LM, Ghajar J, et al. Age-specific cerebral perfusion pressure threshold and survival in children and adolescents with severe traumatic brain injury. Pediatr Crit Care Med 2014;15(1):62–70.

39. Zweifel C, Lavinio A, Steiner LA, et al. Continuous monitoring of cerebrovascular pressure reactivity in patients with head injury. Neurosurg Focus 2008;25(4):E2.

40. Aries MJ, Czosnyka M, Budohoski KP, et al. Continuous determination of optimal cerebral perfusion pressure in traumatic brain injury. Crit Care Med 2012;40(8):2456–63.

41. Okonkwo DO, Shutter LA, Moore C, et al. Brain oxygen optimization in severe traumatic brain injury phase-II: a phase II randomized trial. Crit Care Med 2017;45(11):1907–14.

42. Tolias C, Richards D, Bowery N, et al. Investigation of extracellular amino acid release in children with severe head injury using microdialysis. A pilot study. Acta Neurochir Suppl 2002;81:377–9.

43. Tolias CM, Richards D, Bowery N, et al. Extracellular glutamate in the brains of children with severe head injuries: a pilot microdialysis study. Childs Nerv Syst 2002;18(8):368–74.

44. Rohlwink UK, Enslin JM, Hoffman J, et al. Examining cerebral microdialysis in children with traumatic brain injury. Childs Nerv Syst 2017;33:1802–3 [abstract].

45. Waziri A, Claassen J, Stuart RM, et al. Intracortical electroencephalography in acute brain injury. Ann Neurol 2009;66(3):366–77.

46. Vespa PM, Nuwer MR, Juhasz C, et al. Early detection of vasospasm after acute subarachnoid hemorrhage using continuous EEG ICU monitoring. Electroencephalogr Clin Neurophysiol 1997;103(6):607–15.

47. Appavu B, Foldes S, Temkit M, et al. Intracranial electroencephalography in severe pediatric brain trauma. Pediatr Crit Care Med 2020;21:240–7.

48. Appavu B, Riviello JJ. Electroencephalographic patterns in neurocritical care: pathologic contributors or epiphenomena? Neurocrit Care 2018;29:9–19.

49. Scheuer ML. Continuous EEG monitoring in the intensive care unit. Epilepsia 2002;43(Suppl 3):114–27.

50. Foreman B, Claassen J. Quantitative EEG for the detection of brain ischemia. Crit Care 2012;(16):216.

51. Gold CA, Odom N, Srinivasan S, et al. Electrographic correlates of plateau waves in patients with leptomeningeal metastases. Neurohospitalist 2016;6(4):161–6.

52. Kreitzer N, Huynh M, Foreman B. Blood flow and continuous EEG changes during symptomatic plateau waves. Brain Sci 2018;8(1) [pii:E14].

53. Newey CR, Sarwal A, Hantus S. Continuous electroencephalography (cEEG) changes precede clinical changes in a case of progressive cerebral edema. Neurocrit Care 2013;18(2):261–5.

54. Fantaneanu T, Alvarez V, Lee JW. Acute generalized suppression on continuous EEG heralds clinical and radiologic deterioration. Neurology 2015;84(16): e119–20.

55. Fantaneanu T, Sarkis R, Avery K, et al. Delayed deterioration of EEG background rhythm post-cardiac arrest. Neurocrit Care 2017;26(3):411–9.

56. Lothman E. The biochemical basis and pathophysiology of status epilepticus. Neurology 1990;40(5 Suppl 2):13–23.

57. Husain AM, Horn GJ, Jacobson MP. Non-convulsive status epilepticus: usefulness of clinical features in selecting patients for urgent EEG. J Neurol Neurosurg Psychiatry 2003;74:189–91.

58. Payne ET, Zhao XY, Frndova H, et al. Seizure burden is independently associated with short term outcome in critically ill children. Brain 2014;137:1429–38.

59. Chong DJ, Hirsch LJ. Which EEG patterns warrant treatment in the critically ill? Reviewing the evidence for treatment of periodic epileptiform discharges and related patterns. J Clin Neurophysiol 2005;22(2):79–91.

60. Claassen J. How I treat patients with EEG patterns on the ictal-interictal continuum in the neuro ICU. Neurocrit Care 2009;11:437–44.

61. LaRoche SM, Rodriguez V. The Ictal-Interictal continuum. In: LaRoche SM, Haider HA, editors. Handbook of ICU EEG monitoring. 2nd edition. New York: Demos Medical; 2018. p. 186–99.

62. Osman GM, Riviello JJ Jr, Hirsch LJ. EEG in the intensive care unit: anoxia, coma, brain death and related disorders. In: Schomer DL, da Silva L, editors. Niedermeyer's electroencephalography. 7th edition. New York: Oxford; 2018. p. 610–58.

63. Hirsch LJ, Brenner RP, Drislane FW, et al. The ACNS Subcommittee on Research terminology for continuous EEG monitoring: proposed standardized terminology for rhythmic and periodic EEG patterns encountered in critically ill patients. J Clin Neurophysiol 2005;22:128–35.

64. Hirsch LJ, LaRoche SM, Gaspard N, et al. American Clinical Neurophysiology Society's standardized critical care EEG terminology: 2012 version. J Clin Neurophysiol 2013;30(1):1–27.
65. Brenner RP, Schaul N. Periodic EEG patterns: classification, clinical correlation, and pathophysiology. J Clin Neurophysiol 1990;7:249–67.
66. Hirsch LJ, Claassen J, Mayer SA, et al. Stimulus-induced rhythmic, periodic, or ictal discharges (SIRPIDs): a common phenomenon in the critically ill. Epilepsia 2004;45:109–23.
67. Young GB, Jordan KG, Doig GS. An assessment of nonconvulsive seizures in the intensive care unit using continuous EEG monitoring: an investigation of variables associated with mortality. Neurology 1996;47:83–9.
68. Leitinger M, Beniczky S, Rohracher A, et al. Salzburg consensus criteria for non-convulsive status epilepticus-approach to clinical application. Epilepsy Behav 2015;49:158–63.
69. García-Morales I, García MT, Galán-Dávila L, et al. Periodic lateralized epileptiform discharges: etiology, clinical aspects, seizures, and evolution in 130 patients. J Clin Neurophysiol 2002;19(2):172–7.
70. San Juan Orta D, Chiappa KH, Quiroz AZ, et al. Prognosis implications of periodic epileptiform discharges. Arch Neurol 2009;66(8):985–91.
71. Akman CI, Abou Khaled KJ, Segal E, et al. Generalized periodic epileptiform discharges in critically ill children: clinical features and outcome. Epilepsy Res 2013; 106:378–85.
72. Reiher J, Rivest J, Grand'Maison F, et al. Periodic lateralized epileptiform discharges with transitional rhythmic discharges: association with seizures. Electroencephalogr Clin Neurophysiol 1991;78:12–7.
73. Rodriguez Ruiz A, Vlachy J, Lee JW, et al. Association of periodic and rhythmic electroencephalographic patterns with seizures in critically ill patients. JAMA Neurol 2017;74(2):181–8.
74. Gaspard N, Manganas L, Rampal N, et al. Similarity of lateralized rhythmic delta activity to periodic lateralized epileptiform discharges in critically ill patients. JAMA Neurol 2013;70(10):1288–95.
75. Riviello JJ Jr. Digital trend analysis in the pediatric and neonatal intensive care units. J Clin Neurophysiol 2013;30:143–55.
76. Friedman DE, Schevon C, Emerson RG, et al. Cyclic electrographic seizures in critically ill patients. Epilepsia 2008;49(2):281–7.
77. Riviello J, Agadi S, Marx C, et al. Cyclic electrographic seizures in children: A unique EEG pattern of status epilepticus. Abstract 1.068, American Epilepsy Society, Annual Meeting, San Antonio, December, 2010.
78. Struck AF, Westover MB, Hall LT, et al. Metabolic correlates of the ictal-interictal continuum: FDG-PET during continuous EEG. Neurocrit Care 2016;24(3):324–31.
79. Ergun EL, Salanci BV, Erbas B, et al. SPECT in periodic lateralized epileptiform discharges (PLEDs): a case report on PLEDs. Ann Nucl Med 2006;20(3):227–31.
80. Bozkurt MF, Saygi S, Erbas B. SPECT in a patient with postictal PLEDs: is hyperperfusion evidence of electrical seizure? Clin Electroencephalogr 2002;33(4): 171–3.
81. Assal F, Papazyan JP, Slosman DO, et al. SPECT in periodic lateralized epileptiform discharges (PLED): a form of partial status epilepticus? Seizure 2001;10(4): 260–6.
82. Witsch J, Frey HP, Schmidt JM, et al. Electroencephalographic periodic discharges and frequency-dependent brain tissue hypoxia in acute brain injury. JAMA Neurol 2017;74(3):301–9.

83. Subramaniam T, Jain A, Hall LT, et al. Lateralized periodic discharges frequency correlates with metabolism. Neurology 2019;92:e670–4.

84. Alkhachroum A, Meghani M, Terilli K, et al. Hyperemia in subarachnoid hemorrhage patients is associated with an increased risk of seizures. J Cereb Blood Flow Metab 2019. https://doi.org/10.1177/0271678X19863028. 271678 X19863028.

Neurology of Sleep

Samiya F. Ahmad, MD[a],*, Ashura W. Buckley, MD[b],
Daniel G. Glaze, MD[c,d]

KEYWORDS

- Sleep • Pediatric • Childhood • Sleep development • Sleep problems • Insomnia

KEY POINTS

- Sleep problems are common among typically developing children and more frequent among children with neurodevelopmental disabilities, like autism spectrum disorder.
- Sleep disorders contribute not only to problematic sleep but also to daytime challenges with cognition, behavior, and family quality of life.
- Screening for sleep problems, including snoring, should be performed routinely.
- Screening tools, such as the BEARS questionnaire, can identify sleep problems efficiently.
- Many sleep disorders can be evaluated by history and treated with behavior modification; a portion will need further assessment by polysomnography and management with pharmacotherapy and/or surgery.

INTRODUCTION

From the earliest years, differences in the timing, quality, and electrophysiologic architecture of sleep reflect and inform on brain state and overall neurodevelopmental trajectory. More clearly deciphering sleep's contribution in this space seems a natural fit for students of the developing brain. Sleep should be conceptualized as a complex state, behavior, and process without a monolithic function but rather an omniphenomenon differentially focused on the needs of the organism as determined by developmental period. For example, in the earliest years, sleep's major role may be providing the necessary stabilization for building the synapses and refining the essential circuits crucial to the development of motoric fluency, language, and the behavior of socialization. As the individual develops, sleep's role in learning and memory and later in repair may become more important. Dysregulated sleep, in its many forms,

[a] Department of Pediatrics, Baylor College of Medicine, 315 North San Saba Street, Suite 1135, San Antonio, TX 78207, USA; [b] Sleep and Neurodevelopmental Service, Pediatrics and Developmental Neuroscience Branch, National Institute of Mental Health, NIH, Magnuson Clinical Center, Room 1C250, Bethesda, MD 20814, USA; [c] Department of Pediatrics, Baylor College of Medicine, TXCL-1250, Houston, TX 77030, USA; [d] Department of Neurology, Baylor College of Medicine, TXCL-1250, Houston, TX 77030, USA
* Corresponding author.
E-mail address: Samiya.Ahmad@bcm.edu

Neurol Clin 39 (2021) 867–882
https://doi.org/10.1016/j.ncl.2021.04.007
0733-8619/21/© 2021 Elsevier Inc. All rights reserved.

has the potential to disrupt these essential processes and impact optimal functioning whenever in the life cycle it occurs. Primary disorders of sleep include the apneas, both obstructive and central, the insomnias, the parasomnias, sleep-related movement disorders, and circadian rhythm disorders. Their causes may be related to genetics, anatomic differences, cooccurring medical disorders, environmental factors, or some combination thereof. The practice of clinical sleep medicine requires a deep understanding of both the primary disorder and the subsequent secondary effects of interrupting the sleep process itself. The neurologic and neurodevelopmental consequences of chronic sleep disruption, whether from untreated obstructive sleep apnea (OSA) in a 6 year old with kissing tonsils or from chronic sleep insufficiency in a 17 year old with mismatched sleep need and sleep opportunity, are becoming more apparent as researchers from multiple disciplines more closely examine sleep's contribution to brain health.

DISCUSSION
Development of Sleep and Sleep Requirements

Sleep is a complex process governed by the interaction of circadian and homeostatic processes mitigated by genetic and environmental influences. Sleep cycles are established in utero with the suprachiasmatic nucleus (SCN) setting the circadian rhythm as early as 18 weeks after conception.[1] After 32 weeks' gestation, sleep is divided into active, quiet, and indeterminate sleep.[2] Neonatal sleep is polyphasic, with random intervals of sleep throughout a 24-hour period as the SCN matures and the infant is synchronized to the external environment. The most remarkable changes occur in the first 12 months, with major changes in sleep consolidation and architecture continuing through the preschool period. Unlike in adults outside of pathologic states, the newborn falls directly into active sleep, the predecessor of rapid eye movement (REM) sleep, which occupies fully 50% of the total sleep time in early life. REM versus non–rapid eye movement (NREM) sleep can be clearly differentiated by 2 months of age, when sleep spindles appear on the electroencephalogram (EEG), signaling the onset of N2.[3] Regular sleep-wake rhythms develop by 2 to 4 months of age and mark the transition from neonatal sleep to infant sleep. A diurnal pattern is established by 3 months with consolidation into a major nighttime sleep period and a series of shorter sleep bouts during the day. K-complexes form by 5 to 6 months age, allowing sleep to now be classified with increased certainty into stages N1, N2, N3, and REM.

Infants attain the ability to put themselves to sleep as early as 2 to 4 months of age and can sleep through the night by 6 to 9 months. Many children may require a daytime nap with an average frequency of 2 naps per day, lasting 2 to 4 hours.[4] Individual sleep need is difficult to determine, and the current parameters are consensus and vary by developmental stage, with no consensus reached for under the age of 4 months.[5] **Table 1** lists the sleep requirements for optimal health. Note that consensus recommendations for developmentally appropriate sleep durations are very broad and based on the requirements for typically developing children.

Problematic Sleep

Sleep disorders are reported in 10% to 25% of typically developing children and as many as 40% to 100% of children with neurodevelopmental disorders. Insomnia is the most common sleep complaint, reported in 10% to 30%[6–8] of children, and can stem from behavioral, medical, or psychiatric causes. Insomnia may include difficult initiating or maintaining sleep and must have attendant daytime consequences (International Classification of Sleep Disorders, 3rd edition).[9] In younger age groups, the

Table 1
Sleep requirements for optimal health

Age	Number of Hours per 24-h Period
4–12 mo	12–16
1–2 y	11–14
3–5 y	10–13
6–12 y	9–12
13–18 y	8–10

Data from Paruthi S, Brooks LJ, D'Ambrosio C, et al. Consensus statement of the American Academy of Sleep Medicine on the recommended amounts of sleep for healthy children: methodology and discussion. *J Cl Sleep Med*, 2016 12(11): 1549-1561. Published 2016 Nov 15. https://doi.org/10.5664/jcsm.6288.

clinical presentation may include bedtime refusal or resistance, delaying the actual time to fall asleep, or frequent night awakenings that require parental intervention. Most children outgrow behavioral insomnias, and treatment is based on working with families to set limits and manage expectations. In older age groups, the clinical presentation should be distinguished from delayed sleep phase syndrome, a mismatch between expected developmental changes in sleep propensity and cultural expectations (ie, school start times)[10] that often leads to sleep insufficiency. Importantly, the advent or exacerbation of insomnia in youth warrants special attention for the following reasons: adolescent insomnia is usually chronic, increases the risk for substance abuse and suicide irrespective of cooccurring diagnoses,[8,11,12] and according to a recent meta-analysis, predicts the development of psychopathology.[13] Parasomnias are also very common and may occur in 25% of children. Sleep walking and talking are generally not overly concerning, and most cases can be managed with behavioral support for the parents and attention to safety. Sleep terrors and confusional arousals are likewise not considered developmentally abnormal, although nontypical presentations, such as episodes that occur multiple times a night, should be differentiated from nocturnal epilepsies. Restless legs syndrome (RLS) or Willis-Ekbom disease is a sensorimotor abnormality with a prevalence in pediatric populations of between 2% and 4%,[14,15] and the relationship between genetics, iron stores, and dopamine dysfunction is still being worked out. Children and youth experiencing difficulty with sleep initiation may have RLS or the related periodic limb disorder of sleep (diagnosis is by polysomnography [PSG]), and along with a sensitive sleep history, serum ferritin should be obtained. Restless sleep disorder is a newly described pediatric sleep condition consisting of large body movements that are persistent throughout the night and impact daily behaviors.[16] It is often coexistent with other disorders of sleep, and prevalence is estimated at 7.7%.[16] OSA is estimated to affect 1% to 5%[17] of children, with higher rates among children with obesity, neurodevelopmental disorders, neuromuscular disorders, and certain genetic disorders that affect the anatomy of the head and neck.[18] Weight loss and surgical removal of the tonsils and adenoids are often used, but nasal steroids, continuous positive airway pressure (CPAP), and even watch-and-wait strategies have been used with treatment course dependent on age, cause, and severity. **Table 2** summarizes pediatric sleep disorders.

Children with autism spectrum disorder (ASD) tend to have very high rates of sleep dysfunction with estimates ranging from 53% to 83%.[19,20] Children with attention-deficit/hyperactivity disorder (ADHD) also report higher rates of sleep problems, with some estimates as high as 73%,[21] and because of the relationship between

Table 2
Summary of pediatric sleep disorders

Disorder	Age	Clinical and Diagnostic Features	Diagnostic Evaluation	Treatment
Insomnia Chronic • Behavioral insomnia of childhood • In older children Short term	Infants/toddlers/preschool School age through adolescence >6 mo of age	Difficulty initiating and/or maintaining sleep with daytime consequences, should be distinguished from DSWPD Precipitated by an acute identifiable stressor	History, rule out medical comorbidities, sleep diary, actigraphy, sleep questionnaires Add mental health screen to above History	Behavioral interventions, melatonin, pharmacotherapy
Parasomnias • NREM: confusional arousals, sleep walking, night terrors • REM: nightmares, REM sleep behavior disorder	Any age Confusional arousals: toddlers Sleep terrors: 4–12 y Sleep walking: peaks between 8 and 12 y RBD is rare in children; has been noted in narcolepsy, ASD, Tourette syndrome, and other NDD	1st third of night; increased sympathetic activity, confusion, difficult to awaken, no memory Last third of night; easily awakened, dream recall	History, caregiver video recording; PSG/full EEG montage for atypical presentations	Parent education, sleep extension, safety precautions, scheduled awakenings, benzodiazepine
Sleep-related movement disorder • Restless legs syndrome • Periodic limb movement disorder	Early childhood to adolescence; RLS diagnosed retrospectively to ≤6 mo of age	Urge to move legs, which is worse at rest and in the evenings, relieved by movement, and causes distress Sleep disturbance or daytime fatigue and PSG with ≥5 PLMS/hour of sleep	History, serum ferritin PSG, serum ferritin	Iron (oral or intravenous), warm compresses, pharmacotherapy
Obstructive sleep apnea	Any age, peaks between ages 2 and 8 y	Snoring, labored breathing, daytime behavior problems PSG with AHI >1	PSG	T&A, PAP therapy, positional therapy, intranasal steroids, weight reduction

Delayed sleep-wake phase disorder (DSWPD)	Adolescents to young adults	Desired sleep and wake times are significantly delayed compared with desired wake time for at least 3 mo	History, sleep diary, actigraphy	Behavioral intervention, light therapy, strategic melatonin dosing
Narcolepsy	Peaks in 2nd decade of life	Excessive daytime sleepiness, cataplexy, hypnogogic hallucinations, sleep paralysis MSLT with SOL <8 min, ≥2 SOREMPs	PSG + MSLT	Behavioral intervention, stimulants, wake-promoting agents, sodium oxybate

Abbreviations: PAP, positive airway pressure; PLMS, periodic limb movements of sleep; SOL, sleep onset latency; SOREMP, sleep onset REM periods.
Data from Medicine, A.A.o.S., International classification of sleep disorders, 3rd ed. 2014, American Academy of Sleep Medicine: Darien, IL.

chronic sleep disruption and daytime symptoms of hyperactivity and attention deficits, ruling out primary sleep disorders is paramount in this group.

Sleep Evaluation

All children and teenagers should be screened for sleep problems. An example of a short, easy-to-use starting place is The BEARS, a 5-question pediatric sleep screening tool, that helps the clinician cover all the potential problem areas and increases the likelihood that sleep issues will be detected.[22] A practice pathway for identification, evaluation, and management of insomnia in children and adolescents with ASD is delineated by Malow and colleagues.[23]

Overnight PSG is a multiparameter continuous recording encompassing the whole sleep period. It facilitates the objective identification, characterization, and determination of brain activity, breathing, and movement and "unusual" behaviors in relation to awake and sleep states. It is the gold standard for diagnosing OSA and other sleep-related breathing disorders and operationalizes the apnea-hypopnea index (AHI), the number of these events per hour of sleep. In children less than 17 years of age, an obstructive AHI of 1 or less is considered normal, between 1 to 5 is mild OSA, 5 to 10 is moderate OSA, and severe OSA is an AHI of greater than 10.[24] Although suspected OSA is the most common indication for a PSG, it is also indicated in PLMD and narcolepsy and can be beneficial in evaluating sleep-related movements, snoring, restless sleep, and differentiating parasomnias from certain epilepsies.

True disorders of circadian rhythm are rare in prepubescent, typically developing children but may be underdiagnosed in children with NDDs where the complex relationship between cognition, neurologic function, and regulation of circadian rhythmicity may be disturbed.[25] Delayed sleep-wake phase disorder is the most common circadian rhythm disorder in adolescents. Commonly, adolescents may experience a developmentally expected shift in bedtime with the desire to fall asleep falling later in the evening. Because of societal constraints whereby rise time is fixed, these children may develop chronic sleep insufficiency manifesting as daytime sleepiness along with changes in attention, mood, and behavior.[26] Workup for suspected circadian sleep-wake phase rhythm disorders and some types of insomnia can involve the use of actigraphy, a noninvasive, safe, reliable, and validated method for measuring sleep durations, patterns, and efficiency. The actigraphy device is worn on the nondominant wrist and measures sleep in the home environment over days to weeks.

Case Presentations

The authors illustrate the common pediatric sleep complaints through a series of vignettes.

Insomnia: Two cases of sleepy mothers and not-so-sleepy children.

Patient 1

A 15-month-old girl is evaluated for frequent nighttime awakenings. She is habitually rocked to sleep and put to bed at 8 PM For the past 4 months, she has had recurrent night awakenings, requiring her to be rocked back to sleep again. Her parents are frustrated and sleep deprived. She takes 1 to 2 naps per day, has age-appropriate development, and has no medical issues. Her examination reveals a happy child and is entirely normal. She is diagnosed with chronic insomnia, behavioral insomnia of childhood, sleep onset association subtype. After explanation of the problem, a thorough review of sleep expectations for toddlers, and a discussion of various management approaches, the mother opts for a behavioral approach called unmodified extinction, and the following plan is developed: (1) consistent bedtime and morning out of bed time, ensuring developmentally appropriate adequate time for sleep; (2) specified bedtime routine followed by being put to bed awake but drowsy; (3) opportunity to "cry it out"; (4) close follow-up with weekly phone check-in; (5) both parents will be responsible for adherence. After a challenging first weekend, parents report success after 1 full week. Child continues to experience awakenings but is now able to put herself back to sleep without crying or parent intervention, and the family opts to continue the program.

Conditions that are habitually present at the time of sleep onset are termed sleep associations. Similar conditions are thus required for the child to return to sleep following normal, periodic night arousals, which then result in awakenings. These children may also present with difficulty napping, delayed sleep onset, and daytime behavior problems, all of which can lead to family stress. "Crying it out," also known as unmodified extinction, is an efficacious method of treatment, but may not be acceptable for all families. Graduated extinction, bedtime fading, and other positive routines offer an alternative.[27]

Patient 2
A 5-year-old boy with behavior problems and ASD has difficulty attaining and maintaining sleep and is perceived by his mother to sleep less than his neurotypical brothers. His mother is frustrated and sleepy and has difficulty performing her best at work because of the child's chaotic sleep schedule. His nurse practitioner discusses sleep expectations for a child of this age with ASD and makes a diagnosis of chronic insomnia. She also reviews coexisting conditions, such as constipation and gastroesophageal reflux disease, and discusses ways to optimize management to facilitate better sleep. A sleep program is designed with a 24-hour invariant schedule, including a bedtime routine, graduated responses to night awakenings, a reward system, and bedtime passes. A trial of melatonin at bedtime is initiated with follow-up in 1 month.

Sleep problems are ubiquitous in children with ASD, and improving sleep may ameliorate multiple aspects of physical and mental well-being for the patient and family. Practice guidelines by the American Academy of Neurology in 2020 provide recommendations for use of low-dose, pharmaceutical-grade melatonin if behavioral strategies fail and after coexisting medical and pharmacologic factors have been addressed.[28] **Table 3** summarizes medications that can be used to treat insomnia.

Sleep-Disordered Breathing: A Case of Restless Sleep

Patient 3
A 4-year-old girl with Down syndrome (DS) presents with snoring, witnessed apneas, and restless sleep. She often sleeps sitting up with her head bent forward. She has typical Down facies with a short neck, enlarged tongue, and generalized hypotonia. As part of her routine care of children with DS, the pediatrician orders a PSG, which shows severe OSA with 19.6 respiratory-related arousals per hour, 24.9 obstructive respiratory events per hour, an oxygen nadir of 75%, and maximum transcutaneous CO_2 of 53 mm Hg. She is referred to otolaryngology, and an adenotonsillectomy is performed. A repeat PSG shows some improvement but persistent sleep-disordered breathing. Referral is made to sleep medicine clinic for further evaluation and management.

OSA is a constellation of nocturnal and diurnal symptoms with ventilatory irregularities and obstructive events.[17] Peak incidence is between 2 and 8 years, with prevalence especially high in certain populations, ranging from 69% to 76% in children

Table 3
Pharmacologic treatment of insomnia

Medication	Therapeutic Category	Dose at Bedtime	Side Effects	Clinical Pearls
Melatonin	Dietary supplement	Hypnotic dose: 1 mg 30 min before bedtime Increase by 1 mg/wk to maximum 3 mg (<40 kg) or 5 mg (>40 kg) Circadian rhythm adjustment doses: 0.1–0.5 mg, 5–6 h before habitual bedtime	Morning sedation, headache, enuresis, dizziness, mood changes, gastrointestinal complaints, vivid dreaming	Reasonable choice in general and special populations of children with sleep onset insomnia Beneficial in those with circadian phase delay Uncertain reliability of over-the-counter preparations
Gabapentin	Anticonvulsants/mood stabilizers	5 mg/kg, increase weekly by 5 mg/kg to maximum 15 mg/kg	Emotional lability, daytime somnolence	Consider in those with comorbid RLS or PLMD
Clonidine	Alpha-agonist	0.05 mg to 0.3 mg	Morning drowsiness, mid-sleep awakening, hypotension, irritability, rebound hypertension, exacerbation of parasomnias due to increasing N3 sleep	Short half-life supports potential middle-of-the-night dosing Reasonable choice for ADHD-related insomnia
Trazodone	Atypical antidepressant	18 mo to <3 y: 25 mg, increase by 25 mg every 2 wk to maximum 100 mg/dose Ages 3 to adolescents: 50 mg, increase by 25 mg every 2 wk to maximum 150 mg/dose for ages 3–5 y, 200 mg/dose for ages >5 y to adolescents	Sedation, hypotension, arrythmias, serotonin syndrome; risk of priapism in boys (at doses of 100–150 mg)	REM suppressant, rebound may lead to nightmares; likely most useful with comorbid mood disorders ± anxiety
Clonazepam	Benzodiazepine GABA receptor agonist	0.25–0.75 mg	Cognitive impairment, rebound insomnia, anterograde amnesia,	Utility limited to those who may benefit from its anxiolytic and long duration

			disinhibition, dependence, abuse	of action properties; potential for dependence
Ramelteon	Melatonin receptor agonist	2–8 mg	Dizziness, fatigue, increase prolactin/decrease testosterone	Reasonable choice for mild sleep onset insomnia
Mirtazapine	Atypical antidepressant	7.5 mg	Daytime sedation, orthostatic hypotension, weight gain	
Eszopiclone	Non–benzodiazepine receptor agonist	1–3 mg	Headache, dysgeusia, dizziness	Studied in ADHD-related insomnia, limited utility to older adolescents
Zolpidem	Non–benzodiazepine receptor agonist	0.25 mg/kg, maximum 10 mg	Dizziness, headaches, hallucinations	Same as above

No medications are FDA approved in children for insomnia.

with DS.[29] Untreated OSA can have numerous repercussions on overall health with negative impact on neurocognitive and behavioral functioning, cardiovascular health, metabolic morbidity, and increased health care utilization.[30] Adenotonsillectomy remains the first-line treatment in children for moderate to severe OSA, although outcomes postsurgery may not be as favorable as expected, particularly in high-risk children.[31] CPAP therapy should be used in those with moderate to severe residual OSA.

Non–Rapid Eye Movement Parasomnias: Unusual Nighttime Behaviors

Patient 4

A typically developing 8-year-old girl presents with episodes of confusion and wandering an hour after going to bed. Parents are requesting a sleep study, as the child attempted to exit the house on 2 occasions. Her mother reports she herself had sleep walking as a young child but thinks that her daughter's episodes are different. The girl has no memory of the episodes and has been noted to snore. She is doing well academically and socially. Her pediatrician thinks these are parasomnias but orders a sleep study. During the PSG, the child experiences episodes of arousals and sitting up, and must be prevented from getting out of bed by the technologist. She is noted to have significant sleep-disordered breathing with 10.1 obstructive events per hour with an oxygen nadir of 89%. The obstructive events are associated with arousals. EEG findings are normal. A dual diagnosis of NREM parasomnias and OSA is made. The pediatrician advises safety precautions to prevent injury, which include taking her back to bed while not attempting to wake her, as this may prolong confusion and combativeness. Parents are encouraged to maintain a routine sleep/wake schedule that allows her to obtain an age-appropriate amount of sleep and avoid sleep debt. In addition, an ear, nose, and throat specialist referral is made. Following tonsillectomy and adenoidectomy (T&A), repeat PSG demonstrates resolution of sleep-disordered breathing. The episodes of confusional arousals and sleep walking diminish to only monthly and over the following years stop completely.

Parasomnias are undesirable behaviors and movements that occur during sleep and sleep-wake transitions and can be divided into REM, NREM, and other parasomnias.[9] REM-related parasomnias usually occur in the latter third of the night and include nightmares, REM sleep behavior disorder, and sleep paralysis. NREM parasomnias, which happen during the first third of the night, are also known as disorders of partial-arousal and include confusional arousals, sleep walking, and sleep terrors.

Confusional arousals are differentiated from sleep terrors in that they consist of disorientation and crying, whereas the latter is characterized by an abrupt change in physiologic state resulting in an explosion of activity.[32] Provocative factors include sleep deprivation, hypnotic medications, alcohol, and conditions that provoke arousals, in this case, respirator events. History and caregiver recording of events are helpful, and episodes must be distinguished from nocturnal frontal lobe epilepsy. Mainstays of treatment include reassurance, sleep extension, safety measures, and scheduled awakenings before the habitual time of the events. Medications suppressing slow-wave sleep, such as clonazepam, can be used in select cases.[33]

Insufficient Sleep and Delayed Sleep Phase Syndrome: Sleepy Teenagers

Patient 5

A developmentally and socially appropriate 16-year-old young man is seen after failing several classes because he is falling asleep in school. In the afternoons, he is awake and excels in soccer and baseball. He consistently is in bed by 10 PM and gets up each day at 6 AM to be at school by 7:30 AM Although in bed, he is unable to fall asleep at 10 PM and is most likely to be texting on his phone for several hours until sleep onset at around at 1 AM He has difficulty waking in the morning and is sleepy for the first half of the day. When he does sleep, he reports no problems. His examination is normal for a Tanner 4 boy. A urine drug screen is negative, and a 2-week sleep diary confirms the sleep/wake schedule reported. A diagnosis of insufficient sleep syndrome is made. The pediatrician is aware of the school administration's plan to initiate later school start time for teenagers soon. After discussion, a plan of delaying school start time by 1 hour is agreed upon, allowing the patient to extend morning wake time by 90 minutes to 7:30 AM He is instructed to avoid use of electronic media before bedtime, move his bedtime back to 11 PM, and set awake up time of 7:30 AM, including on weekends. A trial of melatonin to advance sleep onset time is considered. As a motivator, he will not start drivers' education until improvement in his sleepiness is verified.

Between 3.3% and 8.4% of teens and young adults experience a delay in circadian phase with intrinsic preferences for later sleep onset.[34,35] When sleep preferences are incongruent with socially acceptable schedules, this can lead to chronic sleep insufficiency and impaired daytime function. Delayed sleep-wake phase syndrome can be treated with behavioral modifications and strategies to advance circadian phase, including strategically timed melatonin and phototherapy.[36]

Narcolepsy: Excessive Daytime Sleepiness

Patient 6
A 16-year-old young woman presents with declining academic performance and difficulty staying awake in school with random daytime sleep attacks of 4 years' duration. She reports buckling of her knees with emotional events and excessive weight gain. Her examination is remarkable for the following: (1) she is witnessed to fall asleep during the evaluation; (2) her body mass index is now 25 vs 18 two years ago; (3) drooping of the eyelids and intermittent twitching of the facial muscles are observed. Her sleep medicine provider requests a 2-week sleep diary and PSG followed by an Multiple sleep latency test (MSLT). Her PSG reveals a total sleep time of 8.2 hours with normal sleep stage distributions and an REM sleep latency of 10 minutes. Awakenings and transitions from all stages of sleep to awake are recorded. There are no significant respiratory findings. During the MSLT, her average sleep latency is 2.3 minutes, and REM sleep is achieved during the nap sessions. Between naps, a humorous story was read to her with video recording documenting episodes of cataplexy (buckling of the knees, falling forward, and dropping of objects held in her hands). A diagnosis of narcolepsy type 1 (with cataplexy) is made. Management options, including scheduled naps, medications, and driving limitations, were discussed.

Narcolepsy with cataplexy, also known as narcolepsy type 1, is a chronic, lifelong condition related to deficiency of the wake-promoting neuropeptide, hypocretin-1 (orexin).[37] It accounts for 50% of cases of narcolepsy and is distinguished from type 2 narcolepsy by the presence of cataplexy.[9] Manifestations of narcolepsy classically include the tetrad of excessive daytime sleepiness, sleep paralysis, cataplexy, and hypnogogic hallucinations, which stem from intrusion of fragments of REM sleep into wakefulness. It is a rare disorder, with a prevalence of 0.025% to 0.05%, presenting most commonly in the second decade of life. Treatment is with lifestyle and behavioral modifications (planned naps, regular exercise, sleep time optimization) and pharmacotherapy. Medications to treat sleepiness include stimulants and wake-promoting agents, such as modafinil and armodafinil.[38] Cataplexy can be addressed with sodium oxybate, atomoxetine, and other classes of medication.[38]

Restless Legs

Patient 7

A typically developing 6-year-old boy is seen by his pediatrician for complaints of hyperactivity and inability to sit still during school. On further history, it is noted that he moves a lot during sleep and has mild snoring. His examination is remarkable for mild enlargement of his tonsils, and that he is frequently out of his chair and his attention must be redirected. A sleep study reveals adequate total sleep and sleep stage distribution, 1.65 respiratory events (all obstructive) per hour, 14.2 periodic limb movements per hour (many of which are associated with arousals), an oxygen nadir of 95%, and a transcutaneous CO_2 maximum 40 mm Hg. After consultation with otolaryngology, T&A is scheduled in 4 months to occur during spring break. He is seen in the sleep clinic where he endorses uncomfortable feelings in his legs during the night that are described as though "bugs are crawling up his legs," requiring him to move his legs or get up out of bed and walk to relieve this feeling. A diagnosis of RLS with periodic limb movements of sleep is made. Notably, his serum ferritin is 20 μg/L. A course of iron supplementation is initiated during the 4 months before the planned T&A. On iron therapy, he begins to sleep better, and his teacher reports that he can sit in the classroom with a longer attention span.

The diagnosis of restless legs is based primarily on a careful history and exclusion of common complaints, such as numbness, positional discomfort, growing pains, and nocturnal leg cramps. Iron deficiency is implicated in the pathogenesis, as suggested by low cerebrospinal fluid ferritin levels in RLS patients compared with healthy controls,[39] and is likely related to the fact that iron is important in cerebral dopamine production.[40] For adolescents 12 years of age and older, 65 mg to 130 mg elemental iron once daily, and for children under 12 years of age, 3 mg/kg/d of elemental iron (maximum 130 mg elemental iron daily) administered once daily, is recommended.[41] Intravenous iron therapy may be considered for refractory cases. No Food and Drug Administration (FDA) -approved drug exists for pediatric RLS, but gabapentin, benzodiazepines, clonidine, and dopamine agonists may be considered.[42]

SUMMARY

The relationship between sleep and neurodevelopment is complex and bidirectional with neurodevelopmental differences likely contributing to dysregulated sleep and the subsequent disruptions in turn interfering with optimal development. As Pediatric Sleep Medicine grows as a field, we are beginning to better understand the importance of identifying salient disruptors of sleep, delineating their potential influence on cognitive development and behavioral health, and thereby moving closer to sleep-mediated interventions. Child neurologists are uniquely situated to meaningfully contribute to the elucidation of mechanisms that will both inform on the mysteries of how sleep shapes the brain and shed light on how best to intervene. General clinicians see mostly typically developing, healthy children with the common sleep complaints of behavioral insomnia of childhood, OSA, parasomnias, and insufficient sleep. The rare and challenging sleep problems can be referred to the sleep specialist.

CLINICS CARE POINTS

Insomnia:
- Chronic insomnia is characterized by problems initiating or maintaining sleep, early morning awakenings, bedtime resistance, and/or difficulty sleeping without parental intervention, as reported by the child or caregivers.

- Management of insomnia in adults and children begins with behavioral programs that have been shown to be effective.
- In some cases, such as children with cognitive impairment, when parents or children are experiencing significant stress, medications may be appropriate. These are frequently prescribed, but there are no approved medications for children with insomnia. When prescribed, medications should always be combined with a behavioral program.
- Insomnia in teens should prompt a careful sleep history and consideration of sleep insufficiency as well as screening for mental health issues.

Excessive sleepiness:
- Insufficient sleep syndrome is a common problem among today's youth and can result in poor academic performance and drowsy driving in adolescents and young adult.
- Narcolepsy is a rare but important cause of excessive daytime sleepiness, but its onset and diagnosis may be missed or delayed because lack of clinical experience with the diagnosis in children, including subtle manifestations of cataplexy.

Obstructive sleep apnea:
- Pediatric sleep-disordered breathing has a prevalence of 1% to 5% and may be more common in children with neurodevelopmental disabilities because of craniofacial dysmorphology, hypotonia, and central nervous system dysregulation of breathing.
- Risk factors for obstructive sleep apnea in neurotypical children are obesity and adenotonsillar hypertrophy.
- All pediatric patients should be screened for snoring.

Nocturnal behaviors:
- Parasomnias are generally benign, although frequent occurrences may cause parental distress and prompt concerns for safety.
- An important differential in atypical presentations is frontal lobe epilepsy.

Restless legs syndrome and PLMD:
- Periodic limb movement disorder (PLMD) is a polysomnography-based diagnosis, whereas restless legs syndrome is a clinical diagnosis. Prevalence in pediatric patients is 2% to 4% and can be associated with nighttime sleep problems and daytime cognitive and behavior dysfunction mainly because of sleep disruption.
- Iron therapy may be effective therapy, which can lead to improved nighttime and daytime symptoms.

FUTURE DIRECTIONS

Given the lack of evidence-based and FDA-approved treatments for many pediatric sleep disorders, research efforts should focus on well-designed pediatric clinical trials. Melatonin is the best-studied agent for pediatric insomnia; however, long-term side effects of chronic use still need investigation. Sleep disorders are well known to cause disruptions in numerous aspects of health and well-being. However, further evaluation is still needed to understand the full impact of early-life sleep disruption on neurodevelopment trajectory.

DISCLOSURE

The authors have nothing to disclose.

REFERENCES

1. Seron-Ferre M, Torres-Farfan C, Forcelledoo ML, et al. The development of the circadian rhythms in the fetus and neonate. Semin Perinatol 2001;25(6):363–70.
2. Carter JC, Wrede JE. Overview of sleep and sleep disorders in infancy and childhood. Pediatr Ann 2017;46(4):e133–8.
3. Kryger MH, Roth T, Dement WC. Principles and practice of sleep medicine. Philadelphia: Saunders/Elsevier.; 2011.
4. Ophoff D, Slaats MA, Boudewyns A, et al. Sleep disorders during childhood: a practical review. Eur J Pediatr 2018;177(5):641–8.
5. Paruthi S, Brooks LJ, D'Ambrosio C, et al. Consensus statement of the American Academy of Sleep Medicine on the recommended amounts of sleep for healthy children: methodology and discussion. J Cl Sleep Med 2016;12(11):1549–61.
6. Burnham MM, Goodlin-Jones BL, Gaylor EE, et al. Nighttime sleep-wake patterns and self-soothing from birth to one year of age: a longitudinal intervention study. J Child Psychol Psychiatry 2002;43(6):713.
7. Calhoun SL, Fernandez-Mendoza J, Vgontzas AN, et al. Prevalence of insomnia symptoms in a general population of young children and preadolescents: gender effects. Sleep Med 2014;15(1):91.
8. Johnson EO, Roth T, Schultz L, et al. Epidemiology of DSM-IV insomnia in adolescence: lifetime prevalence, chronicity, and an emergent gender difference. Pediatrics 2006;117(2):e247.
9. Medicine, A.A.o.S.. International classification of sleep disorders. 3rd edition. Darien (IL): American Academy of Sleep Medicine; 2014.
10. Carskadon MA, Harvey K, Duke P, et al. Pubertal changes in daytime sleepiness. Sleep 1980;2(4):453–60.
11. Roberts RE, Roberts CR, Chan W. Ethnic differences in symptoms of insomnia among adolescents. Sleep 2006;29(3):359–65.
12. Wong MM, Brower KJ, Craun EA. Insomnia symptoms and suicidality in the National Comorbidity Survey - Adolescent Supplement. J Psychiatr Res 2016; 81:1–8.
13. Hertenstein E, Feige B, Gmeiner T, et al. Insomnia as a predictor of mental disorders: a systematic review and meta-analysis. Sleep Med Rev 2019;43:96–105.
14. Picchietti D, Allen RP, Walters AS, et al. Restless legs syndrome: prevalence and impact in children and adolescents–the Peds REST study. Pediatrics 2007;120: 253–66.
15. Picchietti DL, Bruni O, de Weerd A, et al. Pediatric restless legs syndrome diagnostic criteria: an update by the International Restless Legs Syndrome Study Group. Sleep Med 2013;14:1253–9.
16. DelRosso LM, Ferri R. The prevalence of restless sleep disorder among a clinical sample of children and adolescents referred to a sleep centre. J Sleep Res 2019; 28(6):e12870.
17. Rosen CL, Storfer-Isser A, Taylor HG, et al. Increased behavioral morbidity in school-aged children with sleep-disordered breathing. Pediatrics 2004;114(6): 1640–8.
18. Angriman M, Caravale B, Novelli L, et al. Sleep in children with neurodevelopmental disabilities. Neuropediatrics 2015;46(3):199–210.
19. Krakowiak P, Goodlin-Jones B, Hertz-Picciotto I, et al. Sleep problems in children with autism spectrum disorders, developmental delays, and typical development: a population-based study. J Sleep Res 2008;17(2):197–206 [Erratum in: J Sleep Res. 2012 Apr;21(2):231].

20. Richdale AL, Schreck KA. Sleep problems in autism spectrum disorders: prevalence, nature, & possible biopsychological aetiologies. Sleep Med Rev 2009; 13(6):403–11.
21. Sung V, Hiscock H, Sciberras E, et al. Sleep problems in children with attention-deficit/hyperactivity disorder: prevalence and the effect on the child and family. Arch Pediatr Adolesc Med 2008;162(4):336–42.
22. Owens JA, Dalzell V. Use of the 'BEARS' sleep screening tool in a pediatric residents' continuity clinic: a pilot study. Sleep Med 2005;6(1):63–9.
23. Malow B, Byars K, Johnson K, et al. A practice pathway for the identification, evaluation, and management of insomnia in children and adolescents with autism spectrum disorders. Pediatrics 2012;130:S106–24.
24. Roland PS, Rosenfeld RM, Brooks LJ, et al. Clinical practice guideline: polysomnography for sleep-disordered breathing prior to tonsillectomy in children. Otolaryngol Head Neck Surg 2011;145(1 Suppl):S1.
25. Jan JE, Bax MC, Owens JA, et al. Neurophysiology of circadian rhythm sleep disorders of children with neurodevelopmental disabilities. Eur J Paediatr Neurol 2012;16(5):403–12.
26. Owens J. Adolescent Sleep Working Group; Committee on Adolescence. Insufficient sleep in adolescents and young adults: an update on causes and consequences. Pediatrics 2014;134(3):e921–32.
27. Mindell JA, Owens J. Cl Guide to Ped Sleep. 3rd Edition. Wolters Kluwer; 2015.
28. Williams Buckley A, Hirtz D, Oskoui M, et al. Practice guideline: treatment for insomnia and disrupted sleep behavior in children and adolescents with autism spectrum disorder: report of the Guideline Development, Dissemination, and Implementation Subcommittee of the American Academy of Neurology. Neurology 2020;94(9):392–404.
29. Lee CF, Lee CH, Hsueh WY, et al. Prevalence of obstructive sleep apnea in children with Down syndrome: a meta-analysis. J Clin Sleep Med 2018;14(5):867–75.
30. Tan HL, Gozal D, Kheirandish-Gozal L. Obstructive sleep apnea in children: a critical update. Nat Sci Sleep 2013;5:109–23.
31. Tauman R, Gozal D. Obstructive sleep apnea syndrome in children. Expert Rev Respir Med 2011;5(3):425–40.
32. Petit D, Pennestri MH, Paquet J, et al. Childhood sleepwalking and sleep terrors: a longitudinal study of prevalence and familial aggregation. JAMA Pediatr 2015; 169(7):653–8.
33. Attarian J, Zhu L. Treatment options for disorders of arousal: a case series. Int K Neurosci 2013;123(9):623–5.
34. Sivertsen B, Pallesen S, Stormark KM, et al. Delayed sleep phase syndrome in adolescents: prevalence and correlates in a large population based study. BMC Public Health 2013;13:1163.
35. Saxvig IW, Pallesen S, Wilhelmsen-Langeland A, et al. Prevalence and correlates of delayed sleep phase in high school students. Sleep Med 2012;13(2):193–9.
36. Culnan E, McCullough LM, Wyatt JK. Circadian rhythm sleep-wake phase disorders. Neurol Clin 2019;37(3):527–43.
37. Nishino S, Ripley B, Overeem S, et al. Hypocretin (orexin) deficiency inhuman narcolepsy. Lancet 2000;355(9197):39.
38. Morgenthaler TI, Kapur VK, Brown T, et al. Practice parameters for the treatment of narcolepsy and other hypersomnias of central origin. Sleep 2007;30(12):1705.
39. Earley CJ, Connor JR, Beard JL, et al. Ferritin levels in the cerebrospinal fluid and restless legs syndrome: effects of different clinical phenotypes. Sleep 2005;28(9): 1069–75.

40. Allen R. Dopamine and iron in the pathophysiology of restless legs syndrome (RLS). Sleep Med 2004;5(4):385–91.
41. Allen RP, Pichietti DL, Auerbach M, et al. Evidence-based and consensus clinical practice guidelines for the iron treatment of restless legs syndrome/Willis-Ekbom disease in adults and children: an IRLSSG task force report. Sleep Med 2018; 41:27.
42. Garcia-Borreguero D, Larrrosa O, de la Lallave Y, et al. Treatment of restless legs syndrome with gabapentin: a double-blind, cross-over study. Neurology 2002; 59(10):1573.

Evidence-Based Protocols in Child Neurology

James J. Riviello Jr, MD[a],*, Jennifer Erklauer, MD[a,b]

KEYWORDS

- Child neurology • Evidence-based medicine • Treatment guidelines
- Practice parameters

KEY POINTS

- Medical care is delivered across systems that vary in complexity.
- Evidence-based guidelines are based on the scientific method.
- Creating guidelines ensures the delivery of quality care and improves patient outcomes.
- Guidelines in Child Neurology have been created for the major problems encountered: status epilepticus, ICU EEG monitoring, neonatal neurology, stroke, traumatic brain injury, and brain death.

The practice of medicine has advanced but become more complex because of science. In the United States, the science-based foundation of medicine started with the creation of the Johns Hopkins University School of Medicine, modeled on German universities that used a science-based foundation for medical education: the discovery of new knowledge, rather than teaching what was already known.[1] Other schools followed this model. The 1910 Flexner Report led to the standardization of medical training in the United States with the closing of schools that did not adhere to these standards.[2,3]

Yet, these scientific advances have resulted in more complex medical care. More is known about a given disorder: its pathophysiology, pathology, genetics, and treatments, and the addition of basic science research and clinical trials makes it difficult for the individual physician keep up and interpret this.[4] The development of the multiple subspecialties evolved from this. Hospitals have become more complex, moving from a single general hospital to subspecialty units within the individual hospital to hospital systems with inpatient and outpatient care delivered in many locations.

[a] Section of Pediatric Neurology and Developmental Neuroscience, Department of Pediatrics, Baylor College of Medicine, Texas Children's Hospital, 6701 Fannin Street, Suite 1250, Houston, TX 77030, USA; [b] Section of Pediatric Critical Care Medicine, Baylor College of Medicine, Texas Children's Hospital, 6701 Fannin Street, Suite 1250, Houston, TX 77030, USA
* Corresponding author.
E-mail address: riviello@bcm.edu

Neurol Clin 39 (2021) 883–895
https://doi.org/10.1016/j.ncl.2021.04.008
neurologic.theclinics.com

The need to provide quality medical care and improve outcomes has become important. Even remuneration will depend on outcomes in the future. Two initiatives are important in this endeavor: evidence-based medicine (EBM) and quality improvement initiatives. EBM is defined as "the conscientious, explicit, and judicious use of current best evidence in making decisions about the care of individual patients."[5] This evidence is based on research, and EBM has become the foundation of medical care. Quality improvement is defined as "the degree to which health care services for individuals and populations increase the likelihood of desired health outcomes and are consistent with current professional knowledge."[6]

The Neurology and Neurocritical Care Services at Texas Children's Hospital (TCH) provide an example of this situation. TCH has 3 inpatient units, a main campus and 2 satellite campuses, with 55 child neurologists, including 20 epileptologists. Neurology inpatients and intensive care units (ICUs) are present in all 3 locations staffed by different neurologists. We also have a dedicated neurocritical care service that provides the neurology consultations to the various ICUs. The dedicated neurologic ICU is staffed by pediatric critical care medicine specialists interested in the brain and neurologists interested in neurocritical care. Patients with neurologic insults are seen in other dedicated ICUs and multidisciplinary pediatric ICUs in our system. We must ensure that the same quality neurologic care is delivered across the multiple settings within our network; this can only be done by following a standard guideline or treatment protocol for a specific disorder.

Various terms are used for these standardization modalities including practice guidelines, practice parameters, or practice standards. Practice standards are authoritative, whereas guidelines are recommendations. Practice standards are established by an authority or general consent; these are typically done for accreditation and established by an organization. Clinical practice guidelines are systematically developed statements based on evidence and current data, used to help standardize medical care and improve the quality of care.[7,8] Evidence-based refers to using scientifically based research to generate these guidelines. Practice guidelines have also evolved out of national health policy because of 3 major factors: rising health care costs, practice variations, and reports of inappropriate care.[9–11]

The evidence-based process for neurology and child neurology has been driven by the American Academy of Neurology (AAN) and the quality standards committee of the Child Neurology Society (CNS). Guidelines have been created for screening, diagnosis, causation, prognosis, and treatment. Evidence and recommendations are classified, according to the type of study: therapeutic, effectiveness, causation, prognostic accuracy, diagnostic screening, and population screening. Evidence has 4 levels, which refer to its strength. For example, for a therapeutic study, Class I is a randomized controlled trial (RCT) blinded to outcome assessment or has objective outcomes; Class II is a flawed, RCT (nonconcealed) allocation; Class III is a nonrandomized, controlled study; and Class IV has no control group and nonmasked assessment of outcome; this is also referred to as expert opinion. Recommendations have 4 levels, A, B, C, and U, based on the level of evidence for each recommendation.[12]

Individual hospitals can produce evidence-based guidelines for patient care. TCH has an evidence-based outcomes center (EBOC) that produces these guidelines. For neurology, the EBOC has produced guidelines for seizures and status epilepticus (SE), traumatic brain injury (TBI), and stroke, and an autoimmune encephalitis protocol is in preparation.

The typical guideline is also educational, systematically reviewing the data, classifying the evidence, and including references. This article shall review selected guidelines, emphasizing those for inpatient care.

EVIDENCE-BASED PROTOCOLS
Status Epilepticus, Seizures, and Epilepsy

Seizures and SE: Many inpatients seen by our neurology teams have seizures or SE. Treatment guidelines were produced in 1993, by the American Epilepsy Society.[13] These guidelines established a timetable for treatment, recommending lorazepam, at 0.1 mg/kg, or diazepam, at 0.2 mg/kg, by 10 to 20 minutes. A practice parameter for the diagnostic assessment of SE was produced by the AAN/CNS in 2006.[14] The TCH EBOC produced a guideline for SE in 2009, which was updated in 2018.[15] Other national organizations have also developed guidelines for SE, especially the Neurocritical Care Society (NCS) in 2012,[16] and the American Epilepsy Society updated their treatment protocol in an evidence-based guideline in 2016.[17] Both these guidelines recommended the administration of lorazepam or diazepam at 5 minutes. The American Epilepsy Society (AES) reviewed the treatment of refractory convulsive SE in 2020.[18]

For the diagnosis of SE, the evidence shows that electrolytes were abnormal in 6%, blood cultures were abnormal in 2.5%, and a central nervous system infection occurred in 12.8% in those patients in whom these studies were done.[14] Antiepileptic drug (AED) levels were abnormal in 32%. It was observed that 3.6% had evidence of ingestion, 4.2% had inborn errors of metabolism, epileptiform abnormalities occurred in 43% of electroencephalographies (EEGs), and neuroimaging abnormalities occurred in 8% of scans (mostly computerized axial tomography [CAT] scan then). The recommendations were that blood cultures and lumbar puncture should be done when there is a clinical suspicion of a systemic or central nervous system infection (Level U), AED levels should be sent in children with epilepsy who develop SE, toxicology and metabolic studies should be considered when there is a clinical suspicion or when there is no identified cause, and EEG may be helpful in determining if there are focal or generalized features or if there is a concern for nonconvulsive SE or nonepileptic SE. Neuroimaging should be considered, after stabilization, if there are clinical indications or unknown cause. There is insufficient evidence to recommend routine neuroimaging.

Treatment of SE: The Epilepsy Foundation of America (EFA), the NCS, and the AES produced guidelines for the treatment of SE.[13,16,17] All these guidelines recommend a benzodiazepine as the first-line therapy for SE (Table 1). Lorazepam, midazolam, and diazepam are all used, and there is no evidence suggesting that one of these works better than the others. There has been an increasing use of intramuscular or intranasal midazolam, and intramuscular midazolam has been shown to be as effective as intravenous lorazepam. If there is no response to initial benzodiazepine therapy, then second-line medications are used. The AES guideline stated that there is no evidence suggesting the superiority of fosphenytoin, valproic acid, or levetiracetam over each other, but higher doses are recommended than may be typically used (see Table 1). Subsequently, the Established Status Epilepticus Treatment Trial showed equal efficacy among these 3 agents.[19]

For refractory SE, now defined as the failure of the initial benzodiazepine followed by a second-line medication, rather than a strict timeline, there is no data yet to suggest one treatment over the others.

Continuous EEG (CEEG) guidelines: The American Clinical Neurophysiology Society has produced 2 sets of guidelines, the first for CEEG monitoring in the newborn[20] and the second for CEEG monitoring in the older child and the adult.[21] These guidelines are important because they establish the conditions for which CEEG monitoring is needed. Box 1 lists the neonatal indications, and Box 2 lists indications in the older child.

Table 1 Evidence-based initial treatment of seizures and status epilepticus	
First-line treatment, in-patient	IV lorazepam, 0.1 mg/kg, maximum 4 mg/dose, may repeat in 5 min, or IV diazepam, 0.2 mg/kg, maximum 10 mg/dose, may repeat in 5 min, or IV or IM midazolam, 0.2 mg/kg, maximum 10 mg/dose
Second-line treatment, if seizure continues	IV fosphenytoin, 20 mg PE/kg, maximum 1500 mg, or IV valproic acid, 40 mg/kg, maximum 3000 mg/dose, or IV levetiracetam, 60 mg/kg, maximum 4500 mg/dose
First-line treatment, outpatient	Rectal diazepam, 0.2–0.5 (age stratified); maximum dose 20 mg IN midazolam, 0.2 mg/kg

Abbreviations: IM, intramuscular; IN, intranasal; IV, intravenous; PE, fosphenytoin equivalent.
Data from Refs.[13,15–17,19]

CEEG monitoring: There is now the awareness that ongoing clinical and electrographic seizures may aggravate brain injury in the setting of an acute brain insult. The past use of EEG in the ICU was typically done using a short EEG, called a "routine" EEG, or a "snapshot" EEG. These shorter EEGs are less likely to detect actual electrographic seizures, because of the sampling error for a shorter versus a longer study. The introduction of digital technology has permitted longer monitoring times. In all ages, CEEG monitoring is recommended for disorders in which there is a high-risk of seizures. Given the overall relatively high incidence of electrographic seizures in the ICU, CEEG monitoring is preferred.

The guidelines for older children also list the reasons for performing CEEG: detect nonconvulsive seizures or nonconvulsive SE or characterize paroxysmal events in

Box 1 Conditions with a high risk of neonatal seizures that require continuous electroencephalographic monitoring
Acute neonatal encephalopathy: depression from perinatal asphyxia or after cardiopulmonary resuscitation
Cardiac or pulmonary insults with risk of brain injury: pulmonary hypertension, need for extracorporeal membrane oxygenation, critical congenital heart disease requiring early surgery with cardiopulmonary bypass
Infection: meningoencephalitis, sepsis
Trauma: intracranial, subarachnoid, subdural, or intraventricular hemorrhage or encephalopathy and suspicion for central nervous system injury
Inborn errors of metabolism, genetic syndrome involving the central nervous system
Stroke, cerebral sinovenous thrombosis
Premature infants with high-grade intraventricular hemorrhage, encephalopathy
Data from Schellhaas RA, Chang T, Tsuchida T, et al. The American Clinical Neurophysiology Society's guideline on continuous electroencephalographic monitoring in neonates. J Clin Neurophysiol 2011:1–7.

Box 2
Conditions associated with high-likelihood seizures on continuous electroencephalographic recording

Following convulsive SE, especially to detect nonconvulsive SE

Aneurysmal subarachnoid hemorrhage

Intraparenchymal hemorrhage

TBI: moderate to severe

Central nervous system infections

Recent neurosurgical procedures

Brain tumors

Acute ischemic stroke

Hypoxic-ischemic injury following cardiac or respiratory arrest, with or without therapeutic hypothermia

Sepsis-associated encephalopathy

Extracorporeal membrane oxygenation

Patients with epilepsy in the ICU: seizure exacerbation

Modified from Herman ST, Abend NS, Bleck TP, et al. Consensus statement on continuous EEG in critically ill adults and children, Part I: Indications. J Clin Neurophysiol 2015;32:87–95.

---

the ICU; assess the efficacy of therapy for seizures and SE; identify cerebral ischemia; monitor sedation and high-dose suppressant therapy; and assess the severity of encephalopathy and prognostication.[21]

EEG is also an indirect measurement of cerebral blood flow (CBF) and can be used to detect ischemia.[22] EEG frequencies decrease with a decrease in CBF. Early detection of a biomarker of deterioration can result in earlier intervention before an insult becomes irreversible.

The AAN, CNS, AES, and American Academy of Pediatrics (AAP) have produced multiple practice parameters for the care of the patient with epilepsy (**Box 3**).[23–32]

Sudden unexpected death in epilepsy (SUDEP) deserves specific mention because it has been controversial as to how much about SUDEP to discuss. The AAN and AES practice guideline recommends that the families of children with epilepsy should be informed that the rate is 1 of 5000 in children and 1 of 1000 in adults per year.[33] Seizure freedom is greatly associated with a decreased SUDEP risk.

Neuroimaging of seizures: There has been an initial report in 1996 and a reassessment in 2007.[34,35] Emergent neuroimaging is indicated when there is suspicion for a serious structural lesion; these are more likely when there is a new focal deficit; persistent altered mental status, with or without intoxication; fever; recent trauma; persistent headache; history of cancer; anticoagulation; or AIDS. An immediate CAT scan is indicated for patients with a seizure especially with an abnormal examination, predisposing condition, or focal seizure onset.

Neurocritical Care Guidelines

Neonatal neurology
Neuroimaging in the neonate: Head ultrasonography is useful in the management of the preterm infant (less than 3 week postmenstrual age [PMA]) and repeated between 36 and 40 weeks PMA to detect lesions such as intraventricular hemorrhage,

---

Box 3
Practice parameters for epilepsy

The first afebrile seizure[23]

Infantile spasms[24]

"Efficacy and Tolerability of the New Antiepileptic Drugs Part I: Treatment of New Onset Epilepsy"[25] and "Efficacy and Tolerability of the New Antiepileptic Drugs Part II: Treatment of Refractory Epilepsy"[26]

"Practice Guideline Update Summary: Efficacy and Tolerability of the New Antiepileptic Drugs Part I: Treatment of new Epilepsy"[27] and "Practice Guideline Update Summary: Efficacy and Tolerability of the New Antiepileptic Drugs Part II: Treatment-Resistant Epilepsy"[28]

Management of infantile seizures[29]

Febrile seizures: treatment of children with simple febrile seizures[30] and long-term treatment of the child with simple febrile seizure[31]

Neurodiagnostic evaluation of febrile seizures[32]

---

periventricular leukomalacia, and low-pressure ventriculomegaly, which affect prognosis. In encephalopathic term infants, CAT scan is useful to exclude hemorrhage and MRI can be performed after the first postnatal week to establish the pattern of injury and predict neurologic outcome.[36]

Therapeutic hypothermia (TH) for neonatal encephalopathy: TH is now established for the care of the term infant with asphyxia. A Cochrane review including 8 studies of 638 term infants with moderate and severe hypoxic-ischemic injury showed a decreased mortality and major neurodevelopmental disability by 18 months of age. There was an increased need for inotropic agents and thrombocytopenia.[37]

Acute stroke guidelines

Multiple guidelines exist for the management of acute stroke in children including recommendations from the American College of Chest Physicians in 2012,[38] Royal College of Pediatrics and Child Health in 2017,[39] Australian Childhood Stroke Advisory in 2018,[40] and the American Heart Association (AHA) in 2019.[41] The most recent update to the AHA guidelines includes 513 references and more than 60 recommendations for the management of cerebral venous sinus thrombosis, ischemic stroke, and intracerebral hemorrhage in both the neonatal and pediatric age groups. Discussion for each section includes presenting symptoms, risk factors, cause, management, evaluation, and outcome as well as recommendations for clinical practice and identification of knowledge gaps.[41]

In the current AHA guideline, care is mostly supportive for perinatal ischemic stroke. Hyperacute therapies have not been well studied in the neonatal population. Most often, anticoagulation and antithrombotic therapy are not required for secondary stroke prevention but may be considered if there is high risk of stroke recurrence such as thrombophilia or cardiac disease. MRI should be performed with magnetic resonance angiography of the head and neck with inclusion of magnetic resonance venography if there is concern for cerebral venous sinus thrombosis (CVST). For neonatal CVST, anticoagulation can be considered. There is variability among institutions in terms of the use of anticoagulation in this age group because of limited research in this population. If anticoagulation is not initiated, repeat MRI scan with venous imaging is warranted 5 to 7 days later to evaluate for increasing clot burden. For neonatal intracranial hemorrhage (ICH), vitamin K should be administered if there is evidence for coagulation factor deficiencies. Per the AHA guideline, surgical intervention can be considered in the setting of elevated intracranial pressures (ICPs) or hydrocephalus related to hemorrhage. Seizures remain a common presenting symptom for acute stroke from all causes in neonates.

For children with strokes of all types, including ischemic, hemorrhagic, and CVST, the AHA guideline recommends they be treated in an institution with experience in managing childhood stroke including vascular neurology and neurocritical care expertise. The airway, breathing, and circulation should be stabilized, and appropriate supportive care is essential including adequate hydration, avoidance of fever, and maintenance of euglycemia. Close monitoring should occur for change in the examination or evidence of increased ICP. CEEG monitoring can be considered, particularly in patients with altered mental status or if there is a concern for nonconvulsive seizures. Seizures, when present, should be treated.

For acute ischemic stroke, the AHA guideline states that hyperacute stroke therapy remains controversial due to lack of randomized clinical trial data. The use of tissue plasminogen activator (tPA) and endovascular thrombectomy can be considered. This guideline suggests consideration for treatment in children with National Institutes of Health stroke scale (NIHSS) greater than or equal to 6 with radiographically confirmed larger artery occlusion and in larger children in whom the available catheters for acute intervention are appropriately sized. The guideline also recommends consultation and performance of the procedures by endovascular surgeons with experience in treating both children and adults with acute strokes. Special circumstances such as acute stroke in patients with sickle cell disease are also discussed in detail.

These guidelines have also addressed the use of hyperacute therapies in children with slightly modified inclusion criteria. Consideration may be given to use tPA in children aged greater than or equal to 2 years if the following criteria are met: pediatric NIHSS greater than or equal to 4 and less than or equal to 24, treatment can be initiated within 4.5 hours, and hemorrhage has been excluded on neuroimaging. The Royal College of Physicians also includes evidence of a partial or complete occlusion of the intracranial artery corresponding to the clinical or radiologic deficit. All guidelines make reference to evaluation for endovascular therapies for acute stroke in certain situations.

The AHA guidelines recommend consideration for hemicraniectomy if infarct volume is large, defined as at least half of the middle cerebral artery (MCA) territory. Prophylactic hemicraniectomy in the first 24 hours or serial imaging may be required to allow for early intervention. Early decompressive surgery should also be considered in acute cerebellar infarction. The guideline includes detailed recommendations for evaluation of the cause of stroke and secondary stroke prevention.

This latest AHA guideline also includes discussion on the management of hemorrhagic stroke in children. Patients should be stabilized, and coagulopathy, if present, should be corrected. Optimal blood pressure targets are unknown in the pediatric population. Care should be taken to avoid hypotension to maintain adequate cerebral perfusion pressure; however, uncontrolled hypertension can contribute to hematoma expansion and this should be avoided as well. Management of ICP and decompressive craniectomy may be required for posterior fossa or large lobar hemorrhages. Although it is recommended that seizures be treated, there is a lack of evidence to determine if prophylactic seizure medications should be started in pediatric patients with ICH. In adult patients with ICH, prophylactic phenytoin has been associated with higher morbidity and mortality, although studies have been conflicting. AHA guidelines for adult spontaneous ICH do not recommend prophylactic treatment of seizures.[42] Owing to the higher risk of seizures in children and potential secondary brain injury from seizures and their complications, the AHA guideline for pediatric stroke states that prophylactic seizure medication can be considered, but this practice remains controversial. Vascular imaging should be obtained as part of workup for the cause. This guideline includes specific treatment recommendations for various causes including arteriovenous malformations, aneurysms, arteriovenous fistulae, and cavernous malformations.

Finally, management of CVST in pediatric patients is discussed for the first time in the AHA stroke guideline. Recommendations include supportive measures, monitoring for and management of increased ICP, and most often anticoagulation, although the guideline does not recommend using anticoagulation in the setting of otogenic lateral sinus thrombosis. If anticoagulation is not used, repeat venous imaging should be repeated in 3 to 7 days to monitor for extension of thrombus. Children should be evaluated for thrombophilia. Endovascular therapy with thrombolysis and thrombectomy can be considered in severe cases. Close monitoring for increased ICP should occur, as well as close monitoring of visual fields and fundoscopy. Carbonic anhydrase inhibitors, lumbar puncture, optic nerve sheath fenestrations, and ventriculo-peritoneal (VP) shunt may be required if vision is at risk and should be considered on a case-by-case basis with multidisciplinary input. Decompressive craniectomy has been reported in adult patients. Anemia, if present, should be corrected, and infection, if suspected, should be treated.

Pediatric traumatic brain injury

The Brain Trauma Foundation has produced guidelines for the management of severe TBI.[43] Severe TBI is defined as Glasgow Coma Scale score less than 9 in pediatric patients with the most recent update published in 2019 along with a consensus statement and guideline-based algorithm for first- and second-tier therapies. The guideline is divided into 3 major topics: monitoring, thresholds for treatment, and treatments with various subtopics in each category. Level of evidence was graded with each recommendation, and changes from previous editions of the guidelines were highlighted; included articles are summarized in table format. Discussion of the existing evidence is included for each recommendation made.

For neuromonitoring, an ICP monitor is suggested. As in previous editions of the guideline, advanced neuromonitoring including brain oxygenation is addressed; however, there is not enough evidence to support or refute its routine use. Initial neuroimaging should be obtained, but the guidelines neither recommend using computed tomographic (CT) scan alone as a means of determining whether a patient has increased ICP nor do they recommend routine serial neuroimaging studies such as CT.

Treatment thresholds for various parameters are defined in this guideline. For example, target ICP should be less than 20 mm Hg and cerebral perfusion pressure (CPP) targets should be between 40 and 50 mm Hg as to ensure maintaining a CPP >40 mm Hg. Despite no formal recommendation to use cerebral oxygenation monitors, the guideline recommends maintaining brain tissue oxygenation ($PbtO_2$) greater than 10 mm Hg.

To achieve these thresholds, recommendations are made on using hyperosmolar therapy including hypertonic saline (HTS) and mannitol. For patients with intracranial hypertension 3% HTS is recommended, with bolus dosing of 2 to 5 mL/kg over 10 to 20 min and continuous infusion dosed at 0.1 to 1 mL/kg/h, using the minimum dose required to maintain ICP less than 20 mm Hg. For refractory ICP 23.4% HTS can be considered at the dose of 0.5 mL/kg to a maximum of 30 mL. For mannitol, no studies in children met inclusion criteria; however, the guideline recognizes that mannitol is commonly used for ICP management in children. Other measures to control ICP include cerebral spinal fluid drainage via external ventricular device. Although the guideline recommends ensuring adequate sedation analgesia for patients in the ICU with TBI, it cautions against using bolus doses of fentanyl and midazolam for management of ICP because of risks of cerebral hypoperfusion associated with hypotension from these medications. The guideline also recommends against the use of hyperventilation less than 30 mm Hg to treat increased ICP. Normothermia should be targeted. Prophylactic hypothermia is not recommended; however, moderate hypothermia (32°C–34°C) for the management of intracranial hypertension can be considered. High-dose barbiturates and decompressive craniectomy can also be considered for refractory intracranial hypertension. Prophylactic seizure medication is recommended to reduce early posttraumatic seizures. Enteral nutrition within the first 72 hours is preferred.

Post–cardiac arrest management

The most recent pediatric cardiac arrest guidelines are from the AHA and were published 2019[44] and updated in 2020.[45] From a neurology standpoint, this is important as hypoxic-ischemic injury following cardiac arrest is a major determinant of overall outcome. These guidelines address optimal CPR and resuscitation technique, extracorporeal cardiopulmonary resuscitation, CEEG monitoring, and multimodal neurologic prognostication following cardiac arrest.

New in the 2020 guidelines is the recommendation for the use of targeted temperature management to either a goal of 32°C to 34°C followed by 36°C or actively targeting 36°C for 5 days. Regardless of the temperature target, fever must be avoided. CEEG monitoring is recommended. Although there is little randomized data to make a determination, treatment of clinical seizures and electrographic SE is suggested. These guidelines from 2019 and 2020 outline the current data informing post–cardiac arrest neuroprognostication.

The optimal timing to best prognosticate outcome in children is unknown. Adult guidelines suggest to wait at least 72 hours after the patient has been rewarmed to normal temperature and possibly longer. The pediatric guidelines identify a lack of evidence to support reliable evidence-based neuroprognostication in the first 24 to 48 hours postarrest in most cases. Care should be taken to assure that enough time has elapsed before prognostication. Using a multimodal approach is recommended. Ongoing neurologic evaluation is recommended for at least 1 year following cardiac arrest, and all patients should undergo rehabilitation evaluation.

Emergency neurologic life support

Emergency Neurologic Life Support (ENLS), created by the NCS, is a course composed of 14 evidence-based protocols in neurocritical care focusing on immediate care in the first hour of a neurologic emergency.[46] The course includes education on the acute stabilization of the neurocritical care patient as well as the management of specific disease processes including ischemic and hemorrhagic stroke, hypoxic-ischemic injury following cardiac arrest, traumatic injury of the brain and spinal cord, and SE. Participation is open to all health care professionals, and certification is awarded on completion of the course. Many neurocritical care units are requiring this training for their staff, including physicians, nurses, and pharmacists. We have offered ENLS certification to all neurology and critical care providers at our institution and are in the early stages of implementing this certification for the nurses in the pediatric neurocritical care unit. The focus of ENLS has been based on care for adult patients. However, each module includes a section with considerations for the pediatric patient, and this continues to expand with each iteration of the course.

Box 4
Outpatient practice parameters for pediatric neurology

"Practice Parameter, Evaluation of Children and Adolescents with Recurrent Headaches"[49]

"Pharmacologic Treatment of Migraine Headache in Children and Adolescents"[50]

"Practice Parameter: Diagnostic Assessment of the Child with Cerebral Palsy"[51]

"Practice parameter: Evaluation of the Child with Global Developmental Delay"[52]

"Evidence Report: Genetic and Metabolic Testing on Children with Global Developmental Delay"[53]

"Practice Parameter: Screening and Diagnosis of Autism"[54]

"Practice Parameter: Treatment for Insomnia and Disrupted Sleep Behavior in Children and Adolescents with Autism Spectrum Disorder"[55]

"Practice Parameter: Evaluation of the Child with Microcephaly (an Evidence-Based Review)"[56]

"Practice Parameter for the Assessment and Treatment of Children and Adolescents with Attention-Deficit/Hyperactivity Disorder"[57]

"Practice Parameter: Corticosteroid Treatment of Duchenne Dystrophy"[58]

Pediatric brain death

Guidelines for the determination of brain death in infants and children have been published with the most recent version in 2011.[47] The guideline outlines the procedure for determining brain death including prerequisites to testing, the clinical neurologic examination, the apnea test, and ancillary studies. The guideline has been endorsed by multiple professional societies including the AAN, AAP, CNS, Society for Critical Care Medicine, and World Federation of Pediatric Intensive and Critical Care Societies.

Recently, a multidisciplinary subcommittee of the AAN has drafted an updated consensus practice recommendations for the determination of pediatric and adult brain death or death by neurologic criteria. These recommendations are currently open for public comment with finalized recommendations to be published soon. In addition, guidelines for the determination of brain death/death by neurologic criteria were published as part of the World Brain Death Project as an effort to improve standardization in the approach to brain death internationally.[48]

There are other important practice parameters for children that are oriented toward the outpatient practice of child neurology (**Box 4**).[49–58]

CLINICS CARE POINTS

- Evidence-based medicine and clinical practice guidelines help standardize patient care.

- Evidence-based medicine is defined as the conscientious, explicit, and judicious use of current best evidence in making decisions about the care of individual patients. Evidence-based refers to applying the scientific method to acquire this data.

- Clinical practice guidelines are systematically developed based on medical evidence. Evidence-based practice using standard treatment protocols ensures the delivery of quality care across complex medical systems.

- Quality improvement is defined as the degree to which health care services for individuals and populations increase the likelihood of desired health outcomes and are consistent with current professional knowledge.

REFERENCES

1. Barry JM. The great influenza: the story of the deadliest pandemic in history. New York: Penquin Books; 2018.
2. Beck AH. The Flexner Report and the standardization of American medicine. JAMA 2004;291(17):2139–40.
3. Duffy TP. The Flexner Report-100 years later. Yale J Biol Med 2011;84:269–76.
4. Hurwitz BA, Hurwitz KB, Ashwal S. Child neurology practice guidelines: past, present, and future. Pediatr Neurol 2015;52:290–301.
5. Sackett DL, Rosenberg WMC, Gray JAM, et al. Evidence-based medicine: what it is and what it isn't. BMJ 1996;312:71–2.
6. Leviton A, Nichol SM, Allred EN, et al. What is quality improvement and why should neurologists care? J Child Neurol 2012;27(2):251–7.
7. D'Arcy Y. Practice guidelines, standards, consensus statement, position papers: what are they are, how they differ. American Nurse 2017. Available at: https://www.myamericannurse.com/practice-guidelines-standards-consensus-statements-position-papers-what-they-are-how-they-differ/. Accessed October 11, 2007.
8. Clinical Practice Guidelines. Available at: https://www.nccih.nih.gov/health/providers/clinicalpractice.
9. Woolf SH. Practice guidelines: a new reality in medicine. I. Recent developments. Arch Intern Med 1990;150:1811–8.
10. Woolf SH. Practice guidelines: a new reality in medicine. II. Methods of developing guidelines. Arch Intern Med 1992;152:946–52.
11. Woolf SH. Practice guidelines: a new reality in medicine. III. Impact on patient care. Arch Intern Med 1990;153:2646–55.
12. Gronseth GS, Cox J, Gloss D, et al. Clinical practice guideline process manual. American Academy of Neurology; 2017.
13. Working Group on Status Epilepicus. Treatment of convulsive status epilepticus. Recommendations of the Epilepsy Foundation of America's Working group on status epilepticus. JAMA 1993;270:854–9.
14. Riviello JJ, Ashwal S, Hirtz D, et al. Practice parameter: diagnostic assessment of the child with status epilepticus (an evidence based review): report of the Quality Standards Subcommittee of the American Academy of Neurology and the Practice Committee of the Child Neurology Society. Neurology 2006;67:1542–50.
15. Initial management of status epilepticus: evidnce-based guideline. Evidence-based outcomes Center (EBOC), Texas Children's Hospital, 2018.
16. Brophy GM, Bell R, Claassen J, et al. Guidelines for the evaluation and management of status epilepticus. Neurocrit Care 2012;17:3–23.
17. Glauser T, Shinnar S, Gloss D, et al. Evidence-based guideline: treatment of convulsive status epilepticus in children and adults: report of the guideline committee of the American Epilepsy Society. Epilepsy Curr 2016;16(1):48–61.
18. Vossler DG, Bainbridge JL, Boggs JG, et al. Treatment of refractory convulsive status epilepticus: a comprehensive review by the American Epilepsy Society Treatments Committee. Epilepsy Curr 2020;20(5):245–64.
19. Kapur J, Elm J, Chamberlain JM, et al. Randomized trial of three anticonvulsant medications for status epilepticus. N Engl J Med 2019;381:2103–13.
20. Schellhaas RA, Chang T, Tsuchida T, et al. The American Clinical Neurophysiology Society's guideline on continuous electroencephalographic monitoring in neonates. J Clin Neurophysiol 2011;28:611–7.

21. Herman ST, Abend NS, Bleck TP, et al. Consensus statement on continuous EEG in critically ill adults and children, Part I: indications. J Clin Neurophysiol 2015;32: 87–95.

22. Appavu B, Riviello JJ. The neurophysiology of electroencephalographic patterns in neurocritical care- pathologic contributors or epiphenomena? Neurocrit Care 2017;29:9–19.

23. Hirtz D, Ashwal S, Berg A, et al. Practice parameter: evaluating the first afebrile seizure in children. Neurology 2000;55:616–23.

24. Mackay MT, Weiss SK, Adams-Weber T, et al. Practice parameter: medical treatment of infantile spasms. Neurology 2004;62:1668–81.

25. French JA, Kanner AM, Bautista A, et al. Efficacy and tolerability of the new antiepileptic drugs I: treatment of new onset epilepsy. Neurology 2004;62:1252–60.

26. French JA, Kanner AM, Bautista A, et al. Efficacy and tolerability of the new antiepileptic drugs Part II: treatment of refractory epilepsy. Neurology 2004;62: 1261–73.

27. Kanner AM, Ashman E, Gloss D, et al. Practice guideline update summary: efficacy and tolerability of the new antiepileptic drugs I: treatment of new epilepsy. Neurology 2018;91:74–81.

28. Kanner AM, Ashman E, Gloss D, et al. Practice guideline update summary: efficacy and tolerability of the new antiepileptic drugs II: treatment-resistant epilepsy. Neurology 2018;91:82–90.

29. Wilmshurst JM, Gaillard WD, Vinayan KP, et al. Summary of recommendations for the management of infantile seizures: Task Force Report for the ILAE Commission of Pediatrics. Epilepsia 2015;56(8):1185–97.

30. Baumann RJ, Duffner PK. Treatment of children with simple febrile seizures: the AAP practice parameter. Pediatr Neurol 2000;23:11–7.

31. American Academy of Pediatrics. Practice parameter: longterm treatment of the child with simple febrile seizure. Pediatrics 1999;103:1307–9.

32. Clinical practice guideline-Febrile seizures: guideline for the Neurodiagnostic evaluation of the child with a simple febrile seizure. Pediatrics 2011;127:389–94.

33. Harden C, Tomson T, Gloss D, et al. Practice guideline summary: sudden unexpected death in epilepsy incidence rates and risk factors. Neurology 2017;88: 1674–80.

34. Practice parameter: neuroimaging in the emergency patient presenting with seizure-Summary statement. Neurology 1996;47:288–91.

35. Harden CL, Huff JS, Schwartz TH, et al. Reassessment: neuroimaging in the emergency patient presenting with a seizure (an evidence-based review): report of the Therapeutics and Technology Assessment Subcommittee of the American Academy of Neurology. Neurology 2007;69:1772–80.

36. Ment LR, Bada HS, Barnes P, et al. Practice parameter: neuroimaging of the neonate. Neurology 2002;58:1726–38.

37. Jacobs SE, Hunt R, Tarnow-Mordli WO, et al. Cooling for newborns with hypoxic ischemic encephalopathy (Review). Cochrane Database Syst Rev 2007;(4):CD003311.

38. Monagle P, Chan AKC, Goldenberg NA, et al. Antithrombotic therapy in neonates and children. Chest 2012;141(2 Suppl):e737S–801.

39. Royal College of Paediatrics and Child Health. Stroke in childhood: clinical guidelines for diagnosis, management and rehabilitation. London. 2017.

40. Australian Childhood Stroke Advisory Committee. The diagnosis and acute management of childhood stroke: Clinical Guideline 2017. Available at: https://

clicktime.symantec.com/3VVnxm2AexsxmgE2Xy1fmAH7Vc?u=https%3A%2F%2F
www.mcri.edu.au%2Fsites%2Fdefault%2Ffiles%2Fmedia%2Fstroke_guidelines.pdf.

41. Ferriero DM, Fullerton HJ, Bernard TJ, et al. Management of stroke in neonates
    and children. A scientific statement from the American Heart Association/Amer-
    ican Stroke Association. Stroke 2019;50:e51–96.
42. Hemphill JC III, Greenberg SM, Anderson CS, et al. Guidelines for the manage-
    ment of spontaneous intracerebral hemorrhage. A guideline for professionals
    from the American Heart Association/American Stroke Association. Stroke
    2015;46:2032–60.
43. Kochanek PM, Tasker RC, Bell MJ, et al. Management of pediatric severe trau-
    matic brain injury: 2019 consensus and guidelines-based algorithm for first and
    second tier therapies. Pediatr Crit Care Med 2019;20(3):269–79.
44. Topjian AA, de Caen A, Wainwright MS, et al. Pediatric post-cardiac arrest care. A
    scientific statement from the American Heart Association. Circulation 2019;140:
    e194–233.
45. Topjian AA, Raymond TT, Atkins D, et al. Part 4: pediatric basic and advanced life
    support 2020 American Heart Association Guidelines for Cardiopulmonary
    Resuscitation and Emergency Cardiovascular Care. Pediatrics 2020. https://
    doi.org/10.1542/peds.2020-038505D.
46. O'Phelan KH, Miller CM. Emergency neurological life support: third edition, up-
    dates in the approach to early management of a neurological emergency. Neuro-
    crit Care 2017;27:S1–3.
47. Nakagawa TA, Ashwal S, Mathur M, et al. Guidelines for the determination of
    brain death in infants and children: an update of the 1987 task force recommen-
    dations. Crit Care Med 2011;39:2139–55.
48. Greer DM, Shemie SD, Lewis A, et al. Determination of brain death/death by
    neurologic criteria. The World brain death project. JAMA 2020;324(11):1078–97.
49. Lewis DW, Ashwal S, Dahl G, et al. Practice parameter, evaluation of children and
    adolescents with recurrent headaches. Neurology 2002;59:490–8.
50. Lewis DW, Ashwal S, Hershey A, et al. Pharmacological treatment of migraine
    headache in children and adolescents. Neurology 2004;63:2215–24.
51. Ashwal S, Russman BS, Blasco PA, et al. Practice parameter: diagnostic assess-
    ment of the child with cerebral palsy. Neurology 2004;62:851–63.
52. Shevell M, Ashwal S, Donley D, et al. Practice parameter: evaluation of the child
    with global developmental delay. Neurology 2003;60:367–80.
53. Michelson DJ, Shevell MI, Sherr EH, et al. Evidence report: genetic and metabolic
    testing on children with global developmental delay. Neurology 2011;77:1629–35.
54. Filipek PA, Accardo PJ, Ashwal S, et al. Practice parameter: screening and diag-
    nosis of autism. Neurology 2000;55:468–79.
55. Buckley AW, Hirtz D, Oskoui M, et al. Practice guideline: treatment for insomnia
    and disrupted sleep behavior in children and adolescents with autism spectrum
    disorder. Neurology 2020;94:392–404.
56. Ashwal S, Michelson D, Plawner L, et al. Practice parameter: evaluation of the
    child with microcephaly (an evidence-based review). Neurology 2009;73:887–97.
57. Pliszka S, AACP Work Group on Quality. Practice parameter for the assessment
    and treatment of children and adolescents with attention-deficit/hyperactivity dis-
    order. J Am Acad Child Adolesc Psychiatry 2007;46(7):894–921.
58. Moxley RT, Ashwal S, Pandya S, et al. Practice parameter: corticosteroid treat-
    ment of Duchenne dystrophy. Neurology 2005;64:13–20.

Printed and bound by CPI Group (UK) Ltd, Croydon, CR0 4YY

03/10/2024

01040406-0005